# SLEEP DISORDERS
## SOURCEBOOK

**SIXTH EDITION**

# Health Reference Series

# SLEEP DISORDERS
## SOURCEBOOK

### SIXTH EDITION

Provides Basic Consumer Health Information about Sleep Disorders, including Insomnia, Sleep Apnea and Snoring, Jet Lag and Other Circadian Rhythm Disorders, Narcolepsy, and Parasomnias, such as Sleepwalking and Sleep Paralysis, and Features Facts about Other Health Problems That Affect Sleep, Why Sleep Is Necessary, How Much Sleep Is Needed, the Physical and Mental Effects of Sleep Deprivation, and Pediatric Sleep Issues

Along with Tips for Diagnosing and Treating Sleep Disorders, a Glossary of Related Terms, and a List of Resources for Additional Help and Information

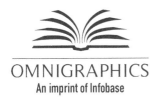

OMNIGRAPHICS
An imprint of Infobase

Bibliographic Note

Because this page cannot legibly accommodate all the copyright notices,
the Bibliographic Note portion of the Preface constitutes an extension
of the copyright notice.

\* \* \*

OMNIGRAPHICS
An imprint of Infobase
132 W. 31st St.
New York, NY 10001
www.infobase.com
James Chambers, *Editorial Director*

\* \* \*

Copyright © 2023 Infobase
ISBN 978-0-7808-2076-0
E-ISBN 978-0-7808-2077-7

Library of Congress Cataloging-in-Publication Data

Names: Chambers, James (Editor), editor.

Title: Sleep disorders sourcebook : provides basic consumer health information about sleep disorders, including insomnia, sleep apnea and snoring, jet lag and other circadian rhythm disorders, narcolepsy, and parasomnias, such as sleepwalking and sleep paralysis, and featuring facts about other health problems that affect sleep, why sleep is necessary, how much sleep is needed, the physical and mental effects of sleep deprivation, and pediatric sleep issues, along with tips for diagnosing and treating sleep disorders, a glossary of related terms, and a list of resources for additional help and information / edited by James Chambers.

Description: Sixth edition. | New York, NY : Omnigraphics, an imprint of Infobase, [2023] | Series: Health reference series | Includes index. | Summary: "Provides basic health information about the diagnosis, treatment, and prevention of sleep disorders in children and adults, along with facts about diseases that affect sleep and the health consequences of sleep deprivation. Includes index, glossary of related terms, and other resources"-- Provided by publisher.

Identifiers: LCCN 2023016505 (print) | LCCN 2023016506 (ebook) | ISBN 9780780820760 (library binding) | ISBN 9780780820777 (ebook)

Subjects: Subjects: LCSH: Sleep disorders. | Consumer education. Classification: LCC RC547 .S536 2023 (print) | LCC RC547 (ebook) | DDC 616.8/498--dc23/eng/20230508

LC record available at https://lccn.loc.gov/2023016505
LC ebook record available at https://lccn.loc.gov/2023016506

The information in this publication was compiled from the sources cited and from other sources considered reliable. While every possible effort has been made to ensure reliability, the publisher will not assume liability for damages caused by inaccuracies in the data, and makes no warranty, express or implied, on the accuracy of the information contained herein.

This book is printed on acid-free paper meeting the ANSI Z39.48 Standard. The infinity symbol that appears above indicates that the paper in this book meets that standard.

Printed in the United States

# Table of Contents

## Part 7. Additional Help and Information

# Preface

## ABOUT THIS BOOK

According to the Centers for Disease Control and Prevention (CDC), a third of U.S. adults report getting less than the recommended amount of sleep. Not getting enough sleep is associated with many chronic diseases and conditions—such as type 2 diabetes, heart disease, obesity, and depression—that pose a threat to public health. It can lead to motor vehicle crashes and mistakes at work, which cause many injuries and disabilities each year. Getting enough sleep is not a luxury but something people need for good health. Sleep disorders can also increase a person's risk of health problems. However, these disorders can be diagnosed and treated, relieving those suffering from them.

*Sleep Disorders Sourcebook, Sixth Edition* offers basic consumer health information about common sleep disorders, including insomnia, sleep apnea, narcolepsy, circadian rhythm disorders, parasomnias, and other health problems that affect sleep, such as cancer, pain, and respiratory disorders. It explains how much sleep is needed, the causes and consequences of sleep deprivation, and the methods used to prevent, diagnose, and treat sleep disorders. Pediatric sleep issues that impact children from infancy through the teen years are also discussed. A glossary of terms related to sleep disorders and a list of resources for further help and information are also included.

## HOW TO USE THIS BOOK

This book is divided into parts and chapters. Parts focus on broad areas of interest. Chapters are devoted to single topics within a part.

*Part 1: Sleep Basics* presents facts about why and how people sleep, explaining circadian rhythms, the physical characteristics of sleep, and the benefits of napping. It offers information on dreams and nightmares and explains how they affect sleep. It also describes sleep in women and men and explains how aging affects sleep patterns and sleep-related myths.

*Part 2: Causes and Consequences of Sleep Deprivation* details sleep deprivation and talks about the people at risk of sleep deprivation. It provides information on why your brain and body need sleep. The part explains how sleep deprivation affects daily activities, such as learning and driving. It also describes the molecular link between lack of sleep and weight gain. The part ends with information on getting enough sleep and how much sleep is needed.

*Part 3: Sleep Disorders* describes conditions that directly affect the ability to sleep. These include disorders such as sleep apnea, snoring, insomnia, circadian rhythm disorders, congenital central hypoventilation syndrome, and parasomnias. Narcolepsy and other disorders associated with excessive sleeping are also discussed.

*Part 4: Other Health Problems That Often Affect Sleep* provides information about health problems that often impact sleep quality, including cancer, chronic disease, stroke, fibromyalgia, headaches, and mental health concerns. The symptoms that disrupt sleep are described, and suggestions for lessening their impact are also provided.

*Part 5: Preventing, Diagnosing, and Treating Sleep Disorders* identifies common sleep disruptors and explains the importance of sleeping habits. It explains the sleep environment, exercises to get proper sleep, and mind and body practices. It describes how sleep studies work and details treatment options for insomnia, including medications, dietary supplements, continuous positive airway pressure, and other complementary and alternative medications.

*Part 6: A Special Look at Pediatric and Teen Sleep Issues* describes sleep disturbances in infancy, childhood, and adolescence; provides sleep information for parents and caregivers; and also discusses about tonsil surgery to improve sleep apnea syndrome in children. It discusses safe sleeping environments for infants and explains sudden infant death syndrome. It provides information on how to get children into bed and offers facts about bed-wetting, sleepwalking, bruxism, and teeth grinding.

*Part 7: Additional Help and Information* includes a glossary of terms related to sleep disorders and a directory of resources offering additional help and support.

## BIBLIOGRAPHIC NOTE

This volume contains documents and excerpts from publications issued by the following U.S. government agencies: Centers for Disease Control and Prevention (CDC); *Eunice Kennedy Shriver* National Institute of Child Health and Human Development (NICHD); Genetic and Rare Diseases Information Center (GARD); Genetics Home Reference (GHR); MedlinePlus; Mental Illness Research, Education and Clinical Centers (MIRECC); Mentalhealth. gov; National Cancer Institute (NCI); National Center for Complementary and Integrative Health (NCCIH); National Center for Posttraumatic Stress Disorder (NCPTSD); National Digestive Diseases Information Clearinghouse (NDDIC); National Heart, Lung, and Blood Institute (NHLBI); National Highway Traffic Safety Administration (NHTSA); National Institute of Arthritis and Musculoskeletal and Skin Diseases (NIAMS); National Institute of General Medical Sciences (NIGMS); National Institute of Justice (NIJ); National Institute of Mental Health (NIMH); National Institute of Neurological Disorders and Stroke (NINDS); National Institute on Aging (NIA); National Institute on Drug Abuse (NIDA); National Institutes of Health (NIH); National Science Foundation (NSF); News and Events; *NIH News in Health*; Office of Disease Prevention and Health Promotion (ODPHP); Office on Women's Health (OWH); Substance Abuse and Mental Health Services Administration (SAMHSA); U.S. Consumer Product Safety Commission (CPSC); U.S. Department of Agriculture (USDA); U.S. Department of Veterans Affairs (VA); and U.S. Food and Drug Administration (FDA).

It also contains original material produced by Infobase and reviewed by medical consultants.

## ABOUT THE *HEALTH REFERENCE SERIES*

The *Health Reference Series* is designed to provide basic medical information for patients, families, caregivers, and the general public. Each volume provides comprehensive coverage on a particular topic. This is especially important for people who may be dealing with a newly diagnosed disease or a chronic disorder in themselves or in a family member. People looking for preventive guidance, information about disease warning signs, medical statistics, and risk factors for health problems will also find answers to their questions in the *Health Reference Series*. The *Series*, however, is not intended to serve as a tool for diagnosing illness, in prescribing treatments, or as a substitute for the physician–patient relationship. All people concerned about medical symptoms or the possibility of disease are encouraged to seek professional care from an appropriate health-care provider.

## A NOTE ABOUT SPELLING AND STYLE

*Health Reference Series* editors use *Stedman's Medical Dictionary* as an authority for questions related to the spelling of medical terms and *The Chicago Manual of Style* for questions related to grammatical structures, punctuation, and other editorial concerns. Consistent adherence is not always possible, however, because the individual volumes within the *Series* include many documents from a wide variety of different producers, and the editor's primary goal is to present material from each source as accurately as is possible. This sometimes means that information in different chapters or sections may follow other guidelines and alternate spelling authorities. For example, occasionally a copyright holder may require that eponymous terms be shown in possessive forms (Crohn's disease vs. Crohn disease) or that British spelling norms be retained (leukaemia vs. leukemia).

## MEDICAL REVIEW

Infobase contracts with a team of qualified, senior medical professionals who serve as medical consultants for the *Health Reference Series*. As necessary, medical consultants review reprinted and originally written material for currency and accuracy. Medical consultation services are provided to the *Health Reference Series* editors by:

Dr. Vijayalakshmi, MBBS, DGO, MD
Dr. Senthil Selvan, MBBS, DCH, MD
Dr. K. Sivanandham, MBBS, DCH, MS (Research), PhD

## *HEALTH REFERENCE SERIES* UPDATE POLICY

The inaugural book in the *Health Reference Series* was the first edition of *Cancer Sourcebook* published in 1989. Since then, the *Series* has been enthusiastically received by librarians and in the medical community. In order to maintain the standard of providing high-quality health information for the layperson, the editorial staff felt it was necessary to implement a policy of updating volumes when warranted.

Medical researchers have been making tremendous strides, and it is the purpose of the *Health Reference Series* to stay current with the most recent advances. Each decision to update a volume is made on an individual basis.

Some of the considerations include how much new information is available and the feedback we receive from people who use the books. If there is a topic you would like to see added to the update list, or an area of medical concern you feel has not been adequately addressed, please write to: custserv@infobaselearning.com.

# Part 1 | **Sleep Basics**

# Chapter 1 | **Understanding Sleep**

## **Chapter Contents**

## ABOUT SLEEP

Sleep is a complex biological process that helps people process new information, stay healthy, and reenergize. Periods of sleep and wakefulness are part of how our bodies function.

Although you are resting while you sleep, your brain remains highly active. Sleep consists of different stages that repeat several times each night. During sleep, the brain cycles through two distinct phases: rapid eye movement (REM) sleep and non-REM sleep. Not completing the full sleep process can stress your body.

## WHY IS SLEEP IMPORTANT?

Each sleep phase and stage is important to ensure that the mind and body are completely rested. Certain stages help you feel rested and energetic the next day, while other stages help you learn information and form memories. Sleep is important in the function of your body's other systems, such as your metabolism and immune system. Sleep may also help your body clear toxins from your brain that build up while you are awake.

Not getting enough or enough quality sleep contributes, in the short term, to problems with learning and processing information, and it can have a harmful effect on long-term health and well-being. According to the Centers for Disease Control and Prevention (CDC), many U.S. adults report that they do not get the recommended number of hours of sleep each night.

Sleep affects how well you do your daily tasks, your mood, and your health in the following ways:

- **Performance**. Cutting back on sleep by as little as one hour can make it difficult to focus the next day and can slow your response time. Insufficient sleep can also make you more likely to take risks and make poor decisions according to the National Heart, Lung, and Blood Institute (NHLBI).
- **Mood**. Sleep affects your mood. Insufficient sleep can make you more easily annoyed or angry, and that

can lead to trouble with relationships, particularly for children and teens. Also, people who do not get enough sleep are more likely to become depressed according to the NHLBI.

- **Health.** Sleep is important for good health. Research in adults has shown that lack of sleep or lack of quality sleep increases a person's risk for high blood pressure, heart disease, and other medical conditions. Your environment can affect the quality of your sleep by causing disturbances that prevent you from sleeping through the night. Also, during sleep, the body produces hormones that help the body grow and, throughout life, build muscle, fight illnesses, and repair damage to the body. Growth hormone, for example, is produced during sleep, and it is essential for growth and development. Other hormones produced during sleep affect how the body uses energy, which may explain why lack of sleep contributes to obesity and diabetes.[1]

## HOW MUCH SLEEP DO ADULTS NEED?

It is important to get enough sleep. Sleep helps keep your mind and body healthy. Most adults need seven or more hours of good-quality sleep on a regular schedule each night.

Getting enough sleep is not only about total hours of sleep. It is also important to get good-quality sleep on a regular schedule, so you feel rested when you wake up. If you often have trouble sleeping—or if you often still feel tired after sleeping—talk with your doctor.

## HOW MUCH SLEEP DO CHILDREN NEED?

Kids need even more sleep than adults:

- Teens need 8–10 hours of sleep each night.
- School-aged children need 9–12 hours of sleep each night.

---

[1] "About Sleep," *Eunice Kennedy Shriver* National Institute of Child Health and Human Development (NICHD), April 29, 2019. Available online. URL: www.nichd.nih.gov/health/topics/sleep/conditioninfo. Accessed March 8, 2023.

- Preschoolers need to sleep between 10 and 13 hours a day (including naps).
- Toddlers need to sleep between 11 and 14 hours a day (including naps).
- Babies need to sleep between 12 and 16 hours a day (including naps).
- Newborns need to sleep between 14 and 17 hours a day.

## HEALTH BENEFITS
### Why Is Getting Enough Sleep Important?

Getting enough sleep has many benefits. It can help you:

- get sick less often
- stay at a healthy weight
- lower your risk for serious health problems, such as diabetes and heart disease
- reduce stress and improve your mood
- think more clearly and do better in school and at work
- get along better with people
- make good decisions and avoid injuries—for example, drowsy drivers cause thousands of car accidents every year

## SLEEP SCHEDULE
### Does It Matter When You Sleep?

Yes. Your body sets your "biological clock" according to the pattern of daylight where you live. This helps you naturally get sleepy at night and stay alert during the day.

If you have to work at night and sleep during the day, you may have trouble getting enough sleep. It can also be hard to sleep when you travel to a different time zone.

## TROUBLE SLEEPING
### Not Asleep?

Many things can make it harder for you to sleep, including the following:

- stress or anxiety
- pain

- certain health conditions, such as heartburn or asthma
- some medicines
- caffeine (usually from coffee, tea, and soda)
- alcohol and other drugs
- untreated sleep disorders, such as sleep apnea or insomnia

If you are having trouble sleeping, try making changes to your routine to get the sleep you need. You may want to:
- change what you do during the day—for example, get your physical activity in the morning instead of at night
- create a comfortable sleep environment—for example, make sure your bedroom is dark and quiet
- set a bedtime routine—for example, go to bed at the same time every night[2]

## Section 1.2 | **Anatomy of Sleep**

## BRAIN BASICS: UNDERSTANDING SLEEP

Sleep is an important part of your daily routine—you spend about one-third of your time doing it. Quality sleep—and getting enough of it at the right times—is as essential to survival as food and water. Without sleep, you cannot form or maintain the pathways in your brain that let you learn and create new memories, and it is harder to concentrate and respond quickly.

Sleep is important to a number of brain functions, including how nerve cells (neurons) communicate with each other. In fact, your brain and body stay remarkably active while you sleep. Recent findings suggest that sleep plays a housekeeping role that removes toxins in your brain that build up while you are awake.

[2] Office of Disease Prevention and Health Promotion (ODPHP), "Get Enough Sleep," U.S. Department of Health and Human Services (HHS), July 15, 2022. Available online. URL: https://health.gov/myhealthfinder/healthy-living/mental-health-and-relationships/get-enough-sleep. Accessed March 8, 2023.

Everyone needs sleep, but its biological purpose remains a mystery. Sleep affects almost every type of tissue and system in the body—from the brain, heart, and lungs to metabolism, immune function, mood, and disease resistance. Research shows that a chronic lack of sleep, or getting poor-quality sleep, increases the risk of disorders, including high blood pressure, cardiovascular disease, diabetes, depression, and obesity.

Sleep is a complex and dynamic process that affects how you function in ways scientists are now beginning to understand. This chapter describes how your need for sleep is regulated and what happens in the brain during sleep.

## BRAIN AND SLEEP

Several structures within the brain are involved with sleep. The hypothalamus, a peanut-sized structure deep inside the brain, contains groups of nerve cells that act as control centers affecting sleep and arousal. Within the hypothalamus is the suprachiasmatic nucleus (SCN)—clusters of thousands of cells that receive information about light exposure directly from the eyes and control your behavioral rhythm. Some people with damage to the SCN sleep erratically throughout the day because they are not able to match their circadian rhythms with the light–dark cycle. Most blind people maintain some ability to sense light and are able to modify their sleep–wake cycle.

The brain stem, at the base of the brain, communicates with the hypothalamus to control the transitions between wake and sleep. (The brain stem includes structures called the "pons," "medulla," and "midbrain.") Sleep-promoting cells within the hypothalamus and the brain stem produce a brain chemical called "gamma-aminobutyric acid" (GABA), which acts to reduce the activity of arousal centers in the hypothalamus and the brain stem. The brain stem (especially the pons and medulla) also plays a special role in rapid eye movement (REM) sleep; it sends signals to relax muscles essential for body posture and limb movements so that we do not act out our dreams.

The thalamus acts as a relay for information from the senses to the cerebral cortex (the covering of the brain that interprets and processes information from short- to long-term memory). During most stages of sleep, the thalamus becomes quiet, letting you tune out the external world. But, during REM sleep, the thalamus is active, sending the cortex images, sounds, and other sensations that fill our dreams.

The pineal gland, located within the brain's two hemispheres, receives signals from the SCN and increases the production of the hormone melatonin, which helps put you to sleep once the lights go down. People who have lost their sight and cannot coordinate their natural wake–sleep cycle using natural light can stabilize their sleep patterns by taking small amounts of melatonin at the same time each day. Scientists believe that peaks and valleys of melatonin over time are important for matching the body's circadian rhythm to the external cycle of light and darkness.

The basal forebrain, near the front and bottom of the brain, also promotes sleep and wakefulness, while part of the midbrain acts as an arousal system. Release of adenosine (a chemical by-product of cellular energy consumption) from cells in the basal forebrain and probably other regions supports your sleep drive. Caffeine counteracts sleepiness by blocking the actions of adenosine.

The amygdala, an almond-shaped structure involved in processing emotions, becomes increasingly active during REM sleep.

## SLEEP STAGES AND MECHANISMS
### Sleep Stages

There are two basic types of sleep: REM sleep and non-REM sleep (which has three different stages). Each is linked to specific brain waves and neuronal activity. You cycle through all stages of non-REM and REM sleep several times during a typical night, with increasingly longer, deeper REM periods occurring toward morning.

- **Stage 1.** Non-REM sleep is the changeover from wakefulness to sleep. During this short period (lasting several minutes) of relatively light sleep, your heartbeat, breathing, and eye movements slow, and your muscles relax with occasional twitches. Your brain waves begin to slow from their daytime wakefulness patterns.

- **Stage 2.** Non-REM sleep is a period of light sleep before you enter deeper sleep. Your heartbeat and breathing slow, and your muscles relax even further. Your body temperature drops, and your eye movements stop. Brain wave activity slows but is marked by brief bursts of electrical activity. You spend more of your repeated sleep cycles in stage 2 sleep than in other sleep stages.
- **Stage 3.** Non-REM sleep is the period of deep sleep that you need to feel refreshed in the morning. It occurs in longer periods during the first half of the night. Your heartbeat and breathing slow to their lowest levels during sleep. Your muscles are relaxed, and it may be difficult to awaken you. Brain waves become even slower.

REM sleep first occurs about 90 minutes after falling asleep. Your eyes move rapidly from side to side behind closed eyelids. Mixed-frequency brain wave activity becomes closer to that seen in wakefulness. Your breathing becomes faster and irregular, and your heart rate and blood pressure increase to near-waking levels. Most of your dreaming occurs during REM sleep although some can also occur in non-REM sleep. Your arm and leg muscles become temporarily paralyzed, which prevents you from acting out your dreams. As you age, you sleep less of your time in REM sleep. Memory consolidation most likely requires both non-REM and REM sleep.

## Sleep Mechanisms

Two internal biological mechanisms—circadian rhythm and homeostasis—work together to regulate when you are awake and sleep. Circadian rhythms direct a wide variety of functions, from daily fluctuations in wakefulness to body temperature, metabolism, and the release of hormones. They control your timing of sleep and cause you to be sleepy at night and your tendency to wake up in the morning without an alarm. Your body's biological clock, which is based on a roughly 24-hour day, controls most circadian rhythms. Circadian rhythms synchronize with environmental cues (light, temperature) about the actual time of the day, but they continue even in the absence of cues.

Sleep–wake homeostasis keeps track of your need for sleep. The homeostatic sleep drive reminds the body to sleep after a certain time and regulates sleep intensity. This sleep drive gets stronger every hour you are awake and causes you to sleep longer and more deeply after a period of sleep deprivation.

Factors that influence your sleep–wake needs include medical conditions, medications, stress, sleep environment, and what you eat and drink. Perhaps the greatest influence is the exposure to light. Specialized cells in the retinas of your eyes process light and tell the brain whether it is day or night and can advance or delay our sleep–wake cycle. Exposure to light can make it difficult to fall asleep and return to sleep when awakened.

Night shift workers often have trouble falling asleep when they go to bed and also have trouble staying awake at work because their natural circadian rhythm and sleep–wake cycle are disrupted. In the case of jet lag, circadian rhythms become out of sync with the time of the day when people fly to a different time zone, creating a mismatch between their internal clock and the actual clock.

## HOW MUCH SLEEP DO YOU NEED?

Your need for sleep and your sleep patterns change as you age, but this varies significantly across individuals of the same age. There is no magic "number of sleep hours" that works for everybody of the same age. Babies initially sleep as much as 16–18 hours per day, which may boost growth and development (especially of the brain). School-aged children and teens, on average, need about 9.5 hours of sleep per night. Most adults need seven to nine hours of sleep a night, but after the age of 60, nighttime sleep tends to be shorter, lighter, and interrupted by multiple awakenings. Older people are also more likely to take medications that interfere with sleep.

In general, people are getting less sleep than they need due to longer work hours and the availability of round-the-clock entertainment and other activities. Many people feel they can "catch up" on missed sleep during the weekend, but depending on how sleep-deprived they are, sleeping longer on the weekends may not be adequate.

## DREAMING AND SLEEP TRACKING
### Dreaming

Everyone dreams. You spend about two hours each night dreaming but may not remember most of your dreams. Its exact purpose is not known, but dreaming may help you process your emotions. Events from the day often invade your thoughts during sleep, and people suffering from stress or anxiety are more likely to have frightening dreams. Dreams can be experienced in all stages of sleep but usually are most vivid in REM sleep. Some people dream in color, while others only recall dreams in black and white.

### Tracking Sleep through Smart Technology

Millions of people are using smartphone apps, bedside monitors, and wearable items (including bracelets, smartwatches, and head-bands) to informally collect and analyze data about their sleep. Smart technology can record sounds and movement during sleep, journal hours slept, and monitor heartbeat and respiration. Using a companion app, data from some devices can be synced to a smart-phone or tablet or uploaded to a personal computer (PC). Other apps and devices make white noise, produce light that stimulates melatonin production, and use gentle vibrations to help us sleep and wake.

## THE ROLE OF GENES AND NEUROTRANSMITTERS
### Chemical Signals to Sleep

Clusters of sleep-promoting neurons in many parts of the brain become more active as we get ready for bed. Nerve-signaling chem-icals called "neurotransmitters" can "switch off" or dampen the activity of cells that signal arousal or relaxation. GABA is associated with sleep, muscle relaxation, and sedation. Norepinephrine and orexin (also called "hypocretin") keep some parts of the brain active while we are awake. Other neurotransmitters that shape sleep and wakefulness include acetylcholine, histamine, adrenaline, cortisol, and serotonin.

## Genes and Sleep

Genes may play a significant role in how much sleep we need. Scientists have identified several genes involved with sleep and sleep disorders, including genes that control the excitability of neurons and "clock" genes such as *Per*, *tim*, and *Cry*, that influence our circadian rhythms and the timing of sleep. Genome-wide association studies have identified sites on various chromosomes that increase our susceptibility to sleep disorders. Also, different genes have been identified with such sleep disorders as familial advanced sleep-phase disorder, narcolepsy, and restless legs syndrome (RLS). Some of the genes expressed in the cerebral cortex and other brain areas change their level of expression between sleep and wake.

Several genetic models—including the worm, fruit fly, and zebra fish—are helping scientists to identify molecular mechanisms and genetic variants involved in normal sleep and sleep disorders. Additional research will provide a better understanding of inherited sleep patterns and risks of circadian and sleep disorders.

## Sleep Studies

Your health-care provider may recommend a polysomnogram or other test to diagnose a sleep disorder. A polysomnogram typically involves spending the night at a sleep lab or sleep center. It records your breathing, oxygen levels, eye and limb movements, heart rate, and brain waves throughout the night. Your sleep is also video- and audio-recorded. The data can help a sleep specialist determine if you are reaching and proceeding properly through the various sleep stages. Results may be used to develop a treatment plan or determine if further tests are needed.[3]

---

[3] "Brain Basics: Understanding Sleep," National Institute of Neurological Disorders and Stroke (NINDS), March 17, 2023. Available online. URL: www.ninds.nih.gov/health-information/public-education/brain-basics/brain-basics-understanding-sleep. Accessed March 24, 2023.

## Section 1.3 | **What Makes Us Sleep?**

Sleep and wakefulness are generally regulated by our brains working with input from our senses and our circadian clock. This system pushes us to wake up and remain awake at certain times and pushes us to sleep at certain times. Research has helped us begin to understand this system at the level of the cells in the brain. More work is needed to understand exactly how the brain, senses, and our body's clockwork in waking and sleeping and what can happen to disturb this cycle.

## SLEEP DRIVE

The need for sleep is driven by the length of time you are awake. The longer you are awake, the greater your "drive" or need to sleep. The drive to sleep continues to build within your body until you are able to sleep.

## CIRCADIAN CLOCK

Your body has a natural clock, called a "circadian clock," that helps you regulate your sleep. The word "circadian" refers to rhythmic biological cycles that repeat about every 24 hours. These cycles are also called "circadian rhythms." Your circadian clock is strongly influenced by light, which is the reason why people living in different regions have different sleeping schedules. This is also the reason why people who work night shifts can have difficulty falling asleep or staying awake.

At bedtime, when your drive to sleep is greatest, your sleep drive and circadian clockwork together to allow you to fall asleep. After you have slept for some time, when your drive to sleep is lower, your circadian clock allows you to stay asleep until the end of the night.

## Circadian Rhythms

Circadian rhythms regulate changes in the brain and body that occur over the course of a day. Your body's biological clock controls most circadian rhythms. This clock is found in a region of the brain called the "hypothalamus." The hypothalamus affects sleep and arousal.

Light detected by special neurons in the eye sends signals to many areas of the brain, including the hypothalamus. Signals from the hypothalamus travel to different regions of the brain, including the pineal gland. In response to light, such as sunlight, the pineal gland turns off the production of melatonin, a hormone that causes a feeling of drowsiness. The levels of melatonin in the body normally increase after darkness, which makes you feel drowsy.

The change in melatonin during the sleep–wake cycle reflects circadian rhythms. During sleep, the hypothalamus also controls changes in body temperature and blood pressure. Because circadian rhythms are controlled by light, people who have some degree of blindness in both eyes may have trouble sleeping.[4]

Many factors play a role in preparing your body to fall asleep and wake up. You have an internal "body clock" that manages when you are awake and when your body is ready for sleep.

## YOUR BODY CLOCK

The body clock typically has a 24-hour repeating rhythm (called the "circadian rhythm"). Two processes interact to control this rhythm:

- The first is a pressure to sleep that builds with every hour that you are awake. This drive for sleep peaks in the evening when most people fall asleep. A compound called "adenosine" seems to be one factor linked to this drive for sleep. While you are awake, the level of adenosine in your brain continues to rise. The increasing level of this compound signals a shift toward sleep. While you sleep, your body breaks down adenosine.

[4] "What Makes Us Sleep?" *Eunice Kennedy Shriver* National Institute of Child Health and Human Development (NICHD), April 29, 2019. Available online. URL: www.nichd.nih.gov/health/topics/sleep/conditioninfo/causes. Accessed March 10, 2023.

- A second process involves your internal body clock. This clock is in sync with certain cues in the environment. Light, darkness, and other cues help determine when you feel awake and when you feel sleepy.

For example, light signals received through your eyes tell your brain that it is daytime. This area of your brain helps align your body clock with periods of the day and night.

## HORMONES
Your body releases chemicals in a daily rhythm that your body clock controls.

### Melatonin
When it gets dark, your body releases a hormone called "melatonin." Melatonin signals your body that it is time to prepare for sleep, and it helps you feel sleepy. The amount of melatonin in your bloodstream peaks as the evening passes. Researchers believe this peak is an important part of preparing your body for sleep. Exposure to bright artificial light late in the evening can disrupt this process, making it hard to fall asleep. Examples of bright artificial light include the light from a TV screen, computer screen, or a very bright alarm clock.

### Cortisol
As the sun rises, your body releases cortisol. This hormone naturally prepares your body to wake up.

## CHANGES IN BODY CLOCK WITH AGING
The rhythm and timing of the body clock change with age. Teens fall asleep later at night than younger children and adults. One reason for this is that melatonin is released and peaks later in the 24-hour cycle for teens. As a result, it is natural for many teens to prefer later bedtimes at night and sleep later in the morning than adults.

People also need more sleep early in life when they are growing and developing. For example, newborns may sleep more than 16 hours a day, and preschool-aged children need to take naps. Young children tend to sleep more in the early evening. Teens tend to sleep more in the morning. Also, older adults tend to go to bed earlier and wake up earlier.

The patterns and types of sleep also change as people mature. For example, newborn infants spend more time in rapid eye movement (REM) sleep. Dreaming typically occurs during REM sleep. The amount of deep or slow-wave sleep (non-REM sleep) peaks in early childhood and then drops sharply after puberty. It continues to decline as people age.[5]

## Section 1.4 | Circadian Rhythms

### WHAT ARE CIRCADIAN RHYTHMS?

Circadian rhythms are physical, mental, and behavioral changes that follow a 24-hour cycle. These natural processes respond primarily to light and dark and affect most living things, including animals, plants, and microbes. Chronobiology is the study of circadian rhythms. One example of a light-related circadian rhythm is sleeping at night and being awake during the day.

### WHAT ARE BIOLOGICAL CLOCKS?

Biological clocks are organisms' natural timing devices regulating the cycle of circadian rhythms. They are composed of specific molecules (proteins) that interact with cells throughout the body. Nearly every tissue and organ contains biological clocks. Researchers have identified similar genes in people, fruit flies, mice, plants, fungi, and several other organisms that make the clocks' molecular components.

[5] "What Makes You Sleep?" National Heart, Lung, and Blood Institute (NHLBI), March 24, 2022. Available online. URL: www.nhlbi.nih.gov/health/sleep-deprivation/body-clock. Accessed March 10, 2023.

## WHAT IS THE MASTER CLOCK?

A master clock in the brain coordinates all the biological clocks in a living thing, keeping the clocks in sync. In vertebrate animals, including humans, the master clock is a group of about 20,000 nerve cells (neurons) that form a structure called the "suprachiasmatic nucleus," or "SCN." The SCN is in a part of the brain called the "hypothalamus" and receives direct input from the eyes. Figure 1.1 shows how the SCN controls circadian rhythms.

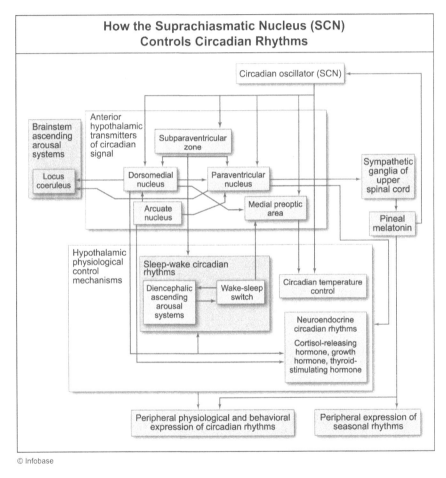

© Infobase

**Figure 1.1.** How the Suprachiasmatic Nucleus Controls Circadian Rhythms

*Infobase*

## DOES THE BODY MAKE AND KEEP ITS OWN CIRCADIAN RHYTHMS?

Yes, natural factors in your body produce circadian rhythms. For humans, some of the most important genes in this process are the *Period* and *Cryptochrome* genes. These genes code for proteins that build up in the cell's nucleus at night and lessen during the day. Studies in fruit flies suggest that these proteins help activate feelings of wakefulness, alertness, and sleepiness. However, signals from the environment also affect circadian rhythms. For instance, exposure to light at a different time of day can reset when the body turns on *Period* and *Cryptochrome* genes.

## HOW DO CIRCADIAN RHYTHMS AFFECT HEALTH?

Circadian rhythms can influence important functions in our bodies, such as:

- hormone release
- eating habits and digestion
- body temperature

However, most people notice the effect of circadian rhythms on their sleep patterns. The SCN controls the production of melatonin, a hormone that makes you sleepy. It receives information about incoming light from the optic nerves, which relay information from the eyes to the brain (refer to Figure 1.2). When there is less light—for example, at night—the SCN tells the brain to make more melatonin, so you get drowsy.

## WHAT FACTORS CAN CHANGE CIRCADIAN RHYTHMS?

Changes in our body and environmental factors can cause our circadian rhythms and the natural light–dark cycle to be out of sync:

- Mutations or changes in certain genes can affect our biological clocks.
- Jet lag or shift work causes changes in the light–dark cycle.
- Light from electronic devices at night can confuse our biological clocks.

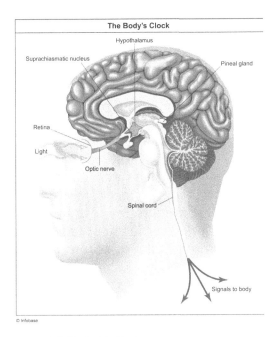

**Figure 1.2.** The Body's Clock

*Infobase*

These changes can cause sleep disorders and may lead to other chronic health conditions, such as obesity, diabetes, depression, bipolar disorder, and seasonal affective disorder.

## HOW ARE CIRCADIAN RHYTHMS RELATED TO JET LAG?

When you pass through different time zones, your biological clock will be different from the local time. For example, if you fly east from California to New York, you "lose" three hours. When you wake up at 7:00 a.m. on the East Coast, your biological clock is still running on West Coast time, so you feel the way you might at 4:00 a.m. Your biological clock will reset, but it will do so at a different rate. It often takes a few days for your biological clock to align with a new time zone. Adjusting after "gaining" time may be slightly easier than after "losing" time because the brain adjusts differently in the two situations.

## HOW DO RESEARCHERS STUDY CIRCADIAN RHYTHMS?

Scientists learn about circadian rhythms by studying humans and by using organisms with similar biological clocks' genes, such as fruit flies and mice. Researchers doing these experiments control the subject's environment by altering light and dark periods. Then they look for changes in gene activity or other molecular signals. Scientists also study organisms with irregular circadian rhythms to identify which genetic components of biological clocks may be broken.

Understanding what makes biological clocks tick may lead to treatments for jet lag, sleep disorders, obesity, mental health disorders, and other health problems. It can also improve ways for people to adjust to nighttime shift work. Learning more about the genes responsible for circadian rhythms will also help us understand more about the human body.[6]

## WHY ARE SLEEP PATTERNS SOMETIMES THROWN OFF AFTER TRAVELING ACROSS TIME ZONES?

Circadian rhythms are disrupted when people travel from one time zone to another. The feeling that you experience when your circadian rhythms (biological cycles) are disrupted is called "jet lag." The reason for jet lag is the change in time zones. For example, traveling from California to New York makes your body's biological clock "lose" three hours. When you are in New York and your alarm rings at 8:00 a.m., you will feel tired and groggy because your body is still on California time, which would be 5:00 a.m. It will take your body a few days to adjust to the new time zone, but the adjustment will eventually take place. After a couple of days, you will find that 8:00 a.m. feels like the correct time to wake up if that is part of your normal schedule and you have had an adequate sleep.

Some studies have shown that supplements of melatonin, a hormone that is produced by the body and sold as a treatment for insomnia, can help treat jet lag. This supplement has been especially effective for people crossing five or more time zones and for those

---

[6] "Circadian Rhythms," National Institute of General Medical Sciences (NIGMS), May 4, 2022. Available online. URL: www.nigms.nih.gov/education/fact-sheets/Pages/circadian-rhythms.aspx. Accessed March 8, 2023.

traveling east. However, additional studies are needed to test the safety and effectiveness of melatonin for insomnia and jet lag; few studies are available, and it has not been tested for long-term use. Before you take any kind of supplement, be sure to check with your health-care provider.[7]

Section 1.5 | Sleep Myths

## MYTHS AND FACTS ABOUT SLEEP

Sleep is a basic necessity of life, as important to our health and well-being as air, food, and water. When we sleep well, we wake up feeling refreshed, alert, and ready to face daily challenges. When we do not, every part of our lives can suffer. Our jobs, relationships, productivity, health, and safety (and that of those around us) are all put at risk. There are many common myths about sleep. We hear them frequently and may even experience them far too often. Sometimes, they can be characterized as "old wives' tales," but there are other times the incorrect information can be serious and even dangerous. The National Sleep Foundation (NSF) has compiled this list of common myths about sleep and the facts that dispel them.

### Turning Up the Radio, Opening the Window, and Turning On the Air Conditioner Are Effective Ways to Stay Awake When Driving

These "aids" are ineffective and can be dangerous to the person who is driving while feeling drowsy or sleepy. If you are feeling tired while driving, the best thing to do is to pull off the road in a safe rest area and take a nap for 15–45 minutes. Caffeinated beverages can help overcome drowsiness for a short period of time; however, it takes about 30 minutes before the effects are felt. The best prevention for drowsy driving is a good night's sleep the night before your trip.

---

[7] "Other Sleep FAQs," *Eunice Kennedy Shriver* National Institute of Child Health and Human Development (NICHD), April 29, 2019. Available online. URL: www.nichd.nih.gov/health/topics/sleep/more_information/other-faqs. Accessed March 9, 2023.

## Daytime Sleepiness Always Means a Person Is Not Getting Enough Sleep

Excessive daytime sleepiness is a condition in which an individual feels very drowsy during the day and has the urge to fall asleep when he/she should be fully alert and awake. The condition, which can occur even after getting enough nighttime sleep, can be a sign of an underlying medical condition or sleep disorder such as narcolepsy or sleep apnea. These problems can often be treated, and symptoms should be discussed with a physician. Daytime sleepiness can be dangerous and puts a person at risk of drowsy driving, injury, and illness and can impair mental abilities, emotions, and performance.

## You Can "Cheat" on the Amount of Sleep You Get

Sleep experts say most adults need between seven and nine hours of sleep each night for optimum performance, health, and safety. When we do not get adequate sleep, we accumulate a sleep debt that can be difficult to "pay back" if it becomes too big. The resulting sleep deprivation has been linked to health problems such as obesity and high blood pressure, negative mood and behavior, decreased productivity, and safety issues at home, on the job, and on the road.

## During Sleep, Your Brain Rests

The body rests during sleep; however, the brain remains active, gets "recharged," and still controls many body functions, including breathing. When we sleep, we typically drift between two sleep states, rapid eye movement (REM) and non-REM, in 90-minute cycles. Non-REM sleep has four stages with distinct features, ranging from stage 1 drowsiness, when one can be easily awakened, to "deep sleep" stages 3 and 4, when awakenings are more difficult and where the most positive and restorative effects of sleep occur; however, even in the deepest non-REM sleep, our minds can still process information. REM sleep is an active sleep where dreams occur, breathing and heart rate increase and become irregular, muscles relax, and eyes move back and forth under the eyelids.

### If You Wake Up in the Middle of the Night, It Is Best to Lie in Bed, Count Sheep, or Toss and Turn Until You Eventually Fall Back Asleep

Waking up in the middle of the night and not being able to go back to sleep is a symptom of insomnia. Relaxing imagery or thoughts may help induce sleep more than counting sheep, which some research suggests may be more distracting than relaxing. Whichever technique is used, most experts agree that if you do not fall back asleep within 15–20 minutes, you should get out of bed, go to another room, and engage in a relaxing activity such as listening to music or reading. Return to bed when you feel sleepy. Avoid watching the clock.

### The Older You Get, the Fewer Hours of Sleep You Need

Sleep experts recommend a range of seven to nine hours of sleep for the average adult. While sleep patterns change as we age, the amount of sleep we need generally does not. Older people may wake more frequently through the night and may actually get less nighttime sleep, but their sleep need is no less than younger adults. Because they may sleep less during the night, older people tend to sleep more during the day. Naps planned as part of a regular daily routine can be useful in promoting wakefulness after the person awakens. According to sleep experts, teens need at least 8.5–9.25 hours of sleep each night, compared to an average of seven to nine hours each night for most adults. Their internal biological clocks also keep them awake later in the evening and keep them sleeping later in the morning however, many schools begin classes early in the morning when a teenager's body wants to be asleep. As a result, many teens come to school too sleepy to learn, through no fault of their own.

### Health Problems Such as Obesity, Diabetes, Hypertension, and Depression Are Unrelated to the Amount and Quality of a Person's Sleep

Studies have found a relationship between the quantity and quality of one's sleep and many health problems. For example, insufficient sleep affects growth hormone secretion that is linked to obesity; as the amount of hormone secretion decreases, the chance of weight gain increases. Blood pressure usually falls during the sleep cycle; however, interrupted sleep can adversely affect this normal decline, leading to hypertension and cardiovascular problems. Research has also shown that insufficient sleep impairs the body's ability to use insulin, which can lead to the onset of diabetes. More and more scientific studies are showing correlations between poor and insufficient sleep and disease.

## Snoring Is a Common Problem, Especially among Men, but It Is Not Harmful

Although snoring may be harmless for most people, it can be a symptom of a life-threatening sleep disorder called "sleep apnea," especially if it is accompanied by severe daytime sleepiness. Sleep apnea is characterized by pauses in breathing that prevent air from flowing into or out of a sleeping person's airways. People with sleep apnea frequently awaken during the night, gasping for breath. The breathing pauses reduce blood oxygen levels, can strain the heart and cardiovascular system, and increase the risk of cardiovascular disease. Snoring on a frequent or regular basis has been directly associated with hypertension. Obesity and a large neck can contribute to sleep apnea. Sleep apnea can be treated. Men and women who snore loudly, especially if pauses in the snoring are noted, should consult a physician.[8]

## You Can "Catch Up" on Sleep

Despite popular belief, you cannot regain or catch up on "lost" sleep by sleeping more at another time. Being sleep-deprived means you accumulate a sleep debt that is impossible to "repay" as it gets larger. In addition, long-term sleep deprivation puts you at risk for health problems and may impair your safety and work performance. Sleep

[8] "Safety | Myths and Facts about Sleep," U.S. Department of Agriculture (USDA), September 18, 2021. Available online. URL: www.nrcs.usda.gov/wps/portal/nrcs/detail/ks/people/employees/?cid=nrcs142p2_033304. Accessed March 10, 2023.

deprivation has been linked to obesity, high blood pressure, negative mood and behavior, decreased productivity at work, and safety issues at home, on the job, and on the road. Catching up on sleep may help reduce daytime sleepiness or drowsiness, but it does not reverse the effects of not getting enough sleep or enough quality sleep each night.[9]

---

[9] "What Are Some Myths about Sleep?" *Eunice Kennedy Shriver* National Institute of Child Health and Human Development (NICHD), April 29, 2019. Available online. URL: www.nichd.nih.gov/health/topics/sleep/conditioninfo/sleep-myths. Accessed March 10, 2023.

# Chapter 2 | **Healthy Sleep Habits**

You can take steps to improve your sleep habits. First, make sure that you give yourself enough time to sleep. With enough sleep each night, you may find that you are happier and more productive during the day. Sleep is often the first thing that busy people squeeze out of their schedules. Making time to sleep will help you protect your health and well-being now and in the future.

To improve your sleep habits, doing the following may help:

- Go to bed and wake up at the same time every day. For children, have a set bedtime and a bedtime routine. Do not use the child's bedroom for timeouts or punishment.
- Try to keep the same sleep schedule on weeknights and weekends. Limit the difference to no more than about an hour. Staying up late and sleeping in late on weekends can disrupt your body clock's sleep–wake rhythm.
- Use the hour before bed for quiet time. Avoid intense exercise and bright artificial light, such as from a TV or computer screen. The light may signal the brain that it is time to be awake.
- Avoid heavy or large meals within a few hours of bedtime. (Having a light snack is okay.) Also, avoid alcoholic drinks before bed.
- Avoid nicotine (i.e., cigarettes) and caffeine (including caffeinated soda, coffee, tea, and chocolate). Nicotine and caffeine are stimulants, and both substances can interfere with sleep. The effects of caffeine can last up

to eight hours. Therefore, a cup of coffee in the late afternoon can make it hard for you to fall asleep at night.

- Spend time outside every day (when possible) and be physically active.
- Keep your bedroom quiet, cool, and dark (a dim night light is fine if needed).
- Take a hot bath or use relaxation techniques before bed.

Napping during the day may boost your alertness and performance. However, if you have trouble falling asleep at night, limit naps or take them earlier in the afternoon. Adults should nap for no more than 20 minutes. Napping in preschool-aged children is normal and promotes healthy growth and development.[1]

## WHY YOU NEED A GOOD NIGHT'S SLEEP

We have so many demands on our time—jobs, family, errands—not to mention finding some time to relax. To fit everything in, we often sacrifice sleep. But sleep affects both mental and physical health. It is vital to your well-being.

Of course, sleep helps you feel rested each day. But, while you are sleeping, your brain and body do not just shut down. Internal organs and processes are hard at work throughout the night.

"Sleep services all aspects of our body in one way or another: molecular, energy balance, as well as intellectual function, alertness, and mood," says Dr. Merrill Mitler, a sleep expert and neuroscientist at the National Institutes of Health (NIH).

When you are tired, you cannot function at your best. Sleep helps you think more clearly, have quicker reflexes, and focus better. "The fact is, when we look at well-rested people, they are operating at a different level than people trying to get by on one or two hours less nightly sleep," says Dr. Mitler.

"Loss of sleep impairs your higher levels of reasoning, problem-solving, and attention to detail," Dr. Mitler explains. Tired people

---

[1] "Healthy Sleep Habits," National Heart, Lung, and Blood Institute (NHLBI), March 24, 2022. Available online. URL: www.nhlbi.nih.gov/health/sleep-deprivation/healthy-sleep-habits. Accessed March 9, 2023.

tend to be less productive at work. They are at a much higher risk for traffic accidents. Lack of sleep also influences your mood, which can affect how you interact with others. A sleep deficit over time can even put you at a greater risk of developing depression.

But sleep is not just essential for the brain. "Sleep affects almost every tissue in our bodies," says Dr. Michael Twery, a sleep expert at the NIH. "It affects growth and stress hormones, our immune system, appetite, breathing, blood pressure, and cardiovascular health."

Research shows that lack of sleep increases the risk of obesity, heart disease, and infections. Throughout the night, your heart rate, breathing rate, and blood pressure rise and fall, a process that may be important for cardiovascular health. Your body releases hormones during sleep that help repair cells and control the body's use of energy. These hormone changes can affect your body weight.

"Ongoing research shows a lack of sleep can produce diabetic-like conditions in otherwise healthy people," says Dr. Mitler.

Some studies also reveal that sleep can affect the efficiency of vaccinations. Dr. Twery described research showing that well-rested people who received the flu vaccine developed stronger protection against the illness.

A good night's sleep consists of four to five sleep cycles. Each cycle includes periods of deep sleep and rapid eye movement (REM) sleep when we dream. "As the night goes on, the portion of that cycle that is in REM sleep increases. It turns out that this pattern of cycling and progression is critical to the biology of sleep," Dr. Twery says.

Although personal needs vary, on average, adults need seven to eight hours of sleep per night. Babies typically sleep about 16 hours a day. Young children need at least 10 hours of sleep, while teenagers need least nine hours. To attain the maximum restorative benefits of sleep, getting a full night of quality sleep is important, says Dr. Twery.

Sleep can be disrupted by many things. Stimulants such as caffeine or certain medications can keep you up. Distractions such as electronics—especially the light from TVs, cell phones, tablets, and e-readers—can prevent you from falling asleep.

As people get older, they may not get enough sleep because of illness, medications, or sleep disorders. By some estimates, about 70 million Americans of all ages suffer from chronic sleep problems. The two most common sleep disorders are insomnia and sleep apnea.

People with insomnia have trouble falling or staying asleep. Anxiety about falling asleep often makes the condition worse. Most of us have occasional insomnia. But chronic insomnia—lasting at least three nights per week for more than a month—can trigger serious daytime problems such as exhaustion, irritability, and difficulty concentrating.

Common therapies include relaxation and deep-breathing techniques. Sometimes, medicine is prescribed. But consult a doctor before trying even over-the-counter (OTC) sleep pills, as they may leave you feeling unrefreshed in the morning.

People with sleep apnea have a loud, uneven snore (although not everyone who snores has apnea). Breathing repeatedly stops or becomes shallow. If you have apnea, you are not getting enough oxygen, and your brain disturbs your sleep to open your windpipe.

Apnea is dangerous. "There is little air exchange for 10 seconds or more at a time," explains Dr. Phyllis Zee, director at the Center for Circadian and Sleep Medicine at Northwestern University—The Feinberg School of Medicine. "The oxygen goes down, and the body's fight or flight response is activated. Blood pressure spikes, your heart rate fluctuates, and the brain wakes you up partially to start your breathing again. This creates stress."

Apnea can leave you feeling tired and moody. You may have trouble thinking clearly. "Also, apnea affects the vessels that lead to the brain, so there is a higher risk of stroke associated with it," Dr. Zee adds.

If you have mild sleep apnea, you might try sleeping on your side, exercising, or losing weight to reduce symptoms. A continuous positive airway pressure (CPAP) machine, which pumps air into your throat to keep your airway open, can also help. Another treatment is a bite plate that moves the lower jaw forward. In some cases, however, people with sleep apnea need surgery.

"If you snore chronically and wake up choking or gasping for air and feel that you are sleepy during the day, tell your doctor and get evaluated," Dr. Zee advises.

The NIH is funding several studies to gain deeper insights into sleep apnea and other aspects of sleep. One five-year study of 10,000 pregnant women is designed to gauge the effects of apnea on the mother's and baby's health. Dr. Zee says that this study will shed more light on apnea and the importance of treatment.

Good sleep is critical to your health. To make each day a safe, productive one, take steps to make sure you regularly get a good night's sleep.[2]

## DAYTIME HABITS
Making small changes to your daily routine can help you get the sleep you need.

### Change What You Do during the Day
- Try to spend some time outdoors in the daylight—earlier in the day is best.
- Plan your physical activity for earlier in the day, not right before you go to bed.
- Stay away from caffeine (including coffee, tea, and soda) late in the day.
- If you have trouble sleeping at night, limit daytime naps to 20 minutes or less.
- If you drink alcohol, drink only in moderation (less than one drink in a day for women and less than two drinks in a day for men)—alcohol can keep you from sleeping well.
- Do not eat a big meal close to bedtime.
- If you smoke, make a plan to quit—the nicotine in cigarettes can make it harder for you to sleep.

[2] *NIH News in Health*, "The Benefits of Slumber," National Institutes of Health (NIH), April 2013. Available online. URL: https://newsinhealth.nih.gov/2013/04/benefits-slumber. Accessed March 9, 2023.

## NIGHTTIME HABITS
## Create a Good Sleep Environment

- Make sure your bedroom is dark—if there are streetlights near your window, try putting up light-blocking curtains.
- Keep your bedroom quiet.
- Consider keeping electronic devices—such as TVs, computers, and smartphones—out of your bedroom.

## Set a Bedtime Routine

- Go to bed at the same time every night.
- Try to get the same amount of sleep each night.
- Avoid eating, talking on the phone, or reading in bed.
- Avoid using computers or smartphones, watching TV, or playing video games at bedtime.
- If you find yourself up at night worrying about things, use these tips to help manage stress.
- If you are still awake after staying in bed for more than 20 minutes, get up. Do something relaxing, such as reading or meditating, until you feel sleepy.

## SEE A DOCTOR
## If You Are Concerned about Your Sleep, See a Doctor

Talk with a doctor or nurse if you have any of the following signs of a sleep disorder:

- trouble falling or staying asleep
- still feeling tired after a good night's sleep
- sleepiness during the day that makes it difficult to do everyday activities, such as driving or concentrating at work
- frequent loud snoring
- pauses in breathing or gasping while sleeping
- tingling or crawling feelings in your legs or arms at night that feel better when you move or massage the area
- trouble staying awake during the day
- feeling like it is hard to move when you first wake up

Even if you do not have these problems, talk with a doctor if you feel like you often have trouble sleeping. Keep a sleep diary for a week and share it with your doctor. A doctor can suggest different sleep routines or medicines to treat sleep disorders. Talk with a doctor before trying over-the-counter (OTC) sleep medicine.

## WHAT ARE SOME TIPS FOR A GOOD NIGHT'S SLEEP?

Sleep experts at the National Institute of Neurological Disorders and Stroke recommend that you try several approaches if you have trouble falling asleep:

- **Set a schedule**. Go to bed at the same time each night and wake up at the same time each morning.
- **Exercise 20–30 minutes each day**. Regular daily exercise can help people sleep, as long as it is not done too close to bedtime.
- **Avoid caffeine, nicotine, and alcohol**. Caffeine acts as a stimulant and can keep you awake. Caffeine can be found in coffee, chocolate, soft drinks, certain teas, diet drugs, and pain relievers. Nicotine affects how deeply you sleep, and smokers tend to sleep very lightly. Alcohol prevents people from entering deep sleep (sleep stage 3) and REM sleep.
- **Relax before bed**. Try taking a warm bath, reading, or drinking warm herbal tea before falling asleep. You can train yourself to associate these types of restful activities with sleep, particularly if you make them part of your nighttime ritual.
- **Sleep until sunlight**. Try to wake up with the sunrise, if possible. If this is not possible, use bright lights in the morning. Sunlight (or bright light) helps the body's internal biological clock reset itself each day. Experts recommend an hour of exposure to morning sunlight for people having problems falling asleep.
- **Do not lie in bed awake**. If you are unable to fall asleep, try doing something else, such as reading, watching television, or listening to music, until you feel tired. The anxiety you feel when you are unable to fall

asleep further contributes to insomnia. Therefore, lying in bed waiting to fall asleep can worsen insomnia.

- **Control your room temperature**. Maintain a comfortable temperature in your bedroom. Temperature extremes can disrupt sleep or prevent you from falling asleep.
- **Know when it is time to see a health-care provider**. You should visit your doctor or a sleep specialist if you continue to have problems sleeping. If you have trouble falling asleep night after night or if you always feel tired the next day, you may have a sleep disorder and should see a health-care provider.[3]

[3] Office of Disease Prevention and Health Promotion (ODPHP), "Get Enough Sleep," U.S. Department of Health and Human Services (HHS), July 15, 2022. Available online. URL: https://health.gov/myhealthfinder/healthy-living/mental-health-and-relationships/get-enough-sleep. Accessed March 8, 2023.

# Chapter 3 | **Phases of Sleep**

## WHAT HAPPENS DURING SLEEP?

In broad terms, the brain of someone who is sleeping cycles through two basic phases: rapid eye movement (REM) sleep and non-REM sleep. Non-REM sleep includes three different stages. A person cycles through REM sleep and non-REM sleep several times a night. Each phase of sleep helps the mind and body stay rested. Certain stages help you feel rested and energetic the next day, while both phases help you learn information and form memories.

Sleep progresses in a cycle: from non-REM sleep stage 1 to non-REM sleep stage 2, to non-REM sleep stage 3, to REM sleep. Then the process starts over again with non-REM sleep stage 1. The length of sleep stages changes during a given night's sleep. For example, near the beginning of sleep, the body cycles through relatively short periods of REM sleep and long periods of deep sleep. As the night goes on, periods of REM sleep increase, and those of deep sleep decrease. Near the end of a night of sleep, a person spends nearly all of their time in stages 1 and 2 and REM.

Some of the characteristics of each phase include the following.

## NON-RAPID EYE MOVEMENT SLEEP

As you begin to fall asleep, you enter non-REM sleep, which consists of stages 1 through 3, as follows:

- Stage 1:
  - You are in between being awake and being asleep.
  - Your heartbeat and breathing slow, and your muscles relax.
- Stage 2:
  - You are in a light sleep.
  - Your brain waves slow down.

- Your body temperature lowers.
- Stage 3:
  - Your deepest and most restorative sleep happens.
  - Your heartbeat and breathing slow to their lowest levels.
  - Your muscles relax.
  - Your body increases the supply of blood to your muscles.
  - Your body performs tissue growth and repair.
  - Your energy is restored.
  - Your body releases hormones.

## RAPID EYE MOVEMENT SLEEP

You first enter REM sleep about 90 minutes after you fall asleep. REM sleep becomes longer later into the night. REM is characterized as follows:
- Your brain and body are energized.
- Your breathing becomes fast and irregular.
- Your brain is active, and dreaming occurs.
- Your eyes dart back and forth.
- Your body becomes immobile and relaxed, preventing you from acting out your dreams.
- Your body temperature is not as tightly regulated.

REM sleep begins in response to signals sent to and from different regions of the brain. Signals are sent to the brain's cerebral cortex, which is responsible for learning, thinking, and organizing information. Signals are also sent to the spinal cord to shut off the movement, creating a temporary inability to move the muscles ("paralysis") in the arms and legs. If this temporary paralysis is disrupted, people might move while they are dreaming ("sleepwalking"). A person who sleepwalks is at risk of injury.

REM sleep is thought to be involved in storing memories, learning, and balancing mood. REM sleep stimulates regions of the brain that are used for learning. Studies have shown that when people are deprived of REM sleep, they are not able to remember what they were taught before going to sleep. Lack of REM sleep has also been linked to certain health conditions, such as migraines. However, insufficient sleep, regardless of the sleep stage, can interfere with learning, memory, and performance. If you have any concerns about your sleep quality and habits, speak with your health-care provider.

## DREAMING

Scientists are not sure why we dream. While some of the signals sent to the cortex during sleep are important for learning and memory, some signals seem to be random. Dreams are generally most vivid during REM sleep, but dreaming can also occur during non-REM sleep.

Through research, we are learning more about dreaming. One study, for example, found that a pattern of brain activity from a part of the cortex near the back of the brain is a good predictor of whether an individual is dreaming and whether the individual was in REM or non-REM sleep.[1]

---

[1] "What Happens during Sleep?" *Eunice Kennedy Shriver* National Institute of Child Health and Human Development (NICHD), April 29, 2019. Available online. URL: www.nichd.nih.gov/health/topics/sleep/condition-info/what-happens. Accessed March 9, 2023.

# Chapter 4 | **What Happens during Sleep?**

## Chapter Contents

## Section 4.1 | **How Sleep Resets the Brain**

People spend about a third of their lives asleep. When we get too little shut-eye, it takes a toll on attention, learning, and memory, not to mention our physical health. Virtually, all animals with complex brains seem to have this same need for sleep. But exactly what is it about sleep that is so essential?

Two studies funded by the National Institutes of Health (NIH) in mice now offer a possible answer. The two research teams used entirely different approaches to reach the same conclusion: The brain's neural connections grow stronger during waking hours but scale back during snooze time. This sleep-related phenomenon apparently keeps neural circuits from overloading, ensuring that mice (and quite likely humans) awaken with brains that are refreshed and ready to tackle new challenges.

The idea that sleep is required to keep the brain wiring sharp goes back more than a decade. While a fair amount of evidence has emerged to support the hypothesis, its originators Chiara Cirelli, M.D., Ph.D., professor, Department of Psychiatry at the University of Wisconsin-Madison, and Giulio Tononi, M.D., Ph.D., professor of psychiatry at the University of Wisconsin-Madison, set out in their new study to provide some of the first direct visual proof that it is indeed the case.

As published in the journal *Science*, the researchers used a painstaking, cutting-edge imaging technique to capture high-resolution pictures of two areas of the mouse's cerebral cortex, a part of the brain that coordinates incoming sensory and motor information. The technique, called "serial scanning three-dimensional (3D) electron microscopy," involves repeated scanning of small slices of the brain to produce many thousands of images, allowing the researchers to produce detailed 3D reconstructions of individual neurons.

Their goal was to measure the size of the synapses, where the ends of two neurons connect. Synapses are critical for one neuron to pass signals on to the next, and the strength of those neural connections corresponds to their size.

The researchers measured close to 7,000 synapses in all. Their images show that synapses grew stronger and larger as these nocturnal mice scurried about at night. Then, after six to eight hours of sleep during the day, those synapses shrank by about 18 percent as the brain reset for another night of activity. Importantly, the effects of sleep held when the researchers switched the mice's schedule, keeping them up and engaged with toys and other objects during the day.

In the second science report, Richard L. Huganir, Ph.D., director, Department of Neuroscience, professor of neuroscience, and his colleagues at Johns Hopkins University School of Medicine, Baltimore, measured changes in the levels of certain brain proteins with sleep to offer biochemical evidence for this weakening of synapses. Their findings show that levels of protein receptors found on the receiving ends of synapses dropped by 20 percent while their mice slept.

The researchers also show that the protein Homer1a—important in regulating sleep and wakefulness—rises in synapses during a long snooze, playing a critical role in the resetting process. When the protein was lacking, the brain did not reset properly during sleep. This suggests that Homer1a responds to chemical cues in the brain that signal the need to sleep.

These studies add to prior work that suggests another function of sleep is to allow glial lymphatics in the brain to clear out proteins and other toxins that have deposited during the day. All of this goes to show that a good night's sleep can really bring clarity. Therefore, the next time you are struggling to make a decision and someone tells you to "sleep on it," that might be really good advice.[1]

[1] "How Sleep Resets the Brain," National Institutes of Health (NIH), February 14, 2017. Available online. URL: https://directorsblog.nih.gov/2017/02/14/how-sleep-resets-the-brain. Accessed March 9, 2023.

## Section 4.2 | **Brain May Flush Out Toxins during Sleep**

A good night's rest may literally clear the mind. Using mice, researchers showed for the first time that the space between brain cells may increase during sleep, allowing the brain to flush out toxins that build up during waking hours. These results suggest a new role for sleep in health and disease. The study was funded by the National Institute of Neurological Disorders and Stroke (NINDS), part of the National Institutes of Health (NIH).

"Sleep changes the cellular structure of the brain. It appears to be a completely different state," said Maiken Nedergaard, M.D., D.M.Sc., co-director of the Center for Translational Neuromedicine at the University of Rochester Medical Center in New York and leader of the study.

For centuries, scientists and philosophers have wondered why people sleep and how it affects the brain. Only recently, scientists have shown that sleep is important for storing memories. In this study, Dr. Nedergaard and her colleagues unexpectedly found that sleep may also be the period when the brain cleanses itself of toxic molecules.

Their results, published in *Science*, show that during sleep, a plumbing system called the "glymphatic system" may open, letting fluid flow rapidly through the brain. Dr. Nedergaard's lab recently discovered that the glymphatic system helps control the flow of cerebrospinal fluid (CSF), a clear liquid surrounding the brain and spinal cord.

"It is as if Dr. Nedergaard and her colleagues have uncovered a network of hidden caves, and these exciting results highlight the potential importance of the network in normal brain function," said Roderick Corriveau, Ph.D., program director at the NINDS.

Initially, the researchers studied the system by injecting dye into the CSF of mice and watching it flow through their brains while simultaneously monitoring electrical brain activity. The dye flowed rapidly when the mice were unconscious, either asleep or anesthetized. In contrast, the dye barely flowed when the same mice were awake.

"We were surprised by how little flow there was into the brain when the mice were awake," said Dr. Nedergaard. "It suggested that the space between brain cells changed greatly between conscious and unconscious states."

To test this idea, the researchers inserted electrodes into the brain to directly measure the space between brain cells. They found that the space inside the brains increased by 60 percent when the mice were asleep or anesthetized.

"These are some dramatic changes in extracellular space," said Charles Nicholson, Ph.D., professor at New York University's Langone Medical Center and an expert in measuring the dynamics of brain fluid flow and how it influences nerve cell communication.

Certain brain cells, called "glia," control flow through the glymphatic system by shrinking or swelling. Noradrenaline is an arousing hormone that is also known to control cell volume. Similar to using anesthesia, treating awake mice with drugs that block noradrenaline-induced unconsciousness and increased brain fluid flow and the space between cells, further supporting the link between the glymphatic system and consciousness.

Previous studies suggest that toxic molecules involved in neurodegenerative disorders accumulate in the space between brain cells. In this study, the researchers tested whether the glymphatic system controls this by injecting mice with labeled beta-amyloid, a protein associated with Alzheimer disease (AD), and measuring how long it lasted in their brains when they were asleep or awake. Beta-amyloid disappeared faster in mice brains when the mice were asleep, suggesting sleep normally clears toxic molecules from the brain.

"These results may have broad implications for multiple neurological disorders," said Jim Koenig, Ph.D., program director at the NINDS. "This means the cells regulating the glymphatic system may be new targets for treating a range of disorders."

The results may also highlight the importance of sleep. "We need sleep. It cleans up the brain," said Dr. Nedergaard.[2]

---

[2] News and Events, "Brain May Flush Out Toxins during Sleep," National Institutes of Health (NIH), October 17, 2013. Available online. URL: www.nih.gov/news-events/news-releases/brain-may-flush-out-toxins-during-sleep. Accessed March 9, 2023.

## Section 4.3 | **Sleep and Your Hormones**

When you were young, your parent may have told you that you need to get enough sleep to grow strong and tall. He or she may have been right! Deep sleep (stage 3 non-rapid eye movement (non-REM) sleep) triggers more release of growth hormone, which contributes to growth in children and boosts muscle mass and the repair of cells and tissues in children and adults. Sleep's effect on the release of sex hormones also contributes to puberty and fertility. Consequently, women who work at night and tend to lack sleep may be at an increased risk of miscarriage.

Your parent was also probably right if he or she told you that getting a good night's sleep on a regular basis would help keep you from getting sick and help you get better if you do get sick. During sleep, your body creates more cytokines—cellular hormones that help the immune system fight various infections. Lack of sleep can reduce your body's ability to fight off common infections. Research also reveals that a lack of sleep can reduce the body's response to the flu vaccine. For example, sleep-deprived volunteers given the flu vaccine produced less than half as many flu antibodies as those who were well-rested and given the same vaccine.

Although lack of exercise and other factors also contribute, the current epidemic of diabetes and obesity seems to be related, at least in part, to chronically short or disrupted sleep or not sleeping during the night. Evidence is growing that sleep is a powerful regulator of appetite, energy use, and weight control. During sleep, the body's production of the appetite suppressor leptin increases, and the appetite stimulant ghrelin decreases. Studies find that the less people sleep, the more likely they are to be overweight or obese and prefer eating foods that are higher in calories and carbohydrates. People who report an average total sleep time of five hours a night, for example, are much more likely to become obese than people who sleep seven to eight hours a night.

A number of hormones released during sleep also control the body's use of energy. A distinct rise and fall of blood sugar levels during sleep appears to be linked to sleep stages. Not sleeping at the right time, not getting enough sleep overall, or not enough of each stage of sleep disrupts this pattern. One study found that when healthy young men slept only four hours a night for six nights in a row, their insulin and blood sugar levels matched those seen in people who were developing diabetes. Another study found that women who slept less than seven hours a night were more likely to develop diabetes over time than those who slept between seven and eight hours a night.[3]

## Section 4.4 | How Snoozing Strengthens Memories

When you learn something new, the best way to remember it is to sleep on it. That is because sleeping helps strengthen memories you have formed throughout the day. It also helps link new memories to earlier ones. You might even come up with creative new ideas while you slumber.

What happens to memories in your brain while you sleep? And how does lack of sleep affect your ability to learn and remember? NIH-funded scientists have been gathering clues about the complex relationship between sleep and memory. Their findings might eventually lead to new approaches to help students learn or help older people hold onto memories as they age.

"We have learned that sleep before learning helps prepare your brain for the initial formation of memories," says Dr. Matthew Walker, sleep scientist at the University of California, Berkeley. "And then, sleep after learning is essential to help save and cement that new information into the architecture of the brain, meaning that you are less likely to forget it."

---

[3] "Your Guide to Healthy Sleep," National Heart, Lung, and Blood Institute (NHLBI), January 8, 2011. Available online. URL: www.nhlbi.nih.gov/resources/your-guide-healthy-sleep. Accessed March 9, 2023.

## What Happens during Sleep?

While you snooze, your brain cycles through different phases of sleep, including light sleep, deep sleep, and REM sleep, when dreaming often occurs. The cycles repeat about every 90 minutes.

The non-REM stages of sleep seem to prime the brain for good learning the next day. If you have not slept, your ability to learn new things could drop by up to 40 percent. "You cannot pull an all-nighter and still learn effectively," Dr. Walker says. Lack of sleep affects a part of the brain called the "hippocampus," which is key for making new memories.

You accumulate many memories, moment by moment, while you are awake. Most will be forgotten during the day. "When we first form memories, they are in a very raw and fragile form," says professor of psychiatry Dr. Robert Stickgold of Harvard Medical School.

But when you doze off, "sleep seems to be a privileged time when the brain goes back through recent memories and decides both what to keep and what not to keep," Dr. Stickgold explains. "During a night of sleep, some memories are strengthened." Research has shown that memories of certain procedures, such as playing a melody on a piano, can actually improve while you sleep.

Memories seem to become more stable in the brain during the deep stages of sleep. After that, REM—the most active stage of sleep—seems to play a role in linking together related memories, sometimes in unexpected ways. That is why a full night of sleep may help with problem-solving. REM sleep also helps you process emotional memories, which can reduce the intensity of emotions.

It is well known that sleep patterns tend to change as we age. Unfortunately, the deep memory-strengthening stages of sleep start to decline in our late 30s. A study by Dr. Walker and colleagues found that adults older than 60 had a 70 percent loss of deep sleep compared to young adults aged 18–25. Older adults had a harder time remembering things the next day, and memory impairment was linked to reductions in deep sleep. The researchers are now exploring options for enhancing deep stages of sleep in this older age group.

"While we have limited medical treatments for memory impairment in aging, sleep actually is a potentially treatable target,"

Dr. Walker says. "By restoring sleep, it might be possible to improve memory in older people."

For younger people, especially students, Dr. Stickgold offers additional advice. "Realize that the sleep you get the night after you study is at least as important as the sleep you get the night before you study." When it comes to sleep and memory, he says, "you get very little benefit from cutting corners."[4]

[4] *NIH News in Health*, "Sleep on It," National Institutes of Health (NIH), April 2013. Available online. URL: https://newsinhealth.nih.gov/2013/04/sleep-it. Accessed March 9, 2023.

# Chapter 5 | **Napping: A Healthy Habit**

## Chapter Contents

## Section 5.1 | **What Is Napping?**

Most mammals are polyphasic sleepers, which means they sleep—or nap—multiple times during a 24-hour period. Humans, on the other hand, are monophasic sleepers since they have distinct, alternate phases of sleeping and waking. Whether this forms the natural sleep pattern for humans has not been clearly established; however, napping is an integral part of many cultures globally.

The United States is fast becoming a nation of deprived sleepers due primarily to a culture that often promotes a hectic lifestyle. Napping could be a solution since sleeping for 20–30 minutes during normal waking hours has been shown to result in remarkable improvements in mood, alertness, and performance.

## THE TYPES OF NAPPING

The following are the three different ways that we usually nap:

- **Planned napping**. Also known as "preparatory napping," this involves taking a nap before you are sleepy in anticipation of going to bed late. This helps you avoid feeling tired because of inadequate sleep later on.
- **Emergency napping**. You may take an emergency nap when you feel tired and unable to continue the task you were engaged in. This type of napping is very useful when you have been driving and are feeling drowsy or when you need to counter fatigue when operating dangerous machinery.
- **Habitual napping**. This is the practice of taking naps as a regular routine at a particular time of the day. Young children nap this way, and it is not uncommon in many cultures for adults to nap after lunch.

## RECOMMENDATIONS FOR NAPPING

- A nap of 20–30 minutes is optimal. It tends not to interfere with your regular sleep pattern and generally does not make you groggy.
- Sleep in a comfortable place with moderate room temperature and without much noise or light filtering in. It is most beneficial to sleep rather than just lie in bed resting.
- Do not take a nap too late in the day because it will affect your regular sleep at night. Do not nap early in the day, either, since you may not be able to sleep well.

## SEVEN STEPS TO HAVE THE PERFECT NAP

Just lying down, closing your eyes, and hoping for the best would not necessarily help you nap. You should think it out and employ a strategy to help you nap better. The following steps will help you get the perfect nap:

### Step One

Decide how long you want to nap. Different durations confer their own benefits:

- **6 minutes**. This nap time provides improvement in memory functions.
- **10-15 minutes**. It improves focus and productivity.
- **20-30 minutes**. This is an optimum nap time, which results in alertness, concentration, and sharp motor skills.
- **40–60 minutes**. Taking a nap for 40–60 minutes boosts brain power; consolidates memory for facts, places, and faces; and improves learning ability.
- **90–120 minutes**. This is a nap time that improves creativity and emotional and procedural memory.

### Step Two
#### NAP BETWEEN 1 P.M. AND 3 P.M.

The body has an inherent biological clock that controls the sleep–wake cycle, known as the "circadian rhythm." Humans experience intense sleep in two periods every 24 hours. One is between 1 and 3 p.m., and the other is from 2 to 4 a.m. Alertness, reaction time, coordination, and mood are decreased during these periods. The lethargy experienced after lunch is actually biological in nature. A nap around this time will put you back on track. Napping between 1 and 3 p.m. will generally not disturb regular sleep. If you work a night shift, the best time to take a nap would be six to eight hours after waking.

## Step Three
### CREATE A CONDUCIVE ATMOSPHERE

If you are unable to fall asleep during the day, you may not be approaching napping the right way. Lighting is an important factor since light inhibits melatonin, the sleep regulation hormone. Darken your room with window shades or use an eye mask. Lie down, rather than sitting, when you take a nap. You will fall asleep 50 percent faster. Many people find that a hammock is the best place to nap because of the gentle swaying motion that promotes sleep.

## Step Four
### USE AN ALARM

You will need to wake up in time to get back to work after a snooze, so set an alarm to wake you up.

## Step Five
### TRY A COFFEE NAP

If you are concerned about becoming sleepy in the afternoon, try having a cup of coffee and taking a nap. Caffeine kicks into the body in 20–30 minutes. This should give you enough time to take a nap and get rejuvenated. Combining coffee and napping can be more beneficial than doing either of them alone.

## Step Six
### AVOID THE BLAHS AFTER NAPPING

Make sure you avoid sleep inertia. If you take a long nap, you may feel groggy after waking up because a full sleep cycle was not completed. Avoid this by having coffee, washing your face, or exposing yourself to bright light. An alternative is to complete a full sleep cycle by taking a nap for at least 90 minutes.

## Step Seven
### GET ADEQUATE SLEEP AT NIGHT

Nothing replaces a good night's sleep, and emergency napping cannot be a long-term substitute for regular, deep sleep. Inadequate sleep on a regular basis can result in hypertension, diabetes, weight gain, depression, and a general feeling of unease.

## PROS OF NAPPING

- Napping improves alertness and performance levels. It reduces mistakes and accidents. A National Aeronautics and Space Administration (NASA) study conducted on military pilots showed that 40 minutes of napping increased alertness by 100 percent and performance by 34 percent.
- Naps improve alertness for some duration after the nap and often increase alertness to some extent over the entire day.
- Napping results in relaxation and rejuvenation. It is a luxurious and pleasant experience, something similar to a mini vacation.
- Taking a nap when you are feeling drowsy behind the wheel can help you regain alertness so that you can continue to drive safely.
- Night-shift workers who nap have been shown to experience improved alertness on the job.
- A 45-minute daytime nap improves memory functioning.
- Napping reduces blood pressure.
- It reduces the risk of cardiovascular diseases.
- Temporary sleep issues due to jet lag, stress, or illnesses can often be remedied by napping.
- A quick nap is very good for mental and physical stamina.
- Napping improves mental acuity and overall health.

## CONS OF NAPPING

- The stigma associated with napping is probably the biggest downside of napping.
- It may be equated with laziness.
- It is often associated with a lack of ambition and low standards.
- Napping may be seen as normal only for children, the sick, and the elderly.
- Napping can be counterproductive for people with sleep disorders or those with irregular sleep patterns.
- Naps are often not recommended for people with sleep apnea.

## References

Belsky, Gail. "The Pros and Cons of Napping," Health, April 8, 2015. Available online. URL: www.health.com/condition/sleep/the-pros-and-cons-of-napping. Accessed April 4, 2023.

Brown, Brendan. "A How-To Guide to the Perfect Nap [Infographic]," Art of Wellbeing, August 7, 2015. Available online. URL: www.artofwellbeing.com/2015/08/07/hack-your-nap. Accessed April 4, 2023.

"Napping," National Sleep Foundation, October 9, 2020. Available online. URL: www.sleepfoundation.org/sleep-topics/napping. Accessed April 4, 2023.

Section 5.2 | **Benefits of Napping**

## SLEEP RESEARCHERS HOME IN ON THE BENEFITS OF NAPPING

Getting a good night's sleep is important for everyone. Good sleep refreshes people, helps them perform better, and contributes significantly to health and happiness. For many veterans, however, getting a good night's sleep is extremely difficult.

Sleep disturbances are common in patients suffering from bipolar disorder, substance abuse, major depression, panic disorder, and chronic pain disorders. Sleep disorders following recent exposure to traumatic events can predict the later development of posttraumatic stress disorder (PTSD).

Disrupted sleep, or the inability to get a full night's sleep without interruption, is a very common negative consequence of PTSD. According to the Veterans Affairs (VA) National Center for PTSD, nightmares are 1 of the 17 symptoms of the disorder, and as many as 71 percent of those with the illness reported experiencing nightmares, sometimes or more frequently, compared to only 3 percent of those who did not serve.

For some who simply cannot get a good night's sleep, there is a way to avoid many of the consequences of sleeplessness. "Napping has been shown to alleviate the negative physical and psychological symptoms of disrupted sleep," says Elizabeth A. McDevitt, a graduate student in the Department of psychology at the University of California, Riverside. At the time the research was conducted, McDevitt was affiliated with the San Diego VA Medical Center and the University of California, San Diego (UCSD).

According to a study published online in the *Journal of Physiology and Behavior* by McDevitt and two colleagues from the San Diego VA and UCSD, napping is especially helpful to manage circadian disruption (problems related either from changes in a person's sleep–wake cycle, such as jet lag, daylight saving time, or between workweeks and weekends, or through the inability to get enough sleep in the time allotted for sleep). In healthy, well-rested subjects, napping has also been shown to improve performance across a range of performance tasks.

Despite the benefits of napping, however, some people report that they simply cannot nap or do not want to nap. In their study, McDevitt and her colleagues set out to determine why some people nap and others do not.

She and her colleagues asked 27 healthy, nonsmoking college students between the ages of 18 and 35 to participate in an experiment. All of them spent between seven and nine hours in bed every night, and none of them had a sleep disorder. They were asked to keep a diary of their sleep habits for a week, including their daily naps if they took them, and wore special actigraph wristwatches (small, wristwatch-shaped devices that record motion and are used to assess sleep by determining whether a person is active or inactive) to verify what they had put down in their diaries.

After a week of measurements, each participant reported to the Laboratory for Sleep and Behavioral Neuroscience at the San Diego VA. Their level of sleepiness was measured at 9 a.m., 11 a.m., 4:30 p.m., and 6:30 p.m. At 1:30 p.m., they were all asked to take a nap and were allowed to sleep for a maximum of 90 minutes—but they were given no more than 120 minutes in bed, whether they napped or not. While they napped, their brain waves were monitored through electrodes to see how deeply they were sleeping.

By correlating the information in the subjects' diaries and analyzing the brain wave information they obtained, the team found that people who nap frequently sleep more lightly during their naps than those who usually never nap at all. In sleep, the body progresses through a series of five stages, from light sleep through dreaming, called the "sleep cycle" (sleep does not progress through these stages in order, however).

Those who had taken three to four naps in the week before the brain wave tests took place had the least amount of slow wave sleep (scientist's term for stage 3, or deep, sleep) and the most amount of stage 1, or light, sleep; those who took one to two naps a week had the most amount of stage 2 sleep, which is somewhat deeper; and those who never napped at all had the highest amount of stage 3 sleep while in the laboratory, meaning they slept most deeply. The naps that people of all groups took did not measurably affect their sleep at night.

Using these data, the team developed two hypotheses. First, some people avoid napping because of the high levels of deep sleep that they fall into when they do nap—meaning that when they wake up, they feel groggy and tired instead of rested and refreshed. And, second, people who choose to nap may just be sleepier people than those who do not.

"Individuals who frequently nap may generally be sleepier people who are self-treating their sleepiness with daytime naps," said McDevitt. "They might be predisposed to be good daytime nappers, or they have learned to become skilled nappers through practice."

The team suggested that future studies should consider the possibility of nap practice or nap training to maximize the benefits of napping and examine how differences in sleep associated with nap behavior may influence changes in performance following a nap.[1]

---

[1] "Sleep Researchers Home In on the Benefits of Napping," U.S. Department of Veterans Affairs (VA), February 11, 2014. Available online. URL: www.research.va.gov/news/features/napping.cfm. Accessed March 9, 2023.

# Chapter 6 | **Dreaming**

## Chapter Contents

## THE BRAIN MAY ACTIVELY FORGET DURING DREAM SLEEP

Rapid eye movement (REM) sleep is a fascinating period when most of our dreams occur. Now, in a study of mice, a team of Japanese and U.S. researchers shows that it may also be a time when the brain actively forgets. Their results suggest that forgetting during sleep may be controlled by neurons found deep inside the brain that were previously known for making an appetite-stimulating hormone. The study was funded by the National Institute of Neurological Disorders and Stroke (NINDS), part of the National Institutes of Health (NIH).

"Ever wonder why we forget many of our dreams?" said Thomas Kilduff, Ph.D., director of the Center for Neuroscience at SRI International, Menlo Park, California, and senior author of the study published in *Science*. "Our results suggest that the firing of a particular group of neurons during REM sleep controls whether the brain remembers new information after a good night's sleep."

REM is one of several sleep stages the body cycles through every night. It first occurs about 90 minutes after falling asleep and is characterized by darting eyes, raised heart rates, paralyzed limbs, awakened brain waves, and dreaming.

For more than a century, scientists have explored the role of sleep in storing memories. While many have shown that sleep helps the brain store new memories, others, including Francis Crick, molecular biologist at Salk Institute for Biological Studies, have raised the possibility that sleep—in particular REM sleep—may be a time when the brain actively eliminates or forgets excess information. Moreover, studies in mice have shown that during sleep—including REM sleep—the brain selectively prunes synaptic connections made between neurons involved in certain types of learning. However, until this study, no one had shown how this might happen.

"Understanding the role of sleep in forgetting may help researchers better understand a wide range of memory-related diseases such as posttraumatic stress disorder and Alzheimer," said Janet He, Ph.D., program director at the NINDS. "This study provides the most direct evidence that REM sleep may play a role in how the brain decides which memories to store."

Dr. Kilduff's lab and that of his collaborator, Akihiro Yamanaka, Ph.D., professor, Research Institute of Environmental Medicine at Nagoya University in Japan, have spent years examining the role of a hormone called "hypocretin/orexin" in controlling sleep and narcolepsy. Narcolepsy is a disorder that makes people feel excessively sleepy during the day and sometimes experience changes reminiscent of REM sleep, such as loss of muscle tone in the limbs and hallucinations. Their labs and others have helped show how narcolepsy may be linked to the loss of hypocretin/orexin-making neurons in the hypothalamus, a peanut-sized area found deep inside the brain.

In this study, Dr. Kilduff worked with the labs of Dr. Yamanaka and Akira Terao, D.V.M., Ph.D. (lab located at Hokkaido University, Sapporo, Japan), to look at neighboring cells that produce melanin-concentrating hormone (MCH), a molecule known to be involved in the control of both sleep and appetite. In agreement with previous studies, the researchers found that a majority (52.8%) of hypothalamic MCH cells fired when mice underwent REM sleep, whereas about 35 percent fired only when the mice were awake and about 12 percent fired at both times.

They also uncovered clues suggesting that these cells may play a role in learning and memory. Electrical recordings and tracing experiments showed that many of the hypothalamic MCH cells sent inhibitory messages, via long stringy axons, to the hippocampus, the brain's memory center.

"From previous studies done in other labs, we already knew that MCH cells were active during REM sleep. After discovering this new circuit, we thought these cells might help the brain store memories," said Dr. Kilduff. To test this idea, the researchers used a variety of genetic tools to turn on and off MCH neurons in mice during memory tests. Specifically, they examined the role that MCH cells played in retention, the period after learning something new but before the new knowledge is stored, or consolidated, into long-term memory. The scientists used several memory tests including one that assessed the ability of mice to distinguish between new and familiar objects.

To their surprise, they found that "turning on" MCH cells during retention worsened memory, whereas turning the cells off improved memories. For instance, activating the cells reduced the time mice spent sniffing around new objects compared to familiar ones, but turning the cells off had the opposite effect.

Further experiments suggested that MCH neurons exclusively played this role during REM sleep. Mice performed better on memory tests when MCH neurons were turned off during REM sleep. In contrast, turning off the neurons while the mice were awake or in other sleep states had no effect on memory.

"These results suggest that MCH neurons help the brain actively forget new, possibly, unimportant information," said Dr. Kilduff. "Since dreams are thought to primarily occur during REM sleep, the sleep stage when the MCH cells turn on, activation of these cells may prevent the content of a dream from being stored in the hippocampus—consequently, the dream is quickly forgotten." In the future, the researchers plan to explore whether this new circuit plays a role in sleep and memory disorders.[1]

## MAPPING THE BRAIN DURING SLEEP YIELDS NEW INSIGHTS ON DREAMING AND CONSCIOUSNESS

A study counters some long-held beliefs on sleep, dreaming, and other consciousness states—such as being under general anesthesia, in a coma, or experiencing an epileptic seizure. The study co-supported by the National Center for Complementary and Integrative Health (NCCIH) was led at the University of Wisconsin-Madison and appears in the journal *Nature Neuroscience*.

---

[1] News and Events, "The Brain May Actively Forget during Dream Sleep," National Institutes of Health (NIH), September 19, 2019. Available online. URL: www.nih.gov/news-events/news-releases/brain-may-actively-forget-during-dream-sleep. Accessed April 4, 2023.

It has long been believed that the stage of sleep called "REM" owns our dreaming process. However, evidence suggests that dreams also occur during non-REM sleep and at every stage of non-REM, though not as often as in REM. The researchers who conducted this study wanted to gain more clarity on several questions relating to what happens in the brain when we dream (or do not dream) in REM or non-REM, sleep states, as read by high versus low electroencephalogram (EEG) frequencies, and with respect to certain types of remembered dream content such as faces, speech, thoughts, or settings. A key question was whether conscious experiences in sleep have a neural correlate, which is an activity, event, or mechanism in the brain that is associated with a particular experience and makes it possible.

The study was done as a series of experiments. The 32 adults in the first experiment had relatively few awakenings; the seven in the second experiment had relatively large numbers of awakenings and had learned a method to report their dream experiences. In both experiments, participants spent 5–10 nights in a sleep lab; whenever they were awakened, they were asked to describe the last thing they remembered before being awakened. They were also monitored by EEG during the entire sleep time. Each answer was categorized as follows:

- having a dreaming experience for which they could recall the content (This category led to more questioning, for example, about the type of content and degrees of perceptual and/or thought aspects.)
- a dreaming experience for which they could not recall the content
- no experience (The EEG signal patterns were then examined to see if the high- or low-frequency patterns were associated with the presence of dreams or not.)

The researchers then took the results from these experiments and conducted a third experiment (in which seven other participants spent three nights in the sleep lab) to see if the identified EEG patterns could predict the presence or absence of dreaming in real time.

Their major findings are as follows:

- There appears to be a "posterior hot zone" for conscious experiences in sleep (i.e., dreaming) in the parieto-occipital region of the cerebral cortex, and that hot zone could be the neural correlate of dream experiences. This veers from the traditional beliefs that dreaming belongs to REM sleep and is always characterized by waking-state-like, "globally activated," high-frequency EEGs.
- Non-REM sleep did not show an absence of dreaming.
- There was a prominent pattern of reduction in low-frequency EEG activity, which was associated with dreaming, not just the presence of high-frequency EEG patterns.
- In both REM and non-REM sleep, dreaming was correlated with drops in low-frequency EEG activity in posterior cortical regions. In comparison, increases in high-frequency activity in those same regions correlated with specific types of dream content.
- Whether a person had dream-reporting training did not seem to affect the results, and this strengthened support for the concept of a core correlate of dream experience that is not just some other cognitive function.

Future exploration, the authors note, could include examining this paradigm in other types of consciousness states, such as those in epileptic seizures or general anesthesia. This, in turn, might also shed light on whether other brain regions are involved in these various kinds of consciousness experiences.[2]

---

[2] "Mapping the Brain during Sleep Yields New Insights on Dreaming and Consciousness," National Center for Complementary and Integrative Health (NCCIH), April 10, 2017. Available online. URL: www.nccih.nih.gov/research/research-results/mapping-the-brain-during-sleep-yields-new-insights-on-dreaming-and-consciousness. Accessed April 4, 2023.

## Section 6.2 | **World of Dreams: Studying the Human Mind**

### SCIENTISTS BREAK THROUGH THE WALL OF SLEEP TO THE UNTAPPED WORLD OF DREAMS

The researchers supported by the National Science Foundation (NSF) achieve two-way communication with lucidly dreaming people, creating a new method for studying the human mind that might lead to innovative ways of learning and problem-solving.

It is not exactly "one small step for man," but that humble mathematical message is extraordinary in its own way. The first part—"eight minus six"—was transmitted by a scientist to a place just as exotic as the moon yet frequented by each of us. The response—"two"—came from the mind of a sleeping research subject as he snoozed in a neuroscience laboratory outside Chicago.

You see, "eight minus six... two" is a dialogue between two people—one of whom was asleep and dreaming.

"It is authentic communication," says Ken Paller, Ph.D., cognitive neuroscientist at Northwestern University and professor in the Department of Psychology, who oversees the laboratory where this groundbreaking communication took place. "It can be done."

Researchers at Dr. Paller's lab at Northwestern University in Illinois, along with researchers in France, Germany, and the Netherlands, have independently demonstrated two-way communication with people as they are lucidly dreaming during rapid eye movement (REM) sleep. Supported by the U.S. NSF, the breakthrough was achieved in the United States by Karen Konkoly, Dr. Paller's doctoral student, and Christopher Mazurek, a volunteer research participant at the time of the study—and one of the first people to ever engage in a real-time dialogue from within a dream.

This discovery holds tantalizing possibilities for expanding our understanding of how our minds work. It may even lead to methods that could improve our ability to learn difficult skills or solve complex problems. And, with the help of a new smartphone app from Dr. Paller's lab, you could even try it at home.

## The Windows to the Soul (and Dreams)

Research into the fundamental nature of dreams and what the human mind can do while dreaming has been limited by a seemingly unsolvable problem: You cannot get much information about someone's dream while they are actually having the dream. "All we have are the stories people tell when they wake up," says Dr. Paller. That deficiency has left an entire state of consciousness largely unexplored.

The novel methods pioneered by Konkoly, Dr. Paller, and their colleagues are designed to solve this problem and open entirely new areas of research focused on the dreaming mind. Konkoly describes the possibilities: "Right now, we conduct psychology experiments with people who are awake. With two-way communication (during dreams), we could conduct some of the same experiments while people are sleeping. It could really expand our view of consciousness and what the mind is capable of."

But how can a dreaming research subject communicate if they cannot even move, let alone speak, while sleeping? The answer requires some explanation about what happens in our mind during sleep.

Scientists have identified the different stages of sleep by monitoring electrical signals from the brain using electroencephalography (EEG) and from other places in the body. When the electrical signals are recorded and plotted, they chart the course our mind takes as we progress through the stages of sleep.

As you sleep, your mind transitions through several different stages, from light sleep to deep sleep and eventually to REM sleep. REM sleep is notable not just for what is moving—our eyes—but also for what is not. Although our mind is active and dreams often occur during REM sleep, our bodies are almost completely paralyzed. That presents an obvious challenge for communication since we cannot move the body parts we typically use to communicate. As the name "rapid eye movement" suggests, however, there is an exception.

During REM sleep, our eyes move around behind our eyelids in a seemingly random fashion, which often corresponds to the sleeper "looking" at various imagined things in their dream. If you dream that you are looking at something, your closed eyes move correspondingly as if you were looking at something while awake.

That phenomenon led researchers to a key insight: If eye movement were consciously controlled, the dreamer's eyes could become a vehicle for getting a message to the waking world.

## "He Is Lucid! Let's Do Math"

Who among us has not wished we could fly like a bird? Or walk on another planet? So-called lucid dreamers can do these things and more from the comfort of their own bed. Accomplished lucid dreamers have reported being able to regularly achieve awareness in their dreams and even "programming" themselves to have dreams about specific activities or locations.

Christopher Mazurek was not one of those people. "I had no experience with lucid dreaming," says Mazurek, an undergraduate student at Northwestern University and now a research assistant in Dr. Paller's sleep lab. At the time, he was a volunteer research participant. "Before I entered the lab, I never had anything near a lucid dream."

To prepare Mazurek and the other U.S. volunteers, Konkoly wired each participant with electrodes that sense brain activity through the scalp, behind the ears, on the chin, and—critically— near the eyes. Those would allow the researchers to monitor and record even slight eye movements. "When your eyes move in their sockets, it creates an electrical current which is detected by the electrodes and recorded," says Konkoly.

Konkoly also trained each research participant to help them achieve lucidity and instructed them on what to do if they succeeded. That included learning to recognize the specific sound she would play when they entered REM sleep, prompting the participants to realize they are dreaming and thus become lucid. The participants also learned the distinct response signal they should produce from within their dream: moving their eyes from left to right multiple times.

"Repeatedly looking from left to right is a very distinctive eye movement, and it stands out from other eye movements during REM sleep," says Konkoly. As she carefully watched the EEG and saw Mazurek progressing through the stages of sleep and into REM sleep, she spotted the repeating left-right signal on the monitor as Mazurek signaled his awareness.

"He is lucid!" remembers Konkoly. "Let's do the math." Konkoly played a randomly selected audio recording: "eight minus six." Mazurek knew he would be presented with simple math problems but did not know which problems would be selected. Some of the international labs in the study used different methods to send messages to their dreaming subjects, such as flashing lights in Morse code which the sleepers could perceive through their closed eyelids and manifest in their dream. In most of the labs, the research participants were trained to move their "dream eyes" to signal their answer.

A few seconds later, Konkoly saw Mazurek's response written among the peaks and valleys of his eyes' electrical signals: "two." Konkoly sent another randomly selected math problem and once again received a correct response. And what was Mazurek dreaming about during this groundbreaking exchange between two worlds?

"I dreamed I was sleeping in the lab when I heard her question," he says. Despite that rather mundane dreamscape, "It still blew me away how different and intense and odd it all felt. It was different than anything I could have imagined."

To obtain independent verification of their results, Konkoly sent the recorded data to an expert "sleep scorer." Like an astrophysicist who can tell you what elements are in a distant star by deciphering the colored light recorded in a spectrograph, a sleep scorer is trained to "read" the recorded electrical signals and analyze their complex patterns. The sleep scorer confirmed that Mazurek was indeed in REM sleep during the exchange.

While Mazurek was the first in Dr. Paller's lab to achieve two-way communication in a dream, two more participants later accomplished that same feat. Meanwhile, researchers in France, Germany, and the Netherlands were independently testing methods for two-way communication in dreams and reported that three additional individuals were able to provide correct responses while dreaming. The collective results from all the laboratories are now published in the journal *Current Biology*.

## Sleep on It

"Why would you want to do math in your sleep?" quips Konkoly. "I get that comment sometimes."

Joking aside, researchers have a number of ideas for how this discovery could be expanded and applied. "There is evidence that lucid dreaming is a great place to practice skills compared to when you are awake," says Konkoly. "For example, you could slow down time, so you could practice a skill in more detail or practice something without having any fear of the repercussions of failing."

Imagine a surgeon attempting to perfect a technique used in open heart surgery—in a dream.

"There are many unexplored neurobiological aspects to learning and training during REM sleep. But without two-way communication, you cannot conduct a proper controlled experiment to understand it," she adds.

"People say 'sleep on it' when grappling with a hard problem," says Dr. Paller, in reference to his research published in 2019, which showed people who were cued to think about puzzles during sleep exhibited substantial improvement in finding solutions. "There is some sense that sleep can help you find an answer to a problem that is vexing you. Our two-way communication method provides hope for improving that. If you are working on a problem, can you be reminded of that problem during a dream and come up with a creative answer more easily?"

"From run-of-the-mill personal problems to complex global problems, we need creative solutions. If we can help people come up with the answers more easily, we should do that," he says.

Dr. Paller's lab has also developed a smartphone app that aims to make it easier for people to achieve lucidity, which could enable anyone to phone home from the world of dreams without visiting a sleep laboratory.

## Our Full Potential

Although many aspects of the sleeping mind remain a mystery, researchers across a variety of scientific disciplines are utilizing new techniques and analytical methods to better understand it. "Sleep is valuable for our health in ways we have yet to come to grips with," says Dr. Paller. For example, neuroscientists at the University of California, Berkeley, recently uncovered evidence showing that sleep plays a critical role in how our brains flush out beta-amyloid, a toxic substance that contributes to the onset of Alzheimer disease (AD).

"REM sleep is a unique state of consciousness," adds Konkoly. "We spend a lot of time in it, and yet no one really understands its full potential. We want to know how it works."

The pioneering work of Konkoly, Dr. Paller, and their colleagues provides an entirely new method that scientists can use to investigate how sleep and dreams affect health and mental abilities.

And who knows? Perhaps the idea of conversing with someone from within a dream may one day be as routine as sending a text message on your phone: "Can I snooze five more minutes? I have almost figured out this problem..."[3]

---

[3] "Scientists Break through the Wall of Sleep to the Untapped World of Dreams," National Science Foundation (NSF), February 18, 2021. Available online. URL: https://beta.nsf.gov/science-matters/scientists-break-through-wall-sleep-untapped-world. Accessed March 14, 2023.

## Section 6.3 | **Nightmares**

Nightmares are dreams that are threatening and scary. Nearly everyone has had a nightmare from time to time. For trauma survivors, though, nightmares are a common problem. Along with flashbacks and unwanted memories, nightmares are one of the ways in which a trauma survivor may relive the trauma for months or years after the event.

## HOW COMMON ARE NIGHTMARES AFTER TRAUMA?

Among the general public, about 5 percent of people complain of nightmares. Those who have gone through a trauma, though, are more likely to have distressing nightmares after the event. This is true no matter what type of trauma it is.

Trauma survivors who get posttraumatic stress disorder (PTSD) are even more likely to complain of nightmares. Nightmares are 1 of the 17 symptoms of PTSD. For example, a study comparing Vietnam veterans to civilians showed that 52 percent of combat veterans with PTSD had nightmares fairly often. Only 3 percent of the civilians in the study reported that same level of nightmares.

Other research has found even higher rates of nightmares. Of those with PTSD, 71–96 percent may have nightmares. People who have other mental health problems, such as panic disorder, as well as PTSD, are more likely to have nightmares than those with PTSD alone.

Not only are trauma survivors more likely to have nightmares, but also those who do may have them quite often. Some survivors may have nightmares several times a week.

## NIGHTMARES AND CULTURAL DIFFERENCES

Nightmares may be viewed differently in different cultures. For example, in some cultures, nightmares are thought to mean that the dreamer is open to physical or spiritual harm. In other cultures, it is believed that the dreams may contain messages from spirits or may forecast the future. These beliefs may lead those with night-mares to use certain practices in an effort to protect themselves.[4]

## TIPS FOR COPING WITH NIGHTMARES

It is not unusual to have nightmares during times of stress. For combat veterans, these nightmares may include combat scenes. If you have frequent and distressing nightmares, talk to your medical or mental health provider. Frequent nightmares may be a sign of a more serious problem.

- The morning after a nightmare, spend some time thinking about what might be causing increased stress in your life. Even positive stress (such as getting married, a new job, or moving) can cause anxiety that may result in nightmares.
- Practice some form of relaxation every night before bed. Try imagining yourself in a calming or relaxing place, practice deep slow breathing, or listen to soothing music or sounds.
- Make your bedroom as soothing and comfortable as possible. Think about leaving a dim light or nightlight on to help you recognize your surroundings more quickly if you wake up from a nightmare.

## CAUSES OF SLEEP PROBLEMS

- medical problems such as pain, depression, side effects of medicines, or trouble breathing
- circadian rhythm disorder, a shift in the body's normal 24-hour activity cycle

---

[4] National Center for Posttraumatic Stress Disorder (NCPTSD), "Nightmares and PTSD," U.S. Department of Veterans Affairs (VA), October 17, 2019. Available online. URL: www.ptsd.va.gov/understand/related/nightmares. asp. Accessed April 5, 2023.

- lifestyle factors such as a changing sleep schedule, lack of exercise, or too much caffeine
- sleep settings such as a poor mattress, noise, or a room that is too hot or too cold
- stress such as from problems at work, money worries, or family events

## ASSESSMENT AND TREATMENT

The first step in treating sleeping problems is to understand what may be causing the sleep problem. Talk with your doctors. They may suggest a sleep study, an intensive exam of whether medical problems (such as sleep apnea) are part of your sleep problem.

Treatment for sleep disorders can include medicines and working with a sleep specialist to learn ways to improve sleep.

## SLEEP PROBLEMS AND NIGHTMARES

- Ongoing sleep problems can harm relationships and the ability to work and concentrate.
- Nightmares interfere with sleep and can be a sign of other problems.
- There are treatments that can help with sleep problems and nightmares.

## TIPS FOR IMPROVING YOUR SLEEP

Your lifestyle affects your health and your sleep. Here are some healthy sleep habits:

- **Keep a regular sleep schedule**. Go to bed and get up at the same time each day, even on weekends.
- **Have a bedtime routine**. Follow the same routine every night to help your body and mind know when it is time to sleep.
- **Exercise regularly**. Exercise will help you feel more tired at night and will help reduce stress.
- **Relax in the evening**. Avoid things that get you "revved up" for two to four hours before bedtime. Things that tend to do this include heavy meals, strenuous exercise,

heated arguments, paying bills, and action-packed movies.

- **Avoid or limit naps**. Regular naps can set your sleep schedule to include more daytime than nighttime sleep.
- **Use your bed only for sleep and sex**. Keep the television and/or computer out of the bedroom. This will help your mind learn to associate sleeping with the bedroom and sleeping with your bed. Likewise, try to only sleep in your bed, rather than falling asleep on the sofa.
- **Do not spend hours in bed trying to fall asleep**. If you cannot fall asleep within 30 minutes, get up and do something else until you become tired and drowsy. Then try going to bed again.
- **Avoid or limit caffeine and nicotine**. Both can keep you awake at night, and caffeine can stay in the system for as long as 12 hours.
- **Avoid alcohol**. While many people find that it helps them fall asleep, sleep will not be as restful as sleep without alcohol. Regular use of alcohol may also lead to more serious problems. Talk to your doctor about short-term sleep medicines that you might be able to try that will not have harmful side effects.[5]

---

[5] Mental Illness Research, Education and Clinical Centers (MIRECC), "Sleep Problems and Nightmares," U.S. Department of Veterans Affairs (VA), August 15, 2011. Available online. URL: www.mirecc.va.gov/docs/visn6/ Readjustment-brochure-sleep-color-generic-081511.pdf. Accessed April 5, 2023.

## Section 6.4 | Night Terrors

Night terrors, also known as "sleep terrors," are sleep disorders that include episodes of screaming, flailing, or crying while asleep. Night terrors are often paired with sleepwalking. It is most common in children between the ages of 3 and 12, and it affects very few adults. Night terrors in children resolve during the teenage years. Night terror episodes typically last from several seconds to minutes, but some may last longer. Night terrors are not usually a cause for concern, but they may require medical attention if it causes problems with sleep.

## SYMPTOMS OF NIGHT TERRORS

The symptoms of night terrors are similar to a nightmare, but the person who has a night terror episode remains asleep. Night terrors typically occur in the first third to the first half of the sleep cycle. During a night terror episode, the person may:

- suddenly sit up
- have a wide-eyed stare
- sweat
- breathe heavily
- kick and/or move their limbs forcefully
- scream or shout
- be hard to awaken
- be inconsolable

## CAUSES OF NIGHT TERRORS

Night terrors are considered as parasomnia, which is an unusual behavior of the central nervous system (CNS) during sleep. It happens during the deep non-rapid eye movement (non-REM) stage of sleep. There are various factors that contribute to night terrors, such as:

- extreme tiredness
- sleep deprivation
- sleep disruptions
- fever
- headache

A night terror can also be triggered by underlying conditions, such as:

- restless legs syndrome (RLS)
- sleep-disordered breathing
- depression
- anxiety
- medication

A night terror can also occur in members of the same family, as it has a strong genetic link.

## COMPLICATIONS OF NIGHT TERRORS

Complications involved in experiencing night terrors include:

- disrupted sleep
- embarrassment about the condition
- daytime sleepiness
- injury to oneself or others rarely

## WHEN TO SEE A DOCTOR

Night terrors are common in occurrence. However, consult your doctor if night terrors:

- become more frequent
- lead to accidental injury
- periodically disrupt the sleep cycle
- continue beyond teenage years

## DIAGNOSIS OF NIGHT TERRORS

Diagnosis of night terrors begins with reviewing the symptoms and medical history of the patient. The following are a few procedures to diagnose night terrors:

- **A physical examination**. The doctor may perform a physical examination to identify any conditions that may contribute to the night terrors.
- **A discussion of your symptoms**. Night terrors are generally diagnosed based on the description of events. Patients may be asked to complete a questionnaire about their sleep behavior.

- **Nocturnal sleep study (polysomnography)**. The doctor may recommend an overnight sleep study in a lab. Sensors are placed on the patient's body, and their brain waves, heart rate, oxygen level, breathing, and eye and leg movements will be continuously monitored.

## TREATMENT FOR NIGHT TERRORS

Treatment options for night terror include the following:

- **Treating an underlying condition**. If the night terrors are associated with any medical or mental health condition, treatment is focused on that problem.
- **Resolving stress**. Relaxation therapy, biofeedback, hypnosis, and cognitive behavioral therapy (CBT) may help in reducing stress or anxiety.
- **Anticipatory awakening**. This treatment option involves waking a person 15 minutes before he or she experiences a night terror episode.
- **Medication**. Medications are rarely used for night terrors. If necessary, antidepressants may be effective in treating the night terror.

## PREVENTION OF NIGHT TERRORS

Night terrors can be prevented by doing the following:

- Get adequate sleep if you or your child is sleep-deprived. Try to keep a sleep schedule and follow an earlier bedtime.
- Establish a calm activity before bedtime, such as reading a book, solving puzzles, taking a warm bath, meditating, or completing relaxing exercises.
- Keep a sleep diary and take note of your child's sleep pattern. If the night terror episodes are observed to be consistent, they may be used for anticipatory awakening.
- A night terror lasts only for a few minutes. During a night terror, try to calm the person down by using repeated soothing statements and providing physical comfort.

## HOW TO HELP A CHILD DURING A NIGHT TERROR

When your child experiences a night terror episode, do the following:

- Try not to wake your child from sleep. Your child may feel disorientated and confused when you try to wake him or her.
- Make the environment safe before going to bed by locking doors and windows, keeping fragile objects out of reach, and so on.

## References

Newman, Tim. "What Are Night Terrors and Why Do They Happen?" Medical News Today (MNT), December 8, 2017. Available online. URL: https://medicalnewstoday.com/articles/301893.php. Accessed April 4, 2023.

"Night Terrors," KidsHealth, June 2017. Available online. URL: https://kidshealth.org/en/parents/terrors.html. Accessed April 4, 2023.

"Night Terrors," Raising Children Network (Australia) Limited, June 12, 2018. Available online. URL: https://raisingchildren.net.au/preschoolers/sleep/nightmares-night-terrors-sleepwalking/night-terrors. Accessed April 4, 2023.

"Sleep Disorders: Night Terrors," WebMD, November 16, 2018. Available online. URL: https://webmd.com/sleep-disorders/guide/sleep-disorders-night-terrors. Accessed April 4, 2023.

"Sleep Terrors (Night Terrors)," Mayo Clinic, March 9, 2018. Available online. URL: www.mayoclinic.org/diseases-conditions/sleep-terrors/symptoms-causes/syc-20353524. Accessed April 4, 2023.

# Chapter 7 | **How Sleep Affects Your Health**

## HOW DO YOU KNOW IF YOU ARE NOT GETTING ENOUGH SLEEP?

Sleep deficiency can cause you to feel very tired during the day. You may not feel refreshed and alert when you wake up. Sleep deficiency can also interfere with work, school, driving, and social functioning. How sleepy you feel during the day can help you figure out whether you are having symptoms of problem sleepiness.

You might be sleep deficient if you often feel like you could doze off while:

- sitting and reading or watching TV
- sitting still in a public place, such as a movie theater, meeting, or classroom
- riding in a car for an hour without stopping
- sitting and talking to someone
- sitting quietly after lunch
- sitting in traffic for a few minutes

Sleep deficiency can cause problems with learning, focusing, and reacting. You may have trouble making decisions, solving problems, remembering things, managing your emotions and behavior, and coping with change. You may take longer to finish tasks, have a slower reaction time, and make more mistakes.

## SYMPTOMS IN CHILDREN

The symptoms of sleep deficiency may differ between children and adults. Children who are sleep-deficient might be overly active and have problems paying attention. They might also misbehave, and their school performance can suffer. Sleep-deficient children may feel angry and impulsive, have mood swings, feel sad or depressed, or lack motivation.

## SLEEP AND YOUR HEALTH

The way you feel while you are awake depends in part on what happens while you are sleeping. During sleep, your body is working to support healthy brain function and support your physical health. In children and teens, sleep also helps support growth and development.

The damage from sleep deficiency can happen in an instant (such as a car crash), or it can harm you over time. For example, ongoing sleep deficiency can raise your risk of some chronic health problems. It can also affect how well you think, react, work, learn, and get along with others.

### Mental Health Benefits

Sleep helps your brain work properly. While you are sleeping, your brain is getting ready for the next day. It is forming new pathways to help you learn and remember information.

Studies show that a good night's sleep improves learning and problem-solving skills. Sleep also helps you pay attention, make decisions, and be creative.

Studies also show that sleep deficiency changes activity in some parts of the brain. If you are sleep-deficient, you may have trouble making decisions, solving problems, controlling your emotions and behavior, and coping with change. Sleep deficiency has also been linked to depression, suicide, and risk-taking behavior.

Children and teens who are sleep-deficient may have problems getting along with others. They may feel angry and impulsive, have mood swings, feel sad or depressed, or lack motivation. They may also have problems paying attention, and they may get lower grades and feel stressed.

### Physical Health Benefits

Sleep plays an important role in your physical health. Good-quality sleep does the following:

- Heals and repairs your heart and blood vessels.

- Helps support a healthy balance of the hormones that make you feel hungry (ghrelin) or full (leptin). When you do not get enough sleep, your level of ghrelin goes up, and your level of leptin goes down. This makes you feel hungrier than when you are well-rested.
- Affects how your body reacts to insulin. Insulin is the hormone that controls your blood glucose (sugar) level. Sleep deficiency results in a higher-than-normal blood sugar level, which may raise your risk of diabetes.
- Supports healthy growth and development. Deep sleep triggers the body to release the hormone that promotes normal growth in children and teens. This hormone also boosts muscle mass and helps repair cells and tissues in children, teens, and adults. Sleep also plays a role in puberty and fertility.
- Affects your body's ability to fight germs and sickness. Ongoing sleep deficiency can change the way your body's natural defense against germs and sickness responds. For example, if you are sleep-deficient, you may have trouble fighting common infections.
- Decreases your risk of health problems, including heart disease, high blood pressure, obesity, and stroke.

## DAYTIME PERFORMANCE AND SAFETY

Getting enough quality sleep at the right times helps you function well throughout the day. People who are sleep-deficient are less productive at work and school. They take longer to finish tasks, have a slower reaction time, and make more mistakes. After several nights of losing sleep—even a loss of just one to two hours per night—your ability to function suffers as if you have not slept at all for a day or two.

Lack of sleep may also lead to microsleep. Microsleep refers to brief moments of sleep that happen when you are normally awake. You cannot control microsleep, and you might not be aware of it. For example, have you ever driven somewhere and then not remembered part of the trip? If so, you may have experienced microsleep.

Even if you are not driving, microsleep can affect how you function. If you are listening to a lecture, for example, you might miss some of the information or feel like you do not understand the point. You may have slept through part of the lecture and not realized it. Some people are not aware of the risks of sleep deficiency. In fact, they may not even realize that they are sleep-deficient. Even with limited or poor-quality sleep, they may still think they can function well.

For example, sleepy drivers may feel able to drive. Yet studies show that sleep deficiency harms your driving ability as much or more than being drunk. It is estimated that driver sleepiness is a factor in about 100,000 car accidents each year, resulting in about 1,500 deaths.

Drivers are not the only ones affected by sleep deficiency. It can affect people in all lines of work, including health-care workers, pilots, students, lawyers, mechanics, and assembly line workers.[1]

---

[1] "How Sleep Affects Your Health," National Heart, Lung, and Blood Institute (NHLBI), June 15, 2022. Available online. URL: www.nhlbi.nih.gov/health/sleep-deprivation/health-effects. Accessed March 14, 2023.

# Chapter 8 | **What Are Sleep Disorders?**

**Chapter Contents**

## Section 8.1 | Understanding Sleep Disorders

### WHAT IS SLEEP?

Sleep is a complex biological process. While you are sleeping, you are unconscious, but your brain and body functions are still active. They are doing a number of important jobs that help you stay healthy and function at your best. So, when you do not get enough quality sleep, it does more than just make you feel tired. It can affect your physical and mental health, thinking, and daily functioning.

### WHAT ARE SLEEP DISORDERS?

Sleep disorders are conditions that disturb your normal sleep patterns. There are more than 80 different sleep disorders. Some major types include the following:

- **Insomnia**. It is being unable to fall asleep and stay asleep. This is the most common sleep disorder.
- **Sleep apnea**. It is a breathing disorder in which you stop breathing for 10 seconds or more during sleep.
- **Restless legs syndrome (RLS)**. You may feel a tingling or prickly sensation in your legs, along with a powerful urge to move them.
- **Hypersomnia**. It is being unable to stay awake during the day. This includes narcolepsy, which causes extreme daytime sleepiness.
- **Circadian rhythm disorders**. These disorders create problems with the sleep–wake cycle. They make you unable to sleep and wake up at the right times.
- **Parasomnia**. It makes you act in unusual ways while falling asleep, sleeping, or waking from sleep, such as walking, talking, or eating.

Some people who feel tired during the day have a true sleep disorder. But, for others, the real problem is not allowing enough time for sleep. It is important to get enough sleep every night. The amount of sleep you need depends on several factors, including your age, lifestyle, health, and whether you have been getting enough sleep recently. Most adults need about seven to eight hours each night.

## WHAT CAUSES SLEEP DISORDERS?

There are different causes for different sleep disorders, including the following:

- other conditions, such as heart disease, lung disease, nerve disorders, and pain
- mental illnesses, including depression and anxiety
- medicines
- genetics

Sometimes, the cause is unknown.

There are also some factors that can contribute to sleep problems, including the following:

- caffeine and alcohol
- an irregular schedule, such as working the night shift
- aging (As people age, they often get less sleep or spend less time in the deep, restful stage of sleep; they are also more easily awakened.)

## WHAT ARE THE SYMPTOMS OF SLEEP DISORDERS?

The symptoms of sleep disorders depend on the specific disorder. Some signs that you may have a sleep disorder include that:

- you regularly take more than 30 minutes each night to fall asleep
- you regularly wake up several times each night and then have trouble falling back to sleep or you wake up too early in the morning
- you often feel sleepy during the day, take frequent naps, or fall asleep at the wrong times during the day
- your bed partner says that when you sleep, you snore loudly, snort, gasp, make choking sounds, or stop breathing for short periods
- you have creeping, tingling, or crawling feelings in your legs or arms that are relieved by moving or massaging

> them, especially in the evening and when trying to fall asleep
- your bed partner notices that your legs or arms often jerk during sleep
- you have vivid, dreamlike experiences while falling asleep or dozing
- you have episodes of sudden muscle weakness when you are angry or fearful or when you laugh
- you feel as though you cannot move when you first wake up

## HOW ARE SLEEP DISORDERS DIAGNOSED?

To make a diagnosis, your health-care provider will use your medical history, your sleep history, and a physical exam. You may also have a sleep study (polysomnogram). The most common types of sleep studies monitor and record data about your body during a full night of sleep. The data include the following:
- brain wave changes
- eye movements
- breathing rate
- blood pressure
- heart rate and electrical activity of the heart and other muscles

Other types of sleep studies may check how quickly you fall asleep during daytime naps or whether you are able to stay awake and alert during the day.

## WHAT ARE THE TREATMENTS FOR SLEEP DISORDERS?

Treatments for sleep disorders depend on which disorder you have. They may include the following:
- good sleep habits and other lifestyle changes, such as a healthy diet and exercise
- cognitive behavioral therapy (CBT) or relaxation techniques to reduce anxiety about getting enough sleep
- a continuous positive airway pressure (CPAP) machine for sleep apnea

- bright light therapy (in the morning)
- medicines, including sleeping pills (Usually, providers recommend that you use sleeping pills for a short period of time.)
- natural products, such as melatonin (These products may help some people but are generally for short-term use; make sure to check with your health-care provider before you take any of them.)[1]

## Section 8.2 | Key Sleep Disorders

Sleep-related difficulties affect many people. The following is a description of some of the major sleep disorders. If you, or someone you know, are experiencing any of the following, it is important to receive an evaluation by a health-care provider or, if necessary, a provider specializing in sleep medicine.

## INSOMNIA

Insomnia is characterized by an inability to initiate or maintain sleep. It may also take the form of early morning awakening, in which the individual awakens several hours early and is unable to resume sleeping. Difficulty initiating or maintaining sleep may often manifest itself as excessive daytime sleepiness, which characteristically results in functional impairment throughout the day. Before arriving at a diagnosis of primary insomnia, the health-care provider will rule out other potential causes, such as other sleep disorders, side effects of medications, substance abuse, depression, or other previously undetected illness. Chronic psychophysiological insomnia (or "learned" or "conditioned" insomnia) may result from a stressor combined with fear of being unable to sleep. Individuals with this condition may sleep better when not in their own beds. Health-care

---

[1] MedlinePlus, "Sleep Disorders," National Institutes of Health (NIH), January 3, 2020. Available online. URL: https://medlineplus.gov/sleepdisorders.html. Accessed March 14, 2023.

providers may treat chronic insomnia with a combination of the use of sedative-hypnotic or sedating antidepressant medications along with behavioral techniques to promote regular sleep.

## NARCOLEPSY

Excessive daytime sleepiness (including episodes of irresistible sleepiness) combined with sudden muscle weakness is the hallmark sign of narcolepsy. The sudden muscle weakness seen in narcolepsy may be elicited by strong emotion or surprise. Episodes of narcolepsy have been described as "sleep attacks" and may occur in unusual circumstances, such as walking and other forms of physical activity. The health-care provider may treat narcolepsy with stimulant medications combined with behavioral interventions, such as regularly scheduled naps, to minimize the potential disruptiveness of narcolepsy in the individual's life.

## RESTLESS LEGS SYNDROME

Restless legs syndrome (RLS) is characterized by an unpleasant "creeping" sensation, often feeling like it is originating in the lower legs but often associated with aches and pains throughout the legs. This often causes difficulty initiating sleep and is relieved by movement of the leg, such as walking or kicking. Abnormalities in the neurotransmitter dopamine have often been associated with RLS. Health-care providers often combine medication to help correct the underlying dopamine abnormality, along with a medicine to promote sleep continuity in the treatment for RLS.

## SLEEP APNEA

Snoring may be more than just an annoying habit—it may be a sign of sleep apnea. Persons with sleep apnea characteristically make periodic gasping or "snorting" noises, during which their sleep is momentarily interrupted. Those with sleep apnea may also experience excessive daytime sleepiness as their sleep is commonly interrupted and may not feel restorative. Treatment for sleep apnea is dependent on its cause. If other medical problems are present, such as congestive heart failure or nasal obstruction, sleep apnea may resolve with the treatment of these conditions. Gentle air pressure administered during sleep (typically in the form of a nasal continuous positive airway pressure (CPAP) device) may also be effective in the treatment of sleep apnea. As interruption of regular breathing or obstruction of the airway during sleep can pose serious health complications, symptoms of sleep apnea should be taken seriously. Treatment should be sought from a health-care provider.[2]

[2] "Key Sleep Disorders," Centers for Disease Control and Prevention (CDC), December 14, 2022. Available online. URL: www.cdc.gov/sleep/about_sleep/key_disorders.html. Accessed March 14, 2023.

# Chapter 9 | Sleep Disorders in Women

A healthy sleeping pattern is particularly important for women as it has a direct bearing on the quality of their lives. Unlike their predecessors, today's women are faced with the challenge of balancing home and career, and getting adequate sleep—in terms of both quantity and quality—is particularly important in order to recharge depleted energy stores in the body and brain cells and to lay the foundation for a productive day.

Studies have proved that the circadian rhythm, a 24-hour cycle that is internally generated in many organisms, including humans, has a deep impact on the sleep–wake cycle. Clinical evidence points to significant differences in the way men and women sleep, and in recent years, there has been growing interest in how gender influences sleep pathologies. While much is known about the mechanisms that link sleep and circadian rhythms, research on the way gender may affect sleep is still in its nascent stage but is vital to how we understand and treat sleep-related disorders.

Clinical studies across a broad range of ages have shown that women sleep longer but report poorer sleep quality than men. Women may also complain of sleep problems when there is no measurable evidence of sleep disturbance. This reflects a sleep state misperception (SSM), also known as "pseudo-insomnia" or "paradoxical insomnia," a condition recognized as an intrinsic sleep disorder by the International Classification of Sleep Disorders (ICSD), which is a widely accepted tool for clinical practice and research in sleep disorder medicine. The higher incidence of SSM in women may, in part, be attributed to the statistically higher incidence of anxiety, mood, and affective disorders in women.

Despite clinical evidence pointing to a higher incidence of SSM in women than in men, there also exist data that support the fact that women are, in fact, more prone to sleep disorders than men. The risk ratio for sleep problems increases with age and is seen to be more apparent after puberty, indicating that reproductive hormones may affect sleep patterns and circadian rhythms in women. Changes in the ovarian hormonal milieu across the lifespan would also explain how age influences sleep patterns and circadian rhythms in women.

## MENSTRUAL CYCLE AND SLEEP

A report suggests that more than two-thirds of women experience disrupted sleep patterns during their menstrual cycles. These changes in sleep patterns manifest as part of premenstrual syndrome (PMS), a group of symptoms that occur about a week to 10 days before menstruation. Although PMS may affect individuals differently, it is generally associated with mood changes, depression, irritability, fatigue, and insomnia. For some, disturbed sleep patterns may continue even during periods, with abdominal cramping and other symptoms associated with menstruation affecting sleep quality. Studies show a reduction in rapid eye movement (REM) sleep in the first few days of the menstrual cycle while progesterone, the hormone whose levels spike in the latter half of the cycle, has a soporific effect and has been shown to help women sleep better.

## PREGNANCY AND SLEEP

It has been reported that more than three-quarters of women experience sleep problems during pregnancy. While insomnia is common, other sleep-related issues may include sleep apnea, restless legs syndrome, and periodic limb movement disorder (PLMD). Pregnancy places considerable demands on the body, so pregnant women may need a few extra hours of sleep, particularly during the last trimester. But during pregnancy, a number of conditions can impede a good night's sleep. These include increased heart rate, dyspnea (shortness of breath), anxiety, stress, and heartburn.

Women typically gain around 30 pounds of weight during pregnancy, and this puts extra pressure on the pelvis and spine. Consequently, pregnant women frequently experience aches in the legs and back, which often disrupt sleep. The kidneys also overwork during pregnancy since there is a marked increase in the filtration rate, and this results in frequent urination, meaning more trips to the bathroom at night. Unsurprisingly, sleep issues tend to continue for most women even after childbirth. The stress involved in caring for the newborn and waking up frequently to nurse the baby makes it difficult to get through the night without sleep interruptions.

## MENOPAUSE AND SLEEP

Many women face increased sleep issues during and after menopause. In fact, some women begin to experience sleep problems even during perimenopause, the natural transition from a woman's reproductive phase to the cessation of menstrual periods. Sleep issues in menopause are closely linked to altered levels of hormones. A drop in the estrogen level often causes hot flashes and night sweats, which can greatly disrupt sleep, depending on the severity and frequency of symptoms. A decrease in hormone levels can also lead to an increased heart rate and vaginal dryness, and these symptoms may exacerbate anxiety and stress, which may aggravate sleep problems further. There may also be other physical factors that could impact sleep in menopausal women. Arthritis and heartburn, for example, could keep women awake during the night, and the resulting sleep deprivation could lead to fatigue and further aggravate problems such as anxiety and depression.

## MANAGING SLEEP DISORDERS IN WOMEN

The protocol for treating insomnia and other sleep-related disorders is, by and large, the same for men and women and generally includes over-the-counter (OTC) and prescription medications, cognitive behavioral therapy (CBT), complementary and alternative treatments, and recommended lifestyle changes. That said, clinicians need to consider medical, social, and specific biological factors, such as pregnancy and menopause, to determine the type of treatment required for managing sleep disorders in women.

## HEALTHY SLEEP TIPS FOR WOMEN

Lifestyle changes may be particularly useful in dealing with insomnia and sleep issues during pregnancy and menopause. While a balanced diet, adequate physical activity, and effective coping strategies are key recommendations to deal with general sleep-related problems, specific medical conditions—such as osteoarthritis, anxiety, and depression, which may co-occur with sleep disorders, particularly in older women—need to be addressed as well.

Following good nighttime practices can establish a regular wake–sleep pattern and help women deal with sleep issues. Avoiding heavy and spicy food just before bed can help reduce the chances of heartburn and sleep problems precipitated by it. Stimulants such as caffeine, alcohol, and nicotine can make it difficult to fall asleep, so those with sleep issues should avoid these stimulants in the late afternoon and evening. Practicing relaxation techniques during menstruation could help deal with sleep problems associated with menstrual cycles. Exposure to daylight has been shown to release melatonin, a hormone that regulates the sleep and wake cycles and also enhances appetite and mood.

Failure to get a good night's sleep is a common enough problem today, and most people experience it at some time in their lives. These problems may hardly ever require medical attention and may be easily managed by lifestyle modifications. However, serious sleep disorders can have a detrimental effect on your physical, mental, and social well-being and do require medical attention. A sleep specialist can help diagnose sleep problems and develop a treatment plan best suited for you.

## References

Hedaya, Robert J. "PMS and Insomnia: What to Do?" *Psychology Today,* May 4, 2010. Available online. URL: https://psychologytoday.com/blog/health-matters/201005/pms-and-insomnia-what-do. Accessed April 4, 2023.

Mong, Jessica A. et al. "Sleep, Rhythms, and the Endocrine Brain: Influence of Sex and Gonadal Hormones," *Journal of Neuroscience,* 31, no. 45 (2011): 16107–16116. https://doi.org/10.1523/JNEUROSCI.4175-11.2011.

"Sleep and Women," UCLASleepCenter, September 19, 2019. Available online. URL: http://sleepcenter.ucla.edu/sleep-and-women. Accessed April 4, 2023.

"Women and Sleep," The National Sleep Foundation, February 23, 2023. Available online. URL: sleepfoundation.org/sleep-topics/women-and-sleep. Accessed April 4, 2023.

# Chapter 10 | **Sleep Disorders in Men**

Many men consider sleep to be just one more chore on a list of things to do during the course of a 24-hour period. Some may even consider it a waste of time that could be put to better use. But this attitude might be preventing them from harnessing the power of a well-rested mind and body. Sleep should be considered to be one of the body's most valuable daily requirements. A sound investment in sleep provides valuable benefits to many other aspects of life. During sleep, the body recharges itself and prepares for another productive day. A good night's rest allows the human body to feel, think, and perform better, and a well-rested individual will find that he has more time and energy at his disposal during the day.

## CAUSES OF SLEEPLESSNESS IN MEN

A variety of factors may cause sleeplessness in men and prevent them from getting the amount of rest required for the body and mind to recharge. These can include the following.

### Lack of Awareness

Many men simply are not aware of the importance of sleep. Some may even view it as an indication of not working enough and believe they have to fight the urge to sleep. Although the amount of sleep required varies from person to person, in general, adults need at least seven to eight hours of sleep per night. But many people do not get enough sleep and consequently do not have optimal levels of energy and concentration to perform their daily activities. The following are some signs that you are not sleeping enough:

- feeling of tiredness and lack of energy throughout the day
- difficulty concentrating
- slow to get started in the morning
- irritability
- dozing off during the day

Sleeping late is not an option for people who have to be at work early, and most work policies do not allow for naps on the job. The only solution is to go to sleep earlier. Plan to get eight hours of sleep per night and prioritize this to make it a goal.

## Work Demands

Extra hours at work, the need to work during weekends, long commutes to work, and paperwork at home consume much of our time in the modern world. After checking emails and answering mobile phones, it is often past the ideal bedtime. Stress at the workplace and anxiety about the next day can also result in disturbed sleep. The body wants to sleep, but the mind remains awake, and you may toss and turn in bed. Try to leave your work behind when you come home. Maintain boundaries between work and personal time. And working from home—as is common these days—can make the situation even worse. Talking to friends or co-workers about your work life may help relieve stress, as can meditation or physical exercise. Make your bed a place to relax and not worry.

## Full Schedules

Men have busy schedules these days, with many more planned activities in their lives than just work. After work, they might be playing sports or watching their favorite teams in action. They could be doing pet projects or be involved in clubs, civic groups, fraternities, or church activities. Single men could be going out on dates or spending time with friends. Married men might be picking up their kids from school or helping them with their homework.

The key is to prioritize the important things and balance time effectively. Not everything needs to be done each day. Scale back on the number of things you are doing, rearrange tasks, and eliminate less important ones. These can be done when you have free time on other days. When listing and prioritizing activities, make sure sleeping is ranked high on the list.

## Life Changes

Changes in life have the potential to affect your sleep dramatically. These changes may come quite by surprise, or you might have been expecting them. Negative changes tend to be the most disruptive to your sleep, but positive change could have this effect, as well, because of the excitement it causes. Some changes may bring new duties and responsibilities, which could increase stress and keep you up at night. Some negative changes that could affect your sleep include:

- the death of a loved one
- becoming unemployed
- getting divorced
- being involved in an accident
- becoming aware of a major illness
- having a lawsuit filed against you
- an investment that has turned bad

Some positive changes include:
- getting married
- having a baby
- getting a promotion or a new job
- moving or relocating

Some changes may cause men to experience depression, which can have a major impact on sleep patterns. You could toss and turn in bed without sleeping much, or you could sleep longer with little motivation to get out of bed. Depression can also cause men to stop taking care of themselves. They may stop eating, grooming, and exercising. Abuse of alcohol and drugs is common with depression, and there could be a loss of interest in day-to-day activities.

Men often find it difficult to talk about depression and may find it preferable not to seek help from counselors. But they need to be aware that their condition could be hazardous to their health and detrimental to their daily lives. They could begin by talking about the problem to a friend, spouse, doctor, or minister. These people could help them seek help from a counselor when they have made the decision to do so. It is advisable not to face the situation on your own.

## Bad Habits

Poor sleep can be the result of bad habits or routines. These include the consumption of alcohol, nicotine, and coffee in the late afternoon, in the evening, or just before bedtime. Eating big meals or exercising before bedtime can also disturb your sleep. You might tend to have a big meal at night if you were busy during the evening. Instead, try and have a good lunch so that you are satisfied with a smaller dinner. Exercise before work or during your lunch break. Going to sleep at irregular times and waking up at different times daily could disrupt your internal body clock and prevent you from sleeping soundly. To set your body's clock properly, try to wake up at a set time every day, including weekends and holidays. Avoid sleeping late on weekends to catch up on lost sleep. This does not work. Instead, go to bed earlier at night. Also, limit naps to an hour in order to avoid disrupting sleep at night.

## Medical Conditions

Any number of medical conditions may result in poor sleep. The effects could be temporary, as with a sprained ankle, flu, or surgery, while others may be chronic and require long-term treatment. Some medical conditions become more common with increasing age, and they or their medications could begin to interfere with sleep. The following are a few medical conditions that could result in poor sleep patterns:

- epilepsy
- asthma
- other respiratory diseases

- heart disease
- arthritis

Some medications may hinder sleep and keep you jittery through the night. Others may cause sleepiness during the day. Talk to your doctor about your medication; there may be alternatives that could eliminate these types of side effects. The time at which you take your medicine and the dosage could also have a significant effect on the quality of your sleep.

## SLEEP DISORDERS THAT AFFECT MEN

Many people spend enough time lying in bed but do not get quality sleep. Their sleep could be disturbed and broken, or they may sleep through the night but wake up tired. These are indications of an underlying sleep disorder. Sleep disorders are common, but many people who are afflicted with them remain unaware of the condition. And some may shy away from seeking help. But diagnosing and treating sleep disorders can result in a dramatic improvement in sleep, helping to establish healthy sleep patterns and allowing you to be at your best during the day.

The following are some sleep disorders commonly diagnosed among men.

### Obstructive Sleep Apnea

During sleep, muscles in the throat become relaxed. Sometimes, the tissue in the mouth may collapse and prevent air from entering the lungs, or the tongue could fall back and block the airway. This is a disorder known as "obstructive sleep apnea" (OSA), a condition that affects one in four men. This blockage could occur a few times during the night or many hundreds of times. Breathing pauses for a moment when this happens, and you tend to wake up. Someone with OSA often feels very tired during the day. Men are twice as likely as women to have OSA.

Obesity and a larger neck girth increase the likelihood of having OSA since the larger amount of fatty tissue in the neck can block the airway. In addition to sleepiness during the day, another sign of

OSA is loud snoring, which is caused by a partially blocked airway passage. The intensity of snoring could range from mild to severe. Simple snoring is generally normal and harmless, but loud and severe snoring accompanied by gasping for air is a cause for concern. Men are often not aware that they snore. It usually becomes evident when a spouse or sleep partner notices it. Left untreated, sleep apnea carries with it the risk of lung disease, diabetes, and hypertension.

Talk to your doctor if you snore loudly in the night. He or she may refer you to a sleep specialist who can test for sleep apnea. Losing weight and sleeping on the side, rather than the back, are remedies that you can try on your own. But medical treatment is essential for more serious sleep apnea. Continuous positive air pressure (CPAP) is one treatment that can be used to treat sleep apnea. A mask worn on the face during sleep delivers a steady flow of air through the nose. This keeps the airway open and prevents pauses in breathing. The use of an oral device, similar to a mouth guard, could bring relief to people with OSA. And, in some cases, surgery may be recommended.

## Narcolepsy

Narcolepsy is a chronic brain disorder that causes extreme sleepiness during day-to-day activities such as eating, walking, or driving. It causes people to fall asleep suddenly for a few seconds to several minutes. Narcolepsy commonly begins between the ages of 12 and 20 although, in some cases, it may begin later in life. The condition cannot be cured, but it can be controlled with treatment. If you feel as if you could fall asleep at any time, talk to your doctor. He or she may refer you to a sleep specialist who will make a proper diagnosis. Narcolepsy can be treated using medication that will restore your sleep and wakefulness cycle to a normal pattern.

## Delayed Sleep Phase Disorder

Delayed sleep phase disorder (DSPD)—also called "delayed sleep phase syndrome" (DSPS)—is a condition characterized by the tendency to go to sleep and wake up later than what is considered normal, usually by a couple of hours. Every person has an internal clock that prompts the body to sleep and wake up at a given time. Getting into the habit of going to sleep late at night can throw the body clock out of balance, preventing you from falling asleep at the right time. To counteract DSPD, stay away from bright lights during the late afternoon and evening. Use dim lighting in your house and switch off the lights in the bedroom when it is time to sleep. It is also important to get enough daylight in the morning and afternoon. This sends signals to the brain to set the body clock properly.

## Jet Lag Disorder and Shift Work Disorder

Jet lag disorder is caused by traveling long distances by air. This disrupts your body clock because you might reach your destination when your body expects you to sleep, but in reality, it could be daytime there, and you may need to be awake. Your body clock is not able to adjust itself because of the speed of travel involved, and this may make it hard for you to sleep. Shift work disorder can occur in men who work late-night shifts or rotating shifts and often need to work when the body senses that it is time to sleep. After work, these individuals feel that they want to sleep when it is actually time for the body to remain awake. This results in tiredness and the inability to sleep properly.

Melatonin supplements have been shown to improve jet lag among travelers. Melatonin is a hormone that is released by the body at night and helps induce sleep. Light therapy has shown positive benefits for both jet lag disorder and shift work disorder. In light therapy, the eyes are exposed to bright light at a regular time and for a specific duration. This mimics the effect of sunlight on the body's internal clock. Consult your doctor to see if melatonin or light therapy could be beneficial in your case.

## HOW CAN MEN SLEEP BETTER?

Developing good sleep practices is the first step in allowing men to sleep better. You can build these good habits by following some basic tips that will result in healthy sleep patterns and learning counterproductive practices to avoid. One common misconception among men is that alcohol helps them sleep better. Alcohol might help you get to sleep, but it often causes you to wake up during the night. Many men who drink in the evening wake up very early in the morning and experience sleeplessness. To develop good sleep hygiene, refrain from drinking at least six hours before bedtime. Limit how much you drink and how frequently you drink. The heavy use of alcohol is detrimental to overall good health, as well as good sleep. Men sometimes use prescription sleeping pills as a solution to sleep problems. These drugs help to an extent, but they should not be used as a long-term solution. Because of the danger of developing a dependency, doctors generally do not prescribe sleep medication beyond a few weeks at a time.

Over-the-counter (OTC) sleep medicines are readily available at drugstores. These formulations often use antihistamines to induce drowsiness. Even though they allow you to sleep, they can make you groggy during the day and may result in slow response times. They should be used sparingly and with caution. If you have not been sleeping well for more than a month, it is a good idea to consult a doctor. Do not ignore the problem thinking it will disappear. Your physician will likely refer you to a sleep specialist who will diagnose the cause of the problem. Before visiting a sleep specialist, it can be useful to keep a sleep diary for two weeks. This will help the specialist understand your sleep patterns, provide clues about what is hindering your sleep, and assist him or her in suggesting remedies. Sleep is crucial to your well-being, and it touches every other aspect of your life. Do not ignore signs of trouble when there is so much to gain from consulting a doctor for diagnosis and treatment.

## References

"Sleep and Men," UCLA Health. December 28, 2016. Available online. URL: http://sleepcenter.ucla.edu/sleep-and-men. Accessed April 4, 2023.

"Sleep Apnea and Insomnia in Men," BodyLogicMD.com. May 5, 2020. Available online. URL: http://bodylogicmd.com/for-men/sleep-apnea. Accessed April 4, 2023.

"Sleep Disorders," Bon Secours for Men. September 5, 2015. Available online. URL: http://menshealth.bonsecours. com/mens-health-issues/sleep-disorders. Accessed April 4, 2023.

# Chapter 11 | **Sleep and Aging**

Older adults need about the same amount of sleep as all adults—seven to nine hours each night. But older people tend to go to sleep earlier and get up earlier than they did when they were younger.

There are many reasons why older people may not get enough sleep at night. Feeling sick or being in pain can make it hard to sleep. Some medicines can keep you awake. No matter the reason, if you do not get a good night's sleep, the next day you may:

- be irritable
- have memory problems or be forgetful
- feel depressed
- have more falls or accidents

## GET A GOOD NIGHT'S SLEEP

Being older does not mean you have to be tired all the time. You can do many things to help you get a good night's sleep. Here are some ideas:

- Follow a regular sleep schedule. Go to sleep and get up at the same time each day, even on weekends or when you are traveling.
- Avoid napping in the late afternoon or evening if you can. Naps may keep you awake at night.
- Develop a bedtime routine. Take time to relax before bedtime each night. Some people read a book, listen to soothing music, or soak in a warm bath.
- Try not to watch television or use your computer, cell phone, or tablet in the bedroom. The light from these

devices may make it difficult for you to fall asleep. And alarming or unsettling shows or movies, such as horror movies, may keep you awake.

- Keep your bedroom at a comfortable temperature, not too hot or too cold, and as quiet as possible.
- Use low lighting in the evenings and as you prepare for bed.
- Exercise at regular times each day but not within three hours of your bedtime.
- Avoid eating large meals close to bedtime—they can keep you awake.
- Stay away from caffeine late in the day. Caffeine (found in coffee, tea, soda, and chocolate) can keep you awake.
- Remember, alcohol will not help you sleep. Even small amounts make it harder to stay asleep.

## INSOMNIA IS COMMON IN OLDER ADULTS

Insomnia is the most common sleep problem in adults aged 60 and older. People with this condition have trouble falling asleep and staying asleep. Insomnia can last for days, months, and even years. Having trouble sleeping can mean you:
- take a long time to fall asleep
- wake up many times in the night
- wake up early and are unable to get back to sleep
- wake up tired
- feel very sleepy during the day

Often, being unable to sleep becomes a habit. Some people worry about not sleeping even before they get into bed. This may make it harder to fall asleep and stay asleep.

Some older adults who have trouble sleeping may use over-the-counter (OTC) sleep aids. Others may use prescription medicines to help them sleep. These medicines may help when used for a short time. But remember, medicines are not a cure for insomnia. Developing healthy habits at bedtime may help you get a good night's sleep.

## SLEEP APNEA

People with sleep apnea have short pauses in breathing while they are asleep. These pauses may happen many times during the night. If not treated, sleep apnea can lead to other problems, such as high blood pressure, stroke, or memory loss.

You can have sleep apnea and not even know it. Feeling sleepy during the day and being told you are snoring loudly at night could be signs that you have sleep apnea.

If you think you have sleep apnea, see a doctor who can treat this sleep problem. You may need to learn to sleep in a position that keeps your airways open. Treatment using a continuous positive airway pressure (CPAP) device almost always helps people with sleep apnea. A dental device or surgery may also help.

## MOVEMENT DISORDERS AND SLEEP

Restless legs syndrome (RLS), periodic limb movement disorder (PLMD), and rapid eye movement (REM) sleep behavior disorder are common in older adults. These movement disorders can rob you of needed sleep.

People with RLS feel like there is tingling, crawling, or pins and needles in one or both legs. This feeling is worse at night. See your doctor for more information about medicines to treat RLS.

PLMD causes people to jerk and kick their legs every 20–40 seconds during sleep. Medication, warm baths, exercise, and relaxation exercises can help.

REM sleep behavior disorder is another condition that may make it harder to get a good night's sleep. During normal REM sleep, your muscles cannot move, so your body stays still. But, if you have REM sleep behavior disorder, your muscles can move, and your sleep is disrupted.

## ALZHEIMER DISEASE AND SLEEP: A SPECIAL PROBLEM

Alzheimer disease (AD) often changes a person's sleeping habits. Some people with AD sleep too much; others do not sleep enough. Some people wake up many times during the night; others wander or yell at night.

The person with AD is not the only one who loses sleep. Caregivers may have sleepless nights, leaving them tired for the challenges they face.

If you are caring for someone with AD, take the following steps to make him or her safer and help you sleep better at night:

- Make sure the floor is clear of objects.
- Lock up any medicines.
- Attach grab bars in the bathroom.
- Place a gate across the stairs.

## SAFE SLEEP FOR OLDER ADULTS

Try to set up a safe and restful place to sleep. Make sure you have smoke alarms on each floor of your home. Before going to bed, lock all windows and doors that lead outside. Other ideas for a safe night's sleep are as follows:

- Keep a telephone with emergency phone numbers by your bed.
- Have a lamp within reach that is easy to turn on.
- Put a glass of water next to the bed in case you wake up thirsty.
- Do not smoke, especially in bed.
- Remove area rugs so you will not trip if you get out of bed during the night.

## TIPS TO HELP YOU FALL ASLEEP

You may have heard about some tricks to help you fall asleep. You do not really have to count sheep—you could try counting slowly to 100. Some people find that playing mental games makes them sleepy. For example, tell yourself it is five minutes before you have to get up, and you are just trying to get a little more sleep.

Some people find that relaxing their bodies puts them to sleep. One way to do this is to imagine your toes are completely relaxed, then your feet, and then your ankles are completely relaxed. Work your way up the rest of your body, section by section. You may drift off to sleep before getting to the top of your head.

## Sleep and Aging

Use your bedroom only for sleeping. After turning off the light, give yourself about 20 minutes to fall asleep. If you are still awake and not drowsy, get out of bed. When you feel sleepy, go back to bed.

If you feel tired and unable to do your activities for more than two or three weeks, you may have a sleep problem. Talk with your doctor about changes you can make to get a better night's sleep.[1]

[1] National Institute on Aging (NIA), "A Good Night's Sleep," National Institutes of Health (NIH), November 3, 2020. Available online. URL: www.nia.nih.gov/health/good-nights-sleep. Accessed March 14, 2023.

115

# Part 2 | Causes and Consequences of Sleep Deprivation

# Chapter 12 | **Are You Getting Enough Sleep?**

Getting enough sleep is important for people of all ages to stay in good health. Learn how much sleep you need. People often cut back on their sleep for work, for family demands, or even to watch a good show on television. But, if not getting enough sleep is a regular part of your routine, you may be at an increased risk for obesity, type 2 diabetes, high blood pressure, heart disease and stroke, poor mental health, and even early death.

Even one night of short sleep can affect you the next day. Not only are you likely to feel sleepy, but you are also likely to be in a bad mood, be less productive at work, and be involved in a motor vehicle crash.

## HOW MUCH SLEEP DO YOU NEED?
How much sleep you need changes as you age. Table 12.1 shows the recommendations from the Sleep Research Society and the American Academy of Sleep Medicine (AASM).

### Habits to Improve Your Sleep
- Be consistent. Go to bed at the same time each night and get up at the same time each morning, including on the weekends.
- Make sure your bedroom is quiet, dark, relaxing, and at a comfortable temperature.
- Remove electronic devices such as TVs, computers, and phones from the bedroom.

- Avoid large meals, caffeine, and alcohol before bedtime.
- Do not use tobacco.
- Get some exercise. Being physically active during the day can help you fall asleep more easily at night.

**Table 12.1.** Recommended Sleep Duration Based on Age Group

| Age Group | Age | Recommended Hours of Sleep |
|-----------|-----|----------------------------|
| Infant | 4–12 months | 12–16 hours per 24 hours (including naps) |
| Toddler | 1–2 years | 11–14 hours per 24 hours (including naps) |
| Preschool | 3–5 years | 10–13 hours per 24 hours (including naps) |
| School age | 6–12 years | 9–12 hours per 24 hours |
| Teen | 13–18 years | 8–10 hours per 24 hours |
| Adult | 18–60 years | 7 or more hours per night |

## WHAT ABOUT SLEEP QUALITY?

Getting enough sleep is important, but good sleep quality is also essential. Signs of poor sleep quality include feeling sleepy or tired even after getting enough sleep, repeatedly waking up during the night, and having symptoms of a sleep disorder (such as snoring or gasping for air). Better sleep habits may improve the quality of your sleep. If you have symptoms of a sleep disorder, such as snoring or being very sleepy during the day after a full night's sleep, make sure to tell your doctor.[1]

## HOW MUCH SLEEP IS ENOUGH?

The amount of sleep you need each day will change over the course of your life.

---

[1] "Are You Getting Enough Sleep?" Centers for Disease Control and Prevention (CDC), September 19, 2022. Available online. URL: www.cdc.gov/sleep/features/getting-enough-sleep.html. Accessed March 17, 2023.

If you regularly lose sleep or choose to sleep less than needed, the sleep loss adds up. The total sleep lost is called your "sleep debt." For example, if you lose two hours of sleep each night, you will have a sleep debt of 14 hours after a week.

Some people nap to deal with sleepiness. Naps may give a short-term boost in alertness and performance. However, napping does not supply all the other benefits of nighttime sleep, so you cannot really make up for lost sleep. Some people sleep more on their days off than on workdays. They may also go to bed and wake up later on days off.

Sleeping more on days off might be a sign that you are not getting enough sleep. Although extra sleep on days off might help you feel better, it can upset your body's sleep–wake rhythm.[2]

## GET ENOUGH SLEEP

It is important to get enough sleep. Sleep helps keep your mind and body healthy.

### How Much Sleep Do Adults Need?

Most adults need seven or more hours of good-quality sleep on a regular schedule each night. Getting enough sleep is not only about total hours of sleep. It is also important to get good-quality sleep on a regular schedule, so you feel rested when you wake up. If you often have trouble sleeping—or if you often still feel tired after sleeping—talk with your doctor.

### How Much Sleep Do Children Need?

Kids need even more sleep than adults.
- Teens need 8–10 hours of sleep each night.
- School-aged children need 9–12 hours of sleep each night.
- Preschoolers need to sleep between 10 and 13 hours a day (including naps).

---

[2] "How Much Sleep Is Enough," National Heart, Lung, and Blood Institute (NHLBI), March 24, 2022. Available online. URL: www.nhlbi.nih.gov/health/sleep-deprivation/how-much-sleep. Accessed March 17, 2023.

- Toddlers need to sleep between 11 and 14 hours a day (including naps).
- Babies need to sleep between 12 and 16 hours a day (including naps).
- Newborns need to sleep between 14 and 17 hours a day.

## HEALTH BENEFITS
### Why Is Getting Enough Sleep Important?
Getting enough sleep has many benefits. It can help you:
- get sick less often
- stay at a healthy weight
- lower your risk for serious health problems, such as diabetes and heart disease
- reduce stress and improve your mood
- think more clearly and do better in school and at work
- get along better with people
- make good decisions and avoid injuries—for example, drowsy drivers cause thousands of car accidents every year

## SLEEP SCHEDULE
### Does It Matter When You Sleep?
Yes. Your body sets your "biological clock" according to the pattern of daylight where you live. This helps you naturally get sleepy at night and stay alert during the day.

If you have to work at night and sleep during the day, you may have trouble getting enough sleep. It can also be hard to sleep when you travel to a different time zone.

## TROUBLE SLEEPING
### Why Can You Not Fall Asleep?
Many things can make it harder for you to sleep, including the following:
- stress or anxiety
- pain

- certain health conditions, such as heartburn or asthma
- some medicines
- caffeine (usually from coffee, tea, and soda)
- alcohol and other drugs
- untreated sleep disorders, such as sleep apnea or insomnia

If you are having trouble sleeping, try making changes to your routine to get the sleep you need. You may want to:
- change what you do during the day—for example, get your physical activity in the morning instead of at night
- create a comfortable sleep environment—for example, make sure your bedroom is dark and quiet
- set a bedtime routine—for example, go to bed at the same time every night

## SLEEP DISORDERS
## How Can You Tell If You Have a Sleep Disorder?

Sleep disorders can cause many different problems. Keep in mind that it is normal to have trouble sleeping every now and then. People with sleep disorders generally experience these problems on a regular basis.

Common signs of sleep disorders include the following:
- trouble falling or staying asleep
- still feeling tired after a good night's sleep
- sleepiness during the day that makes it difficult to do everyday activities, such as driving or concentrating at work
- frequent loud snoring
- pauses in breathing or gasping while sleeping
- tingling or crawling feelings in your legs or arms at night that feel better when you move or massage the area
- feeling like it is hard to move when you first wake up

If you have any of these signs, talk to a doctor or nurse. You may need testing or treatment for a sleep disorder.

## DAYTIME HABITS

Making small changes to your daily routine can help you get the sleep you need.

Change what you do during the day.

- Try to spend some time outdoors in the daylight— earlier in the day is best.
- Plan your physical activity for earlier in the day, not right before you go to bed.
- Stay away from caffeine (including coffee, tea, and soda) late in the day.
- If you have trouble sleeping at night, limit daytime naps to 20 minutes or less.
- If you drink alcohol, drink only in moderation (less than one drink in a day for women and less than two drinks in a day for men)—alcohol can keep you from sleeping well.
- Do not eat a big meal close to bedtime.
- If you smoke, make a plan to quit—the nicotine in cigarettes can make it harder for you to sleep.

## NIGHTTIME HABITS

Create a good sleep environment.

- Make sure your bedroom is dark—if there are streetlights near your window, try putting up light-blocking curtains.
- Keep your bedroom quiet.
- Consider keeping electronic devices—such as TVs, computers, and smartphones—out of your bedroom.

Set a bedtime routine.

- Go to bed at the same time every night.
- Try to get the same amount of sleep each night.
- Avoid eating, talking on the phone, or reading in bed.
- Avoid using computers or smartphones, watching TV, or playing video games at bedtime.

If you find yourself up at night worrying about things, use these tips to help manage stress.

If you are still awake after staying in bed for more than 20 minutes, get up. Do something relaxing, such as reading or meditating, until you feel sleepy.

## SEE A DOCTOR

If you are concerned about your sleep, see a doctor.

Talk with a doctor or nurse if you have any of the following signs of a sleep disorder:

- trouble falling or staying asleep
- still feeling tired after a good night's sleep
- sleepiness during the day that makes it difficult to do everyday activities, such as driving or concentrating at work
- frequent loud snoring
- pauses in breathing or gasping while sleeping
- tingling or crawling feelings in your legs or arms at night that feel better when you move or massage the area
- trouble staying awake during the day
- feeling like it is hard to move when you first wake up

Even if you do not have these problems, talk with a doctor if you feel like you often have trouble sleeping. Keep a sleep diary for a week and share it with your doctor. A doctor can suggest different sleep routines or medicines to treat sleep disorders. Talk with a doctor before trying over-the-counter (OTC) sleep medicine.[3]

---

[3] Office of Disease Prevention and Health Promotion (ODPHP), "Get Enough Sleep," U.S. Department of Health and Human Services (HHS), July 15, 2022. Available online. URL: https://health.gov/myhealthfinder/healthy-living/mental-health-and-relationships/get-enough-sleep. Accessed March 17, 2023.

# Chapter 13 | **Sleep Deprivation and Deficiency**

## WHAT ARE SLEEP DEPRIVATION AND DEFICIENCY?

Sleep deprivation is a condition that occurs if you do not get enough sleep. Sleep deficiency is a broader concept. It occurs if you have one or more of the following:

- You do not get enough sleep (sleep deprivation).
- You sleep at the wrong time of day.
- You do not sleep well or get all the different types of sleep your body needs.
- You have a sleep disorder that prevents you from getting enough sleep or causes poor-quality sleep

Sleeping is a basic human need, such as eating, drinking, and breathing. Like these other needs, sleeping is vital for good health and well-being throughout your lifetime.

According to the Centers for Disease Control and Prevention (CDC), about one in three adults in the United States reported not getting enough rest or sleep every day. Nearly 40 percent of adults report falling asleep during the day without meaning to at least once a month. Also, an estimated 50–70 million Americans have chronic or ongoing sleep disorders. Sleep deficiency can lead to physical and mental health problems, injuries, loss of productivity, and even a greater likelihood of death. To understand sleep deficiency, understanding what makes you sleep and how it affects your health helps.

Sleep deficiency can interfere with work, school, driving, and social functioning. You might have trouble learning, focusing, and reacting. Also, you might find it hard to judge other people's emotions and reactions. Sleep deficiency can also make you feel frustrated, cranky, or worried in social situations.

The symptoms of sleep deficiency may differ between children and adults. Children who are sleep deficient might be overly active and have problems paying attention. They might also misbehave, and their school performance can suffer.

Sleep deficiency is linked to many chronic health problems, including heart disease, kidney disease, high blood pressure, diabetes, stroke, obesity, and depression. Sleep deficiency is also linked to a higher chance of injury in adults, teens, and children. For example, sleepiness while driving (not related to alcohol) is responsible for serious car crash injuries and death. In older adults, sleep deficiency may be linked to a higher chance of falls and broken bones.

Sleep deficiency has also played a role in human mistakes linked to tragic accidents, such as nuclear reactor meltdowns, the grounding of large ships, and plane crashes. A common myth is that people can learn to get by on little sleep with no negative effects. However, research shows that getting enough quality sleep at the right times is vital for mental health, physical health, quality of life (QOL), and safety.

## HOW IS SLEEP DEPRIVATION TREATED?

If your doctor diagnoses you with a sleep disorder, they may talk to you about healthy sleep habits. Your treatment options will depend on which type you have.

For sleep apnea, the goals of treatment are to help keep your airways open during sleep. This may include a continuous positive airway pressure (CPAP) machine or other breathing devices, therapy, or surgery. For narcolepsy and insomnia, treatment options include medicines and behavior changes.

## HEALTHY SLEEP HABITS

You can take steps to improve your sleep habits. First, make sure that you give yourself enough time to sleep. With enough sleep each night, you may find that you are happier and more productive during the day.

Sleep is often the first thing that busy people squeeze out of their schedules. Making time to sleep will help you protect your health and well-being now and in the future.

To improve your sleep habits, doing the following may also help:

- Go to bed and wake up at the same time every day. For children, have a set bedtime and a standard bedtime routine. Do not use the child's bedroom for time-outs or punishment.
- Try to keep the same sleep schedule on weeknights and weekends. Limit the difference to no more than about an hour. Staying up late and sleeping in late on weekends can disrupt your body clock's sleep–wake rhythm.
- Use the hour before bed for quiet time. Avoid intense exercise and bright artificial light, such as from a TV or computer screen. The light may signal the brain that it is time to be awake.
- Avoid heavy or large meals within a few hours of bedtime. (Having a light snack is okay.) Also, avoid alcoholic drinks before bed.
- Avoid nicotine (i.e., cigarettes) and caffeine (including caffeinated soda, coffee, tea, and chocolate).
- Nicotine and caffeine are stimulants, and both substances can interfere with sleep. The effects of caffeine can last up to eight hours. So a cup of coffee in the late afternoon can make it hard for you to fall asleep at night.
- Spend time outside every day (when possible) and be physically active.
- Keep your bedroom quiet, cool, and dark (a dim night light is fine if needed).
- Take a hot bath or use relaxation techniques before bed.
- Napping during the day may boost your alertness and performance. However, if you have trouble falling asleep at night, limit naps or take them earlier in the

afternoon. Adults should nap for no more than 20 minutes.
- Napping in preschool-age children is normal and promotes healthy growth and development.

## Strategies for Shift Workers

Some people have schedules that conflict with their internal body clocks. For example, shift workers may have trouble getting enough sleep. This can affect how they feel mentally and physically.

If you are a shift worker, you may find it helpful to:
- take naps and raise the amount of time available for sleep
- keep the lights bright at work
- limit shift changes so your body clock can adjust
- limit caffeine use to the first part of your shift
- remove sound and light distractions in your bedroom during daytime sleep (i.e., use light-blocking curtains)

If you are still not able to fall asleep during the day or have problems adapting to a shift-work schedule, talk with your doctor about other options to help you sleep.[1]

---

[1] "Sleep Deprivation and Deficiency," National Heart, Lung, and Blood Institute (NHLBI), March 24, 2022. Available online. URL: www.nhlbi.nih.gov/health/sleep-deprivation. Accessed March 14, 2023.

# Chapter 14 | People at Risk of Sleep Deprivation

**Chapter Contents**

## Section 14.1 | Sleep Deprivation: What Does It Mean for Public Safety Officers?

Scheduling and staffing around the clock require finding a way to balance each organization's unique needs with those of its officers. Questions such as "How many hours in a row should officers work?" and "How many officers are needed on which shift?" need to be balanced against "How much time off do officers need to rest and recuperate properly?" and "What is the best way to schedule those hours to keep employees safe and performing well?" After all, shift work interferes with normal sleep and forces people to work at unnatural times of the day when their bodies are programmed to sleep. Sleep-loss-related fatigue degrades performance, productivity, and safety, as well as health and well-being. Fatigue costs the U.S. economy $136 billion per year in health-related lost productivity alone.

Many managers in policing and corrections have begun to acknowledge—such as their counterparts in other industries—that rotating shift work is inherently dangerous, especially when one works the graveyard shift. Managers in aviation, railroading, and trucking, for example, have had mandated hours-of-work laws for decades. They have begun to use complex mathematical models to manage fatigue-related risks.

All of us experience the everyday stress associated with family life, health, and finances. Most of us also feel work-related stress associated with bad supervisors, long commutes, inadequate equipment, and difficult assignments. But police and corrections officers must also deal with the stresses of working shifts, witnessing or experiencing trauma, and managing dangerous confrontations.

John Violanti, Ph.D., is a 23-year veteran of the New York State Police, a professor in the Department of Social and Preventive Medicine at the University at Buffalo, and an instructor with the Law Enforcement Wellness Association. His research shows that law enforcement officers are dying earlier than they should. The average age of death for police officers in his 40-year study was 66 years of age—a full 10 years sooner than the norm. He and other researchers also found that police officers were much more likely than the general public to have higher-than-recommended cholesterol levels, higher-than-average pulse rates and diastolic blood pressure, and a much higher prevalence of sleep disorders.

So what can be done to make police work healthier? Many things. One of the most effective strategies is to get enough sleep. More than half of police officers fail to get adequate rest, and they have 44 percent higher levels of obstructive sleep apnea (OSA) than the general public. More than 90 percent report being routinely fatigued, and 85 percent report driving while drowsy.

Sleep deprivation is dangerous. Researchers have shown that being awake for 19 hours produces impairments that are comparable to having a blood alcohol concentration (BAC) of 0.05 percent. Being awake for 24 hours is comparable to having a BAC of roughly 10 percent. This means that in just five hours—the difference between going without sleep for 19 hours versus 24 hours—the impact essentially doubles. (It should be noted that in all 50 states and the District of Columbia, it is a crime to drive with a BAC of 0.08 percent or above.)

If you work a 10-hour shift, then attend court, then pick up your kids from school, drive home (hoping you do not fall asleep at the wheel), catch a couple hours of sleep, then get up, and go back to work—and you do this for a week—you may be driving your patrol car while just as impaired as the last person you arrested for driving under the influence (DUI).

Bars and taverns are legally liable for serving too many drinks to people who then drive, have an accident, and kill someone. There is a precedent for trucking companies and other employers being held responsible for drivers who cause accidents after working longer than permitted. It seems very likely that police departments eventually will be held responsible if an officer causes death because he was too tired to drive home safely.

Sleep and fatigue are basic survival issues, just like patrol tactics, firearms safety, and pursuit driving. To reduce risks, stay alive, and keep healthy, officers and their managers have to work together to manage fatigue. Too-tired cops put themselves, their fellow officers, and the communities they serve at risk.

## ACCIDENTAL DEATHS AND FATIGUE

The number of police officer deaths from both felonious assaults and accidents has decreased over the years. Contrary to what most people might think, however, more officers die as a result of accidents than criminal assaults. Ninety-one percent of accidental deaths are caused by car crashes, being hit by vehicles while on foot, aircraft accidents, falls, or jumping.

It is known that the rate of these accidents increases with lack of sleep and time of day. Researchers have shown that the risk increases considerably after a person has been on duty for nine hours or more. After 10 hours on duty, the risk increases by approximately 90 percent; after 12 hours, 110 percent. The night shift has the greatest risk for accidents; they are almost three times more likely to happen during the night shift than the morning shift.

## COUNTERING FATIGUE

Researchers who study officer stress, sleep, and performance have a number of techniques to counteract sleep deprivation and stress. They fall into the following two types:

- things managers can do
- things officers can do

The practices listed below have been well-received by departments that recognize that a tired cop is a danger both to himself or herself and to the public.

### Things Managers Can Do

Review policies that affect overtime, moonlighting, and the number of consecutive hours a person can work. Make sure the policies keep shift rotation to a minimum and give officers adequate rest time. The Albuquerque (N.M.) Police Department, for example, prohibits officers from working more than 16 hours a day and limits overtime to 20 hours per week. This practice earned the Albuquerque team the Healthy Sleep Capital award from the National Sleep Foundation (NSF).

Give officers a voice in decisions related to their work hours and shift scheduling. People's work hours affect every aspect of their lives. Increasing the amount of control and predictability in one's life improves a host of psychological and physical characteristics, including job satisfaction.

Formally assess the level of fatigue officers experience, the quality of their sleep, and how tired they are while on the job, as well as their attitudes toward fatigue and work hours issues. Strategies include administering sleep quality tests, such as those available on the NSF's website (www.sleepfoundation.org), and training supervisors to be alert for signs that officers are overly tired (i.e., falling asleep during a watch briefing) and on how to deal with those who are too fatigued to work safely.

Several Canadian police departments are including sleep screening in officers' annual assessments—something that every department should consider.

Create a culture in which officers receive adequate information about the importance of good sleep habits, the hazards associated with fatigue and shift work, and strategies for managing them. For example, the Seattle Police Department has scheduled an all-day fatigue countermeasures training course for every sergeant, lieutenant, and captain. In the Calgary Police Service, management and union leaders are conducting a long-term, research-based program to find the best shift and scheduling arrangements and to change cultural attitudes about sleep and fatigue.

## Things Officers Can Do

- Stay physically fit. Get enough exercise, maintain a healthy body weight, eat several fruits and vegetables a day, and stop smoking.
- Learn to use caffeine effectively by restricting routine intake to the equivalent of one or two 8-ounce cups of coffee a day. When you need to combat drowsiness, drink only one cup every hour or two; stop doses well before bedtime.
- Exercise proper sleep hygiene. In other words, do everything possible to get seven or more hours of sleep

every day. For example, go to sleep at the same time every day as much as possible, avoid alcohol just before bedtime, use room darkening curtains, and make your bedroom a place for sleep, not for doing work or watching television. Do not just doze off in an easy chair or on the sofa with the television on.

If you have not been able to get enough sleep, try to take a nap before your shift. Done properly, a 20-minute catnap is proven to improve performance, elevate mood, and increase creativity.

If you are frequently fatigued, are drowsy, snore, or have a large build, ask your doctor to check you for sleep apnea. Because many physicians have little training in sleep issues, it is a good idea to see someone who specializes in sleep medicine.[1]

## Section 14.2 | **Sleep Deprivation Affects Athletes**

According to the National Institutes of Health (NIH), although there is still much that is not known about sleep, we do know that sleep is crucial to human physiology and cognition. Lack of sleep may cause autonomic nervous system imbalance, increase stress levels, and decrease glycogen and carbohydrate production. In athletes, reduced sleep can lead to lack of energy, poor focus, fatigue, and slow recovery after a game. Sports place a lot of demand on the muscles and tissues, depleting energy and fluids and breaking down muscles. Sleep helps the body recover quicker, repairs memory, and releases essential hormones. In sports, a split-second decision can make the difference between a win and a loss. And research indicates that poor sleep results in decline in quick decision-making, while the proper amount of sleep shows an increase in this ability.

---

[1] National Institute of Justice (NIJ), "Sleep Deprivation: What Does It Mean for Public Safety Officers?" U.S. Department of Justice (DOJ), March 26, 2009. Available online. URL: https://nij.ojp.gov/topics/articles/sleep-deprivation-what-does-it-mean-public-safety-officers. Accessed April 4, 2023.

## EFFECTS OF SLEEP DEPRIVATION

Reduced sleep can cause a decline in athletic performance, cognition, and immune function and an increase in weight. The amount of sleep required for any given athlete depends on genetic factors, conditioning, and the level of physical activity demanded by the sport. Adolescence is a period of growth in which sleep is vital. However, it has become increasingly clear from research that most teens do not get the proper amount of sleep. Studies suggest that an average of 10 hours of sleep per night can boost athletic performance. Athletes tend to focus on training and practice to achieve success; however, sleep has too often been an overlooked factor. The following are a few effects of lack of sleep:

- **Lower attention span**. Inability to stay focused on the game.
- **Decreased reaction time**. Overall reaction time is vital to athletic performance.
- **Longer recovery**. Some physical activities demand more energy; recovery and healing are slower when sleep is lost.
- **Higher cortisol levels**. High levels of the stress hormone cortisol can hinder tissue repair and growth. Over time, this may prevent an athlete from responding well to heavy training and may also lead to overtraining.
- **Lack of endurance**. Glycogen (stored glucose) is the main source of energy that is needed for endurance. Sleep deprivation causes slower storage of glycogen, preventing athletes from performing well in endurance events.

## HOW SLEEP CAN IMPROVE SPORTS PERFORMANCE

Studies suggest that increased sleep enables better sports performance. Some benefits of proper sleep are as follows:

- In a study, basketball players who got an extra two hours of sleep per night tended to increase their speed by 5 percent and accuracy by 9 percent.

- Athletes who sleep an average of eight to nine hours nightly are better able to perform high-intensity workouts, such as weight lifting, running, or biking.
- Mental strain is a part of any sport. Sleep will help athletes improve their mood, memory, and alertness.
- Players have better reaction time and reflexes.
- Training and practice can cause physical exhaustion. The proper amount of sleep helps the body restore muscle and other tissue.
- Sleep promotes better coordination. While sleeping, the body recalls and consolidates memories linked to the motor skills that were practiced.

## SLEEP TIPS FOR ATHLETES

Athletes have tight schedules when it comes to training and practice. However, experts say that as much as an athlete needs practice, so does he or she need sleep. Since the body is pushed on a regular basis, in order to recover, it needs rest and time. Below are a few tips that can help an athlete get better sleep.

- Establish a regular schedule for going to bed and waking up at the same time every day.
- Since traveling can upset sleep, it is best to get to the place of the competition two or three days early in order to allow the body to adjust.
- Sleep medication should be avoided unless prescribed by a doctor since it can disturb the quality of sleep and hinder performance.
- It is best to avoid caffeine and alcohol because they can disrupt healthful sleep patterns.
- Natural relaxation techniques, such as deep breathing or listening to soft music, can help promote sleep.

## References

Fullagar, Hugh H.K. et al. "Sleep and Athletic Performance: The Effects of Sleep Loss on Exercise Performance, and Physiological and Cognitive Responses to Exercise,"

*Sports Medicine*, 45, no. 2 (2015): 161-186. https://doi. org/10.1007/s40279-014-0260-0.

Griffin, R. Morgan. "Can Sleep Improve Your Athletic Performance?" WebMD, August 13, 2014. Available online. URL: https://webmd.com/fitness-exercise/features/ sleep-athletic-performance. Accessed March 31, 2023.

"How Sleep Affects Athletes' Performance," Sleep.org, April 13, 2022. Available online. URL: https://sleep.org/ articles/how-sleep-affects-athletes. Accessed March 31, 2023.

Sherwood, Chris. "Does a Lack of Sleep Affect an Athlete's Performance?" Livestrong.com, August 14, 2017. Available online. URL: https://livestrong.com/article/372087-does-a-lack-of-sleep-affect-an-athletes-performance. Accessed March 31, 2023.

"Sleep, Athletic Performance, and Recovery," National Sleep Foundation, April 13, 2022. Available online. URL: https://sleepfoundation.org/sleep-news/sleep-athletic-performance-and-recovery. Accessed March 31, 2023.

"Sleep and Athletes," Gatorade Sports Science Institute, July 2017. Available online. URL: https://gssiweb.org/ en/sports-science-exchange/Article/sse-167-sleep-and-athletes. Accessed March 31, 2023.

Quinn, Elizabeth. "Sleep Deprivation and Athletes," Verywell. com, October 5, 2017. Available online. URL: https:// verywell.com/sleep-deprivation-and-athletes-3119144. Accessed March 31, 2023.

## Section 14.3 | **Health and Safety Concerns at Work**

To support optimal health, experts recommend that adults get seven or more hours of sleep per night. However, recent estimates suggest about one-third of adults do not get enough sleep, which can prevent employees from meeting their health and productivity goals and create safety risks at work in the following ways:

- Poor sleep increases a person's risk for a variety of chronic conditions. For example, adults who sleep six or fewer hours per night are more likely to be obese and have diagnoses such as diabetes, coronary heart disease, and stroke than those who report seven to nine hours of sleep.
- In addition, poor sleep slows both physical and cognitive reaction times and accuracy, increasing the risk of injury in the workplace.
- Fatigue and poor sleep also contribute to productivity losses (a measurement of employee efficiency when completing required tasks), costing employers $1,967 per employee per year and adding up to approximately 1.23 million lost working days annually.

Employers of all sizes and industries can help their employees get more and better sleep through evidence-based workplace health programs. This brief introduces strategies employers can adopt to encourage employees to evaluate and address their sleep hygiene, including the practices and habits necessary to achieve the recommended sleep quantity and quality and full alertness at home and work (when appropriate).

## HELPING EMPLOYEES GET THE SLEEP THEY NEED: A GOAL FOR ALL INDUSTRIES

Employees' work and home life can influence the amount and quality of sleep they get. As a result, getting enough sleep can be a problem for anyone, no matter the job. People who work in industries that require shift work or spend long hours on the job are at a higher risk for sleep-related disorders and report getting the least amount of sleep. Their lack of sleep may also put others at risk, especially when their responsibilities involve patient care or transportation. By addressing sleep as part of a workplace health program, companies can increase safety and make employees healthier and safer at home.

There are several promising practices and evidence-based strategies to help employees improve their sleep. Interventions to reduce fatigue or tiredness are associated with decreased self-reported fatigue and increased reaction speed. Examples include encouraging physicians and nurses to take brief naps in the middle of long shifts. Training employees to recognize, report, and help colleagues who show signs of drowsiness can also be beneficial.

Employers should consider whether one or more of the following strategies could benefit their worksite.

## Strategy 1: Start with Education, Training, and Assessment

Providing employees with the information and tools to understand or improve their sleep is a great first step. Over time, a sleep intervention could include the following:

- **Education**. Information about sleep can be incorporated into newsletters or posted in common areas for all employees to see. This may include recommendations from credible health agencies about how much sleep is needed to remain healthy, sleep disorders, and how to achieve quality sleep.
- **Training**. Managers and employees can participate in training to recognize the signs and symptoms of fatigue and learn what to do to reduce fatigue-related accidents.
- **Assessment**. Employers can offer their workers access to tools that evaluate their sleep and provide targeted advice based on their results.

The worker education, training, and assessment can also encourage behavior changes at home, which benefits employees and

142

their families. The report, From Evidence to Practice: Workplace Wellness that Works, by the Institute for Health and Productivity Studies at the Johns Hopkins Bloomberg School of Public Health and the Transamerica Center for Health Studies, and the toolkit, Working on Wellness: Supporting Healthier People, Workplaces and Communities, by the Massachusetts Department of Public Health, both include actionable recommendations for helping employers alert their workers to the importance of sleep and in-depth strategies to better address sleep. Additionally, the American College of Occupational and Environmental Medicine created a detailed overview of these initial strategies to encourage healthy sleep and improve fatigue management in the workplace.

## Strategy 2: Incorporate Dedicated Breaks and Napping Rooms

Sleep does not need to take place at home. When working long shifts and late into the evening, brief naps and dedicated breaks can promote health and reduce accidents and mistakes. For example, medical students who took brief sleep breaks reported decreased tiredness, while nurses who took a one-hour break in a quiet, restful environment were more alert during their shifts and felt less worn out.

Worksites that incorporate napping or extended breaks feature two key attributes:

- dedicated physical spaces with beds or comfortable chairs where employees can rest
- schedules that allow for breaks

It is also important that the company culture supports and actively encourages breaks. A common argument against a napping intervention is that the transition from sleep to wakefulness— known as "sleep inertia"—can be long and initially pose a risk. However, employees can return to their regular routine after a short (15-minute) period of recovery, particularly if naps are no more than 60 minutes.

While the examples described here relate to the health-care sector, they are just as relevant for other industries in which employees work more than 40 hours per week, work in shifts, or work overnight. Various industries, including the U.S. Department of Transportation (DOT), are beginning to publish recommendations or standards which allow for breaks and napping to address driver fatigue.

## Strategy 3: Recognize Tiredness and Pull Over Safely

Alertness is critical for driving safely. One in five fatal motor vehicle crashes involves a drowsy driver. The National Transportation Safety Board (NTSB) reported that drowsy driving is probably the cause of over half of fatal crashes among commercial truck drivers. One of the most effective methods to prevent these accidents is to teach drivers how to recognize tiredness, encourage them to pull over safely, and allow them to take naps. To encourage employees to follow these actions, managers can work with their drivers to effectively plan their trip routes and schedule times for sleep in places that are safe for them to pull over. Instead of taking breaks to rest, some truck drivers rely on caffeine and other stimulants to stay awake. However, this strategy should be used with caution, as there is a lag time between consumption and when the caffeine takes effect. When possible, follow the consumption of a caffeinated beverage immediately with a brief nap to help restore alertness. Lastly, as the stimulating effects from caffeine can last for as long as six to eight hours, experts recommend that individuals not consume caffeinated beverages in the hours before sleep is planned.

## Strategy 4: Modify the Workplace to Increase Alertness

It is important to balance workplace health programming that promotes healthy sleep with environmental interventions that improve alertness. Changes in at least three dimensions of the work environment are recommended to influence how tired or awake employees feel.

- **Lighting**. Adjusting brightness and wavelength can maximize alertness and minimize adverse effects on later sleep quality. For example, increasing brightness to between 750 and 1,000 lux during night shifts can increase alertness and reduce fatigue.

- **Temperature**. Maintaining the temperature at 68 °F promotes wakefulness; as the temperature increases, workers feel drowsier.
- **Noise**. Continuous sound can act as a stimulant for employees and is most effective when music is varied.

Additional information about fatigue risk management in the workplace, including the dangers of fatigue in the worksite and how to address them, is outlined in this statement (www.acoem.org/Guidance-and-Position-Statements/Guidance-and-Position-Statements/Fatigue-Risk-Management-in-the-Workplace) from the Task Force on Fatigue Risk Management of the American College of Occupational and Environmental Medicine (ACOEM).

## MAKE SLEEP A PRIORITY

Workplace health programs can incorporate strategies aimed at improving sleep and reducing fatigue among employees. These interventions can benefit employee health directly by reducing on-the-job safety risks and boosting productivity and indirectly by decreasing the risk of developing chronic health conditions. Employers win because their workers perform better when well-rested, and companies have seen reduced health-care spending costs in the longer term.[2]

---

[2] "Sleep: An Important Health and Safety Concern at Work," Centers for Disease Control and Prevention (CDC), March 9, 2023. Available online. URL: www.cdc.gov/workplacehealthpromotion/initiatives/resource-center/pdf/WHRC-Brief-Sleep-508.pdf. Accessed April 25, 2023.

# Chapter 15 | Drowsy Driving

## Chapter Contents

## DROWSY DRIVING: ASLEEP AT THE WHEEL

Drive alert—protect yourself and others on the road! Learn the risks of drowsy driving and how to prevent it. Drowsy driving is a dangerous combination of driving when sleepy. This usually happens when a driver has not slept enough, but it can also happen because of untreated sleep disorders or shift work. Prescription and over-the-counter medications can also cause drowsiness, and alcohol can interact with sleepiness to increase both impairment and drowsiness.

No one knows the exact moment when sleep will come over their body. Falling asleep at the wheel is clearly dangerous, but being sleepy also affects your ability to drive safely, even if you do not fall asleep. Drowsiness:
* makes you less able to pay attention to the road
* slows your reaction time if you must brake or steer suddenly
* affects your ability to make good decisions

## DID YOU KNOW?
* In a Centers for Disease Control and Prevention (CDC) survey, an estimated 1 in 25 adult drivers (aged 18 years or older) reported having fallen asleep while driving in the previous 30 days.
* In the same CDC survey, adult drivers who snore or usually sleep six or fewer hours per day were more likely to report falling asleep while driving than drivers who do not snore or usually sleep seven or more hours per day, respectively.
* Drowsy driving was involved in 91,000 crashes in 2017—resulting in 50,000 injuries and nearly 800 deaths. In 2020, there were 633 deaths based on police reports. However, these numbers are underestimated, and over 6,000 fatal crashes each year may involve a drowsy driver.

## WHO IS AT GREATER RISK OF DROWSY DRIVING AND RELATED CRASHES AND DEATHS?

Some groups are more prone to drowsy driving than others. These include:

- teen and young adult drivers
- drivers on the road between midnight and 6 a.m. or in the later afternoon
- drivers who do not get enough sleep
- commercial truck drivers
- drivers who work the night shift or long shifts
- drivers with untreated sleep disorders—such as sleep apnea, where breathing repeatedly stops and starts
- drivers who use medicines that make them sleepy

Learn the warning signs of drowsy driving:

- yawning or blinking frequently
- trouble remembering the past few miles driven
- missing your exit
- drifting from your lane
- hitting a rumble strip on the side of the road

## PREVENT DROWSY DRIVING BEFORE TAKING THE WHEEL

- Get enough sleep! Most adults need at least seven hours of sleep a day, and teens need at least eight hours.
- Develop good sleeping habits, such as sticking to a sleep schedule.
- If you have a sleep disorder or have symptoms of a sleep disorder, such as snoring or feeling sleepy during the day, talk to your doctor about treatment options.
- Before you drive, avoid taking medicines that make you sleepy. Be sure to check the label on any medicines you take or talk to your pharmacist.
- Before you drive, avoid drinking alcohol. Alcohol impairs the skills needed for driving and increases drowsiness.[1]

---

[1] "Drowsy Driving: Asleep at the Wheel," Centers for Disease Control and Prevention (CDC), November 21, 2022. Available online. URL: www.cdc.gov/sleep/features/drowsy-driving.html. Accessed March 15, 2023.

## Section 15.2 | **Some Sleep Drugs Can Impair Driving**

### SOME MEDICINES AND DRIVING DO NOT MIX

If you are taking medication, is it safe to drive? Most likely, yes. Still, the U.S. Food and Drug Administration (FDA) advises you to make sure before operating any type of vehicle, whether a car, bus, train, plane, or boat. Although most medications will not affect your ability to drive, some prescription and nonprescription medicines (also called "over-the-counter," or "OTC") can have side effects and cause reactions that may make it unsafe to drive. Side effects can include the following:

- sleepiness/drowsiness
- blurred vision
- dizziness
- slowed movement
- fainting
- inability to focus or pay attention
- nausea
- excitability

Some medicines can affect your driving for a short time after you take them. For others, the effects can last for several hours and even the next day. And some medicines have a warning not to operate heavy machinery—this includes driving a car.

### MEDICINES THAT MIGHT AFFECT DRIVING

Knowing how your medications—or any combination of them—affect your ability to drive is a safety measure. Some drugs that could make it dangerous to drive include the following:

- opioid pain relievers
- prescription drugs for anxiety (e.g., benzodiazepines)
- antiseizure drugs (antiepileptic drugs)
- antipsychotic drugs
- some antidepressants
- products containing codeine

- some cold remedies and allergy products, such as antihistamines (both prescription and OTC)
- sleeping pills
- muscle relaxants
- medicines that treat or control symptoms of diarrhea
- medicines that treat or prevent symptoms of motion sickness
- diet pills, "stay awake" drugs, and other medications with stimulants (e.g., caffeine, ephedrine, pseudoephedrine)

Also, taking cannabidiol (CBD) products and driving can be dangerous. CBD can cause sleepiness, sedation, and lethargy. Because of these side effects, consumers should use caution if planning on operating a motor vehicle after consuming any CBD products.

## SOME SLEEP MEDICINES CAN IMPAIR YOU, EVEN THE NEXT MORNING

People with insomnia have trouble falling or staying asleep. Many take medicines to help them sleep. Come morning, though, some sleep medicines could make you less able to perform activities for which you must be fully alert, including driving.

A common ingredient in a widely prescribed sleep medication is zolpidem, which belongs to a class of medications called "sedative-hypnotics." The FDA has found that medicines containing zolpidem, especially extended-release forms, can impair driving ability and other activities the next morning.

Zolpidem immediate and extended-release forms are marketed as generic drugs under these brand names:
- Ambien and Ambien CR (oral tablet)
- Edluar (tablet placed under the tongue)
- Intermezzo (tablet placed under the tongue)
- Zolpimist (oral spray)

People who take sleep medicines should talk to their health-care professionals about ways to take the lowest effective dose. Do not assume that nonprescription sleep medicines are necessarily safer alternatives. The FDA is also evaluating the risk of next-day impairment with other insomnia drugs, both prescription and OTC versions.

## ALLERGY MEDICINES CAN AFFECT YOUR ABILITY TO DRIVE

For allergy sufferers, medications containing antihistamines can help relieve many different types of allergies, including hay fever. But these medicines may interfere with driving and operating heavy machinery (including driving a car). Antihistamines can slow your reaction time, make it hard to focus or think clearly, and may cause mild confusion even if you do not feel drowsy.

Avoid drinking alcohol or taking sleep medications while using some antihistamines. Those combinations can increase the sedative effects of antihistamines.

## HOW TO AVOID DRIVING WHILE IMPAIRED

You can still drive safely while taking most medications. Talk to your health-care provider about possible side effects. For example, some antihistamines and sleep medications work for longer periods than others. You might feel the sedating effects of these medications for some time after you have taken them and maybe even into the next day.

Doctors and pharmacists can tell you about known side effects of medications, including those that interfere with driving. You can also request printed information about the side effects of any new medicine.

To manage or minimize side effects while driving, your health-care provider may be able to adjust your dose, adjust the timing of when you take the medicine, or change the medicine to one that causes fewer side effects for you.

Here are some more tips:
- Always follow directions for use and read warnings on medication packaging or handouts provided by the pharmacy.
- Do not stop using your medicine unless your prescriber tells you to.

- Tell your health-care provider about all the products you are taking, including prescription, OTC, and herbal products. Also, let them know about any reactions you experience.[2]

---

[2] "Some Medicines and Driving Don't Mix," Centers for Disease Control and Prevention (CDC), September 3, 2021. Available online. URL: www.fda.gov/consumers/consumer-updates/some-medicines-and-driving-dont-mix. Accessed March 15, 2023.

# Chapter 16 | **Jet Lag**

Jet lag is caused by a mismatch between a person's normal daily rhythms and a new time zone. It is a temporary sleep problem that usually occurs when you travel across more than three time zones but can affect anyone who travels across multiple time zones. Jet lag can affect your mood, your ability to concentrate, and your physical and mental performance. Fortunately, you can take steps to minimize the effects of jet lag.

## BEFORE TRAVEL

A few days before you travel, you can begin adjusting your body's natural clock to the time zone at your destination. Depending on where you are traveling, you may want to adjust your sleep patterns to get used to the time change:

- If traveling west, go to bed an hour or two later than usual.
- If traveling east, go to bed an hour or two earlier than usual.

Consider scheduling travel to arrive at your destination at least two days before any important events to give your body time to adjust.

Stomach aches and other stomach problems are a symptom of jet lag; eating smaller meals just before travel may help. If you struggle with jet lag, talk to your doctor about taking medicine or other sleep aids to help you sleep.

## DURING TRAVEL

If you are traveling to a time zone that is more than three hours different from your normal time zone, you should follow the sleep and waking routines of your destination when you arrive. It might help to stay in well-lit areas at your destination during the day. Take any medicine or sleep aids as directed by your health-care provider to help you sleep at night.

Other steps you can take to help you adjust to the new time and avoid jet lag symptoms are as follows:

- Eat small meals to avoid stomach aches or other problems.
- Avoid alcohol as it disrupts sleep.
- Use caffeine and exercise strategically; these may help you stay alert throughout the day, but you should avoid these in the evening.
- Drink plenty of water.
- If you are sleepy during the day, take short naps, no more than 15–20 minutes, to help you feel better during the day yet still sleep at night.

A combination of these steps will help you overcome jet lag more quickly.[1]

## RISK FOR TRAVELERS

Jet lag results from a mismatch between a person's circadian (24-hour) rhythms and the time of day in the new time zone. When establishing risk, clinicians should first determine how many time zones the traveler will cross and what the discrepancy will be between the time of day at home and at the destination. During the first few days after a flight to a new time zone, a person's circadian rhythms are still "anchored" to the time of day at home. Rhythms then adjust gradually to the new time zone. A useful web-based tool for world time zone travel information can be found at www.timeanddate.

---

[1] "Jet Lag," Centers for Disease Control and Prevention (CDC), October 6, 2022. Available online. URL: wwwnc.cdc.gov/travel/page/jet-lag. Accessed March 15, 2023.

com/worldclock/converter.html. If three or more time zones are being crossed, any symptoms such as tiredness are likely due to travel fatigue rather than significant jet lag and will soon abate.

Many people traveling more than three time zones away for a vacation accept the risk of jet lag as a transient and mild inconvenience, while other people who are traveling on business or to compete in athletic events desire clear advice on prophylactic measures and treatments. If two or fewer days are spent in the new time zone, some people may prefer to anchor their sleep–wake schedule to the time of day at home as much as is practical. Thereby, the total "burden" of jet lag resulting from the short round trip is minimized.

## CLINICAL PRESENTATION

The symptomatology of jet lag can often be difficult to define not only because of variation between people but also because the same person can experience different symptoms after each flight. Jet-lagged travelers typically experience one or more of the following symptoms after a flight across three or more time zones:

- poor sleep, including difficulty initiating sleep at the usual time of night (after eastward flights), early awakening (after westward flights), and fractionated sleep (after flights in either direction)
- poor performance in physical and mental tasks during the new daytime
- negative feelings such as fatigue, headache, irritability, anxiety, inability to concentrate, and depression
- gastrointestinal disturbances and decreased interest in, and enjoyment of, meals
- symptoms that are difficult to distinguish from the general fatigue resulting from international travel itself, as well as from other travel factors such as hypoxia in the aircraft cabin

## TREATMENT

Since light and social contacts influence the timing of internal circadian rhythms, a traveler who is staying in the time zone for two or more days should try to follow the local people's sleep–wake habits as much as possible and as quickly as possible. This approach can be supplemented with the following information on specific treatments.

## Light

Exposure to bright light can advance or delay human circadian rhythms depending on when it is received relative to a person's body clock time. Consequently, schedules have been formulated for proposed "good" and "bad" times for exposure to light after arrival in a new time zone

After flights that cross a large number of time zones, the proposed best circadian time for exposure to light immediately after the flight may actually be when it is still dark in the new time zone, which raises the question of whether exposure to supplementary light from a "light box" is helpful. Unfortunately, to date, only one small randomized controlled trial on supplementary bright light for reducing jet lag has been conducted. No clinically relevant effects of supplementary light on jet lag symptoms were detected after a flight across five time zones going west.

## Diet and Physical Activity

Most dietary interventions have not been found to reduce jet lag symptoms. In a recent study, long-haul flight crews showed a small improvement in their general subjective rating of jet lag, but not the separate symptoms of jet lag or alertness, on their days off work when they adopted more regular meal times. Because gastrointestinal disturbance is a common symptom, smaller meals before and during the flight might be better tolerated than larger meals. Caffeine and physical activity may be used strategically at the destination to ameliorate any daytime sleepiness, but little evidence indicates that these interventions reduce overall feelings of jet lag. Any purported treatments that are underpinned by homeopathy, aromatherapy, and acupressure have no scientific basis.

## Hypnotic Medications

Prescription medications such as temazepam, zolpidem, or zopiclone may reduce sleep loss during and after travel but do not necessarily help resynchronize circadian rhythms or improve overall jet lag symptoms. If indicated, the lowest effective dose of a short- to medium-acting compound should be prescribed for the initial few days, bearing in mind the adverse effects of these drugs.

Taking hypnotics during a flight should be considered with caution because the resulting immobility could increase the risk of deep vein thrombosis. Alcohol should not be used by travelers as a sleep aid because it disrupts sleep and can provoke obstructive sleep apnea (OSA).

## Melatonin and Melatonin-Receptor Analogs

Melatonin is secreted at night by the pineal gland and is probably the most well-known treatment for jet lag. Melatonin delays circadian rhythms when taken during the rising phase of body temperature (usually the morning) and advances rhythms when ingested during the falling phase of body temperature (usually the evening). These effects are opposite to those of bright light.

The instructions on most melatonin products advise travelers to take it before nocturnal sleep in the new time zone, irrespective of the number of time zones crossed or the direction of travel. Studies published in the mid-1980s indicated a substantial benefit of melatonin (just before sleep) for reducing overall feelings of jet lag after flights. However, subsequent larger studies did not replicate the earlier findings.

Melatonin is considered a dietary supplement in the United States and is not regulated by the Food and Drug Administration (FDA). Therefore, the advertised concentration of melatonin has not been confirmed for most melatonin products on the market, and the presence of contaminants in the product cannot be ruled out.

Ramelteon, a melatonin-receptor agonist, is an FDA-approved treatment for insomnia. A dose of 1 mg taken just before bedtime can decrease sleep onset latency after eastward travel across five time zones. Higher doses do not seem to lead to further improvements, and the effects of the medication on other symptoms of jet lag and the timing of circadian rhythms are not as clear.

## Combination Treatments

Multiple therapies to decrease jet lag symptoms may be combined into treatment packages. Although marginal gains from multiple treatments may aggregate, evidence from robust randomized controlled trials is lacking for most of these treatment packages. One treatment package offering tailored advice via a mobile application was piloted to be used over several months of frequent flying. Participants reported reduced fatigue compared with the comparator group and improved aspects of health-related behavior such as physical activity, snacking, and sleep quality but not other measures of sleep (latency, duration, use of sleep-related medication).

In conclusion, there is still no "cure" for jet lag. Counseling should focus on the factors that are known, from laboratory simulations, to alter circadian timing. Nevertheless, more randomized controlled trials of treatments prescribed before, during, or after transmeridian flights are needed before the clinician can provide robust, evidence-based advice.[2]

---

[2] "Travel by Air, Land & Sea," Centers for Disease Control and Prevention (CDC), June 24, 2019. Available online. URL: wwwnc.cdc.gov/travel/yellowbook/2020/travel-by-air-land-sea/jet-lag. Accessed April 25, 2023.

# Chapter 17 | **Why Your Body and Brain Need Sleep**

**Chapter Contents**

## GET THE REST YOU NEED

Sometimes, the pace of modern life barely gives you time to stop and rest. It can make getting a good night's sleep on a regular basis seem like a dream. But sleep is as important for good health as diet and exercise. Good sleep improves your brain performance, mood, and health. Not getting enough quality sleep regularly raises the risk of many diseases and disorders. These range from heart disease and stroke to obesity and dementia.

There is more to good sleep than just the hours spent in bed, says Marishka Brown, Ph.D., a sleep expert at the National Institutes of Health (NIH), Program Director for Sleep Disorders at the National Center on Sleep Disorders Research (NCSDR). "Healthy sleep encompasses three major things," she explains. "One is how much sleep you get. Another is sleep quality—that you get uninterrupted and refreshing sleep. The last is a consistent sleep schedule."

People who work the night shift or have irregular schedules may find getting quality sleep extra challenging. And times of great stress—such as the current pandemic—can disrupt our normal sleep routines. But there are many things you can do to improve your sleep.

## SLEEP FOR REPAIR

Why do we need to sleep? People often think that sleep is just "downtime" when a tired brain gets to rest, says Dr. Maiken Nedergaard, who studies sleep at the University of Rochester.

"But that is wrong," she says. While you sleep, your brain is working. For example, sleep helps prepare your brain to learn, remember, and create. Dr. Nedergaard and her colleagues discovered that the brain has a drainage system that removes toxins during sleep. "When we sleep, the brain totally changes function," she explains. "It becomes almost like a kidney, removing waste from the system."

Her team found in mice that the drainage system removes some of the proteins linked with Alzheimer disease (AD). These toxins were removed twice as fast from the brain during sleep.

Everything from blood vessels to the immune system uses sleep as a time for repair, says Dr. Kenneth Wright, Jr., a sleep researcher at the University of Colorado. "There are certain repair processes that occur in the body mostly, or most effectively, during sleep," he explains. "If you do not get enough sleep, those processes are going to be disturbed."

## SLEEP MYTHS AND TRUTHS

How much sleep you need changes with age. Experts recommend school-age children get at least nine hours of sleep a night and teens get between eight and ten hours of sleep. Most adults need at least seven hours or more of sleep each night.

There are many misunderstandings about sleep. One is that adults need less sleep as they get older. This is not true. Older adults still need the same amount. But sleep quality can get worse as you age. Older adults are also likely to take medications that interfere with sleep.

Another sleep myth is that you can "catch up" on your days off. Researchers are finding that this largely is not the case. "If you have one bad night's sleep and take a nap, or sleep longer the next night, that can benefit you," says Dr. Wright. "But if you have a week's worth of getting too little sleep, the weekend is not sufficient for you to catch up. That is not healthy behavior."

In a recent study, Dr. Wright and his team looked at people with consistently deficient sleep. They compared them to sleep-deprived people who got to sleep in on the weekend. Both groups of people gained weight with a lack of sleep. Their bodies' ability to control blood sugar levels also got worse. The weekend catch-up sleep did not help.

On the flip side, more sleep is not always better, says Dr. Brown. For adults, "if you are sleeping more than nine hours a night and you still do not feel refreshed, there may be some underlying medical issue," she explains.

## SLEEP DISORDERS

Some people have conditions that prevent them from getting enough quality sleep, no matter how hard they try. These problems are called "sleep disorders."

The most common sleep disorder is insomnia. "Insomnia is when you have repeated difficulty getting to sleep and/or staying asleep," says Dr. Brown. This happens despite having the time to sleep and a proper sleep environment. It can make you feel tired or unrested during the day.

Insomnia can be short-term, where people struggle to sleep for a few weeks or months. "Quite a few more people have been experiencing this during the pandemic," Dr. Brown says. Long-term insomnia lasts for three months or longer.

Sleep apnea is another common sleep disorder. In sleep apnea, the upper airway becomes blocked during sleep. This reduces or stops airflow, which wakes people up during the night. The condition can be dangerous. If untreated, it may lead to other health problems.

If you regularly have problems sleeping, talk with your health-care provider. They may have you keep a sleep diary to track your sleep for several weeks. They can also run tests, including sleep studies. These look for sleep disorders.

## GETTING BETTER SLEEP

If you are having trouble sleeping, hearing how important it is may be frustrating. But simple things can improve your odds of a good night's sleep.

Treatments are available for many common sleep disorders. Cognitive behavioral therapy (CBT) can help many people with insomnia get better sleep. Medications can also help some people.

Many people with sleep apnea benefit from using a device called a "continuous positive airway pressure" (CPAP) machine. These machines keep the airway open so that you can breathe. Other treatments can include special mouth guards and lifestyle changes. For everyone, "as best you can, try to make sleep a priority," Dr. Brown says. "Sleep is not a throwaway thin—it is a biological necessity."[1]

[1] *NIH News in Health*, "Good Sleep for Good Health," National Institutes of Health (NIH), April 2021. Available online. URL: https://newsinhealth.nih.gov/2021/04/good-sleep-good-health. Accessed March 15, 2023.

## Section 17.2 | **Sleep for a Healthy Heart**

Getting good sleep is not just important for your energy levels—it is critical for your heart health, too. Sleep is not a luxury. It is critical to good health. Sleep helps your body repair itself. Getting enough good sleep also helps you function normally during the day.

## HOW MUCH SLEEP DO YOU NEED?

Most adults need at least seven hours of sleep each night. However, more than one in three American adults say they do not get the recommended amount of sleep. While this may be fine for a day or two, not getting enough sleep over time can lead to serious health problems—and make certain health problems worse.

## WHAT HEALTH CONDITIONS ARE LINKED TO A LACK OF SLEEP?

Adults who sleep less than seven hours each night are more likely to say they have had health problems, including heart attack, asthma, and depression. Some of these health problems raise the risk of heart disease, heart attack, and stroke. These health problems include the following:

- **High blood pressure**. During normal sleep, your blood pressure goes down. Having sleep problems means your blood pressure stays higher for a longer period of time. High blood pressure is one of the leading risks for heart disease and stroke. About 75 million Americans—one in three adults—have high blood pressure.
- **Type 2 diabetes**. Diabetes is a disease that causes sugar to build up in your blood, a condition that can damage your blood vessels. Some studies show that getting enough good sleep may help people improve blood sugar control.
- **Obesity**. Lack of sleep can lead to unhealthy weight gain. This is especially true for children and adolescents, who need more sleep than adults. Not

getting enough sleep may affect a part of the brain that controls hunger.

## WHAT SLEEP CONDITIONS CAN HURT YOUR HEART HEALTH?

Over time, sleep problems can hurt your heart health. Sleep apnea happens when your airway gets blocked repeatedly during sleep, causing you to stop breathing for short amounts of time. Sleep apnea can be caused by certain health problems, such as obesity and heart failure.

Sleep apnea affects how much oxygen your body gets while you sleep and increases the risk for many health problems, including high blood pressure, heart attack, and stroke. It is more common among Blacks, Hispanics, and Native Americans than among Whites.

Insomnia refers to trouble falling asleep, staying asleep, or both. As many as one in two adults experiences short-term insomnia at some point, and one in ten may have long-lasting insomnia. Insomnia is linked to high blood pressure and heart disease. Over time, poor sleep can also lead to unhealthy habits that can hurt your heart, including higher stress levels, less motivation to be physically active, and unhealthy food choices.

## WHAT CAN YOU DO TO GET BETTER SLEEP?

- Stick to a regular sleep schedule. Go to bed at the same time each night and get up at the same time each morning, including on the weekends.
- Get enough natural light, especially earlier in the day. Try going for a morning or lunchtime walk.
- Get enough physical activity during the day. Try not to exercise within a few hours of bedtime.
- Avoid artificial light, especially within a few hours of bedtime. Use a blue light filter on your computer or smartphone.
- Do not eat or drink within a few hours of bedtime; avoid alcohol and foods high in fat or sugar in particular.
- Keep your bedroom cool, dark, and quiet.

Work with your health-care team to identify obstacles to good sleep, including other medical conditions.[2]

## Section 17.3 | **Sleep for Healthy Weight**

### MOLECULAR TIES BETWEEN LACK OF SLEEP AND WEIGHT GAIN

A poor night's sleep can leave you feeling foggy and drowsy throughout the day. Sleep deprivation has also been associated with higher risks of weight gain and obesity in recent years.

A group led by Erin Hanlon Ph.D., a Research Assistant Professor in the Section of Endocrinology, Diabetes, and Metabolism at the University of Chicago, and Eve Van Cauter Ph.D., Professor in the Department of Medicine at the University of Chicago, wanted to better understand how sleep and weight gain interact biologically. They noticed that sleep deprivation has effects in the body similar to the activation of the endocannabinoid (eCB) system, a key player in the brain's regulation of appetite and energy levels. Perhaps most well-known for being activated by chemicals found in marijuana, the eCB system affects the brain's motivation and reward circuits and can spark a desire for tasty foods.

The researchers enrolled 14 healthy, nonobese people—11 men and 3 women—who were 18–30 years old. The participants were placed on a fixed diet and allowed either normal 8.5 hours of sleep or restricted 4.5 hours of sleep for four consecutive days. All participants underwent both sleep conditions in a controlled clinical setting, with at least four weeks in between testing. For both conditions, the researchers collected blood samples from the participants beginning in the afternoon following the second night. The study was supported in part by the National Institutes of Health (NIH) National Center for Research Resources (NCRR) and the National Heart, Lung, and Blood Institute (NHLBI).

---

[2] "How Does Sleep Affect Your Heart Health?" Centers for Disease Control and Prevention (CDC), January 4, 2021. Available online. URL: www.cdc.gov/bloodpressure/sleep.htm. Accessed March 15, 2023.

When sleep-deprived, participants had eCB levels in the afternoons that were both higher and lasted longer than when they had had a full night's rest. This occurred around the same time that they reported increases in hunger and appetite.

After dinner on the fourth night, the participants fasted until the next afternoon. They were then allowed to choose their own meals and snacks for the rest of the day. All food was prepared and served in the clinical setting. Under both sleep conditions, people consumed about 90 percent of their daily calories at their first meal. But, when sleep-deprived, they consumed more and unhealthier snacks in between meals. This was when eCB levels were at their highest, suggesting that eCBs were driving hedonic, or pleasurable, eating.

Dr. Hanlon explains that if you see junk food and you have had enough sleep, you may be able to control some aspects of your natural response. "But if you are sleep deprived, your hedonic drive for certain foods gets stronger, and your ability to resist them may be impaired. So you are more likely to eat it. Do that again and again, and you pack on the pounds."

The authors noted that though the results are based on a small sample size, they are consistent with evidence from other research. Additional studies are needed to look at how changes in eCB levels and timing are affected by other cues, such as the body's internal clock or meal schedules.[3]

---

[3] News and Events, "Molecular Ties between Lack of Sleep and Weight Gain," National Institutes of Health (NIH), March 22, 2016. Available online. URL: www.nih.gov/news-events/nih-research-matters/molecular-ties-between-lack-sleep-weight-gain. Accessed March 16, 2023.

## Section 17.4 | **Making Up Sleep May Not Help**

Catching up on sleep does not reverse damage to the body caused by sleep deprivation according to a study. In fact, so-called recovery sleep may make some things worse. About one of every three adults regularly gets less than seven hours of sleep a night. Over time, lack of sleep can lead to changes in metabolism. These increase the risk of obesity and diabetes.

Some people try to make up for lack of sleep by sleeping more on their days off. A research team studied this strategy for two weeks in 36 men and women. After three nights of normal sleep, the participants were split into three groups. The first group slept up to nine hours a night. The second group was allowed a maximum of five hours of sleep a night. The third group had a maximum of five hours a night for five days but were then allowed to sleep in for two days. They then had two more days of sleep deprivation.

Those who had only five hours of sleep a night gained about three pounds on average during the study. They also had a 13 percent decrease in a key measure of metabolism called "insulin sensitivity." Insulin sensitivity is the body's ability to use insulin properly and control blood sugar levels.

Those who had recovery sleep gained about three pounds but had a 27 percent decrease in insulin sensitivity. Their natural body rhythms were also disrupted. They were more likely to wake up during the nights following the period of recovery sleep. "Catch-up sleep does not appear to be an effective strategy to reverse sleep-loss-induced disruptions of metabolism," says Kenneth P. Wright Jr., Ph.D., Professor in the Department of Integrative Physiology, who led the study at the University of Colorado.[4]

---

[4] *NIH News in Health*, "Making Up Sleep May Not Help," National Institutes of Health (NIH), May 2019. Available online. URL: https://newsinhealth.nih.gov/2019/05/making-up-sleep-may-not-help. Accessed March 16, 2023.

# Chapter 18 | Sleep Health in School Students

**Chapter Contents**

## Section 18.1 | Sleep Duration among Various Age Groups in the United States: Data and Statistics

## DATA AND STATISTICS OF SLEEP AND SLEEP DISORDERS

The amount of sleep you need changes as you age. Several U.S. surveillance systems assess short or insufficient sleep duration among the U.S. population. Understanding more about how short sleep duration and sleep insufficiency vary by demographic and geographic characteristics can help programs prioritize efforts to improve sleep health.

### Children (4 Months to 14 Years) Sleep Data

- Sleep in children aged 4 months to 14 years (refer to Table 18.1) is assessed in the National Survey of Children's Health (NSCH) by asking parents the following questions:
  - **Infants and children aged 0–5 years**. "During the past week, how many hours of sleep did this child get on an average day (count both nighttime sleep and naps)?"
  - **Children and adolescents aged 6–17 years**. "During the past week, how many hours of sleep did this child get on an average weeknight?"
- Short sleep duration is based on age group recommended hours of sleep per day and defined as less than 12 hours for children aged 4–12 months, less than 11 hours for children aged 1–2 years, less than 10 hours for children aged 3–5 years, less than 9 hours for children aged 6–12 years, and less than 8 hours for children aged 13–14 years.

## HIGHLIGHTS

- The prevalence of short sleep among children aged 4 months to 14 years was highest in the following subgroups in 2018–2019: ages 6–12 years (38.4%) and non-Hispanic Black (52.7%).

**Table 18.1.** Sleep Data for Children Aged 4 Months to 14 Years

| Population | Prevalence (%) | 95% Confidence Interval (%) |
|---|---|---|
| Overall | 34.4 | 33.5–35.4 |
| Male | 34.5 | 33.2–35.8 |
| Female | 34.3 | 33.0–35.7 |
| 4 months to 2 years | 34.5 | 32.3–36.8 |
| 3–5 years | 34.7 | 32.6–36.8 |
| 6–12 years | 38.4 | 37.0–39.8 |
| 13–14 years | 20.1 | 18.1–22.3 |
| Hispanic or Latino | 37.6 | 35.0–40.3 |
| Non-Hispanic White | 28.5 | 27.6–29.4 |
| Non-Hispanic Black or African American | 52.7 | 49.7–55.6 |
| Non-Hispanic American Indian or Alaska Native | 37.1 | 29.1–45.8 |
| Non-Hispanic Asian | 31.3 | 27.9–34.9 |
| Non-Hispanic Native Hawaiian | 36.1 | 22.7–52.1 |
| Non-Hispanic two or more races | 33.3 | 30.3–36.5 |

Source: The National Survey of Children's Health (NSCH), 2018–2019.
Note: For four months to two years, short sleep duration was defined as less than 12 hours for children aged 4–12 months and less than 11 hours for children aged one to two years.

## High School Students Sleep Data

- The Youth Risk Behavior Survey (YRBS) assesses sleep in high school students using the question: "On an average school night, how many hours of sleep do you get?"
- Short sleep duration for high school students is defined as less than 8 hours of sleep per 24-hour period as per age group recommendations.

## HIGHLIGHTS
- The prevalence of short sleep duration among high school students increased between 2009 and 2019 (refer to Table 18.2).
- Short sleep duration prevalence was higher among female students than male students across the years.

**Table 18.2.** Short Sleep Duration among U.S. High School Students, 2009–2019

| Year | Overall (%) | Overall 95% Confidence Interval (%) | Female (%) | Female 95% Confidence Interval (%) | Male (%) | Male 95% Confidence Interval (%) |
|------|-------------|-------------------------------------|------------|------------------------------------|----------|----------------------------------|
| 2009 | 69.1 | 67.5–70.7 | 71.8 | 70.1–73.4 | 66.7 | 64.9–68.4 |
| 2011 | 68.6 | 67.3–69.9 | 70.9 | 69.2–72.5 | 66.4 | 64.6–68.2 |
| 2013 | 68.3 | 66.8–69.8 | 71.1 | 69.5–72.7 | 65.5 | 63.5–67.5 |
| 2015 | 72.7 | 70.4–74.9 | 75.6 | 73.3–77.7 | 69.9 | 67.0–72.8 |
| 2017 | 74.6 | 73.1–76.0 | 75.4 | 73.5–77.2 | 73.7 | 71.8–75.4 |
| 2019 | 77.9 | 76.3–79.4 | 79.7 | 77.6–81.6 | 76.2 | 74.5–77.7 |

*Source: The CDC National Youth Risk Behavior Survey (YRBS), 2009–2019.*

## HIGHLIGHTS
- The prevalence of short sleep among high school students was highest in the following subgroups in 2019: female (79.7%), non-Hispanic Asian (82.8%), and 12th grade (83.0%; refer to Table 18.3).

**Table 18.3.** Short Sleep Duration among U.S. High School Students, 2019

| Population | Prevalence (%) | 95% Confidence Interval (%) |
|------------|----------------|-----------------------------|
| Overall | 77.9 | 77.9–77.9 |
| Male | 76.2 | 76.2–76.2 |

**Table 18.3.** Continued

| Population | Prevalence (%) | 95% Confidence Interval (%) |
|---|---|---|
| Female | 79.7 | 79.7–79.7 |
| 9th grade | 71.1 | 71.1–71.1 |
| 10th grade | 75.5 | 75.5–75.5 |
| 11th grade | 82.8 | 82.8–82.8 |
| 12th grade | 83.0 | 83.0–83.0 |
| Hispanic or Latino | 78.1 | 78.1–78.1 |
| Non-Hispanic American Indian or Alaska Native | 76.9 | 76.9–76.9 |
| Non-Hispanic Asian | 82.8 | 82.8–82.8 |
| Non-Hispanic Black | 80.5 | 80.5–80.5 |
| Non-Hispanic White | 76.8 | 76.8–76.8 |
| Non-Hispanic two or more races | 79.5 | 79.5–79.5 |

*Source: The CDC National Youth Risk Behavior Survey (YRBS), 2009–2019.*
*Note: Data were statistically unreliable for non-Hispanic Native Hawaiian or Other Pacific Islander.*

## Adults

- The Behavioral Risk Factor Surveillance System (BRFSS) assesses sleep in adults using the question: "On average, how many hours of sleep do you get in a 24-hour period?"
- Short sleep duration is based on age group recommended hours of sleep per day and is defined as less than seven hours for adults.

## HIGHLIGHTS

- Age-adjusted prevalence of adults who reported short sleep duration remained unchanged from 2013 to 2020 (refer to Table 18.4).
- Short sleep duration prevalence was higher among males than females across the years.

**Table 18.4.** Short Sleep Duration among U.S. Adults, 2013–2020

| Year | Overall (%) | Overall 95% Confidence Interval (%) | Female (%) | Female 95% Confidence Interval (%) | Male (%) | Male 95% Confidence Interval (%) |
|---|---|---|---|---|---|---|
| 2013 | 37.2 | 35.1–39.0 | 37.2 | 34.8–38.7 | 37.6 | 36.1–38.8 |
| 2014 | 37.2 | 34.8–38.3 | 35.9 | 33.9–37.9 | 37.5 | 35.6–38.9 |
| 2016 | 36.5 | 35.1–38.1 | 35.9 | 34.3–37.3 | 37 | 35.5–38.7 |
| 2018 | 37.4 | 36.0–39.6 | 36.3 | 34.5–38.5 | 38.9 | 37.5–39.8 |
| 2020 | 34.8 | 33.8–36.1 | 34 | 32.5–35.3 | 35.4 | 34.6–36.4 |

*Source: The CDC Behavioral Risk Factor Surveillance System (BRFSS), 2013, 2014, 2016, 2018, 2020.*
*Note: The sleep module is not part of the core survey in the following years: 2015, 2017, and 2019.*

## HIGHLIGHTS

- The crude prevalence of adults who reported short sleep duration was highest in the following subgroups: men (33.4%), adults aged 25–44 years (36.4%), non-Hispanic Native Hawaiian and Other Pacific Islander (47.0%), and non-Hispanic Black or African American (43.5%; refer to Table 18.5).

**Table 18.5.** Short Sleep among U.S. Adults, 2020

| Population | Prevalence (%) | 95% Confidence Interval (%) |
|---|---|---|
| Overall | 32.8 | 32.4–33.1 |
| Male | 33.4 | 32.9–33.9 |
| Female | 32.2 | 31.7–32.7 |
| 18–24 years | 29.7 | 28.6–30.9 |
| 25–44 years | 36.4 | 35.7–37.0 |
| 45–64 years | 34.5 | 33.9–35.1 |
| 65 or older | 26.1 | 25.5–26.8 |

**Table 18.5.** Continued

| Population | Prevalence (%) | 95% Confidence Interval (%) |
|---|---|---|
| Hispanic or Latino | 32.3 | 31.2–33.4 |
| Non-Hispanic White | 30.7 | 30.4–31.1 |
| Non-Hispanic Black or African American | 43.5 | 42.3–44.6 |
| Non-Hispanic American Indian or Alaska Native | 38.2 | 35.2–41.1 |
| Non-Hispanic Asian | 30.5 | 28.2–32.7 |
| Non-Hispanic Native Hawaiian | 47.0 | 42.0–52.0 |
| Non-Hispanic multiracial | 39.5 | 37.2–41.9 |
| Non-Hispanic others | 38.0 | 33.8–42.3 |

*Source: The CDC Behavioral Risk Factor Surveillance System (BRFSS), 2020.*[1]

## Section 18.2 | Sleep and Health of Middle and High School Students

Adequate sleep contributes to a student's overall health and well-being. Students should get the proper amount of sleep at night to stay focused, improve concentration, and improve academic performance. Children and adolescents who do not get enough sleep have a higher risk for many health problems, including obesity, diabetes, poor mental health, and injuries. They are also likely to have attention and behavior problems, which can contribute to poor academic performance in school.

---

[1] "Data and Statistics," Centers for Disease Control and Prevention (CDC), September 12, 2022. Available online. URL: www.cdc.gov/sleep/data_statistics.html. Accessed April 25, 2023.

## HOW MUCH SLEEP DO STUDENTS NEED?

How much sleep someone needs depends on their age. The recommendations made by the American Academy of Sleep Medicine (AASM) for children and adolescents are shown in Table 18.6.

**Table 18.6.** Recommended Hours of Sleep per Day for Children and Adolescents

| Age Group | Recommended Hours of Sleep per Day |
| --- | --- |
| Children (6–12 years) | 9–12 hours per 24 hours |
| Adolescents (13–18 years) | 8–10 hours per 24 hours |

## INSUFFICIENT SLEEP AMONG STUDENTS

The data from the 2015 national and state Youth Risk Behavior Surveys, a Centers for Disease Control and Prevention (CDC) study, shows that a majority of middle and high school students reported getting less than the recommended amount of sleep for their age.

### Middle School Students (Grades 6–8)
- Students in nine states were included in the study.
- About 6 out of 10 students (57.8%) did not get enough sleep on school nights.

### High School Students (Grades 9–12)
- A national sample was used.
- About 7 out of 10 students (72.7%) did not get enough sleep on school nights.

## WHAT CAN SCHOOLS DO?
### Provide Sleep Education

Schools can add sleep education to the K–12 curriculum to help children and adolescents learn why sleep is important to maintain a healthy lifestyle. Lessons in sleep patterns and sleep disorders, snoring, drowsy driving, and insomnia are among the topics teachers can cover in the classroom to help students develop healthy sleep habits.

Sleep education programs in school may result in significantly longer weekday and weekend total sleep time and improved sleep hygiene (habits that support good sleep) after completion. However, more research is needed to determine how best to maintain these improvements in the long term. One possible strategy is to incorporate refresher sessions for students.

## Review School Start Times

The combination of late bedtimes and early school start times results in most adolescents not getting enough sleep. In recent years, evidence has accumulated that later school start times for adolescents result in more students getting enough sleep.

School officials can learn more about the research connecting sleep and school start times. School districts can support adequate sleep among students by implementing delayed school start times as recommended by the American Academy of Pediatrics (AAP), the American Medical Association (AMA), and the AASM.

In 2014, the AAP recommended that middle schools and high schools start no earlier than 8:30 a.m. in order to allow adolescents to get the sleep they need. The AMA, the AASM, and other medical associations have since expressed support for delaying school start times for adolescents.

Good sleep hygiene in combination with later school times will enable adolescents to be healthier and better academic achievers.

## WHAT CAN PARENTS DO?
- Model and encourage habits that help promote good sleep.
- Setting a regular bedtime and rise time, including on weekends, is recommended for everyone—children, adolescents, and adults alike. Adolescents with parent-set bedtimes usually get more sleep than those whose parents do not set bedtimes.
- Dim lighting. Adolescents who are exposed to more light (such as room lighting or light from electronics) in the evening are less likely to get enough sleep.

- Implement a media curfew. Technology use (computers, video gaming, or mobile phones) may also contribute to late bedtimes. Parents should consider banning technology use after a certain time or removing these technologies from the bedroom.

## WHAT CAN HEALTH-CARE PROFESSIONALS DO?

- Health-care professionals can educate adolescent patients and their parents about the importance of adequate sleep and the factors that contribute to insufficient sleep among adolescents.[2]

## Section 18.3 | Sleep Deprivation and Learning

## THE LEARNING PROCESS AND SLEEP

Getting good-quality sleep is important for learning and memory. Studies on animals and humans have shown that sleep plays a crucial role in how well we learn and remember new information. When we do not get enough sleep, focusing and learning efficiently is harder. On the other hand, getting enough sleep helps our brains consolidate memories and make connections between new and old information.

Memory consolidation happens during both rapid eye movement (REM) and non-REM stages of sleep. During these stages, our brains are working to preserve important memories and eliminate unnecessary information. Getting enough sleep helps us lock in the things we learn throughout the day and link them to our existing knowledge.

While researchers are continuing to investigate the precise mechanisms through which sleep influences learning and memory, the evidence suggests that getting enough sleep is critical for

---

[2] "Sleep and Health," Centers for Disease Control and Prevention (CDC), May 29, 2019. Available online. URL: www.justice.gov/ovw/domestic-violence. Accessed March 16, 2023.

these cognitive processes. Inadequate sleep can make it harder to focus and learn, while getting the recommended amount of sleep can promote good physical health and enable our brains to function correctly.

## SLEEP STAGES AND TYPES OF MEMORY

Sleep and memory are closely related, and getting enough sleep can help your brain process and store new information. When you sleep, your brain goes through different stages (refer to Figure 18.1), and each stage helps with memory in different ways.

The first three stages of sleep prepare your brain to learn new information the next day, and not getting enough sleep can affect your ability to learn by as much as 40 percent. In these stages, your brain sorts out memories from the preceding day, distinguishing significant ones and eliminating insignificant ones.

The final stage of sleep, REM sleep, is when most dreaming occurs. During this stage, your brain processes emotional memories, and the thalamus sends cues from your senses to the cerebral cortex, which is responsible for interpreting and processing information from your memories. Slow-wave sleep (SWS), on the other hand, which is deep and restorative, may be important for consolidating newly learned knowledge.

The process of learning and remembering new information also happens in three stages, namely, acquisition, consolidation, and recall. Acquisition and recall happen while you are awake, but consolidation appears to happen during sleep, as neural connections that help develop lasting memories become stronger.

## IMPACT OF SLEEP DEPRIVATION ON LEARNING

Sleep deprivation can impair our capacity to recall things, learn new things, and make sound decisions. The quantity of sleep we require depends on our age, but both too little and too much sleep can impair our cognitive capacities. When we are sleep-deprived, we have difficulties paying attention, and our neurons do not function as well, which might cause us to forget information and make poor decisions. Chronic sleep deprivation can also have an effect

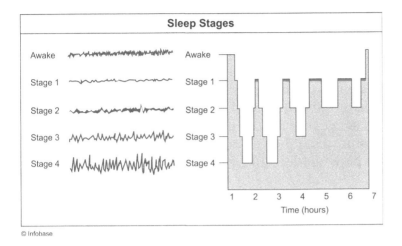

© Infobase

**Figure 18.1.** Sleep Stages

*Infobase*

on our emotions, making it difficult to learn and remember new knowledge. Sleep deprivation can also have negative impacts on our health, such as changes in appetite and weight. Overall, getting enough sleep is critical for keeping our brains operating properly.

Without proper rest, the body can feel tired to the extreme point of exhaustion. At such a stage, the muscles can weaken from lack of sleep; the body's organs are not synchronized; and neurons do not function optimally.

## TIPS TO IMPROVE LEARNING THROUGH SLEEP

To improve your sleep quality, you can incorporate some adjustments to your bedtime routine, also known as "sleep hygiene." It is recommended to stick to a consistent sleep schedule by sleeping and waking up at the same time each day to minimize daytime drowsiness. Creating a cozy sleep atmosphere with comfortable bedding and calming scents can aid in relaxation. Additionally, indulging in a warm bath, light yoga, or meditation before bedtime can help you unwind. Lastly, reducing the use of electronic devices before sleeping can be beneficial, as blue light can activate the brain and disrupt the sleep cycle. By integrating these practices, you can prepare yourself for a more restful and rejuvenating sleep.

Scientists are still studying how sleep affects our ability to learn and remember things, but one thing is certain—lack of sleep may impair our brains and bodies in a variety of ways. We may feel sleepy and have difficulties recalling what we learned during the day if we do not get enough sleep. However, this is still a developing field of study, and there is much more to discover about the relationship between sleep and learning.

## References

Cappello, Kelly. "The Impact of Sleep on Learning and Memory," University of Pennsylvania, December 21, 2020. Available online. URL: www.med.upenn.edu/csi/the-impact-of-sleep-on-learning-and-memory.html. Accessed April 12, 2023.

Mona, Breanna. "Can Sleep Help You Learn? Here's What Research Has to Say," Healthline Media, October 17, 2021. Available online. URL: www.healthline.com/health/sleep/sleep-learning. Accessed April 12, 2023.

Pacheco, Danielle. "Memory and Sleep," Sleep Foundation, February 8, 2023. Available online. URL: www.sleepfoundation.org/how-sleep-works/memory-and-sleep. Accessed April 12, 2023.

"Sleep, Learning, and Memory," Harvard Medical School, December 18, 2007. Available online. URL: https://healthysleep.med.harvard.edu/healthy/matters/benefits-of-sleep/learning-memory. Accessed April 12, 2023.

# Part 3 | **Sleep Disorders**

# Chapter 19 | **Breathing Disorders of Sleep**

## Chapter Contents

## WHAT IS SLEEP APNEA?

Sleep apnea is a common condition in which your breathing stops and restarts many times while you sleep. This can prevent your body from getting enough oxygen. You may want to talk to your health-care provider about sleep apnea if someone tells you that you snore or gasp during sleep or if you experience other symptoms of poor-quality sleep, such as excessive daytime sleepiness.

The following are the two types of sleep apnea:

- **Obstructive sleep apnea (OSA)**. It happens when your upper airway becomes blocked many times while you sleep, reducing or completely stopping airflow. This is the most common type of sleep apnea. Anything that could narrow your airway, such as obesity, large tonsils, or changes in your hormone levels, can increase your risk for OSA.
- **Central sleep apnea**. It happens when your brain does not send the signals needed to breathe. Health conditions that affect how your brain controls your airway and chest muscles can cause central sleep apnea.

To diagnose sleep apnea, your provider may have you do a sleep study. Breathing devices such as continuous positive air pressure (CPAP) machines and lifestyle changes are common sleep apnea treatments. If these treatments do not work, surgery may be recommended to correct the problem that is causing your sleep apnea. If your sleep apnea is not diagnosed or treated, you may not get enough good-quality sleep. This can lead to trouble concentrating, making decisions, remembering things, or controlling your behavior. Sleep apnea is also linked to serious health problems.

## SYMPTOMS OF SLEEP APNEA

Your partner may alert you to some of the symptoms of sleep apnea, such as:

- breathing that starts and stops during sleep
- frequent loud snoring
- gasping for air during sleep

You may also notice the following symptoms yourself:

- daytime sleepiness and tiredness, which can lead to problems learning, focusing, and reacting
- dry mouth or headaches
- sexual dysfunction or decreased libido
- waking up often during the night to urinate

Children who have sleep apnea may be overactive and may experience bedwetting, worsening asthma, and trouble paying attention in school.

Talk to your health-care provider about your symptoms. You may need a sleep study to help diagnose the condition.

## CAUSES AND RISK FACTORS OF SLEEP APNEA
### What Causes Sleep Apnea?

Obstructive sleep apnea is caused by conditions that block airflow through your upper airways during sleep. For example, your tongue may fall backward and block your airway. Central sleep apnea is caused by problems with the way your brain controls your breathing while you sleep. Your age, family history, lifestyle habits, other medical conditions, and some features of your body can raise your risk of sleep apnea. Healthy lifestyle changes can help lower your risk.

### What Raises the Risk of Obstructive Sleep Apnea?

Many conditions can cause OSA. Some factors, such as unhealthy lifestyle habits, can be changed. Other factors, such as age, family history, race and ethnicity, and sex, cannot be changed.

- **Age**. Sleep apnea can occur at any age, but your risk increases as you get older. As you age, fatty tissue can build up in your neck and tongue and raise your risk of OSA.

- **Endocrine disorders or changes in hormone levels**. Your hormone levels can affect the size and shape of your face, tongue, and airway. People who have low levels of thyroid hormones or high levels of insulin or growth hormone have a higher risk of OSA.
- **Family history and genetics**. Sleep apnea can be inherited. Your genes help determine the size and shape of your skull, face, and upper airway. Also, your genes can raise your risk of other health conditions, such as cleft lip, cleft palate, and Down syndrome, that can lead to OSA.
- **Heart or kidney failure**. These conditions can cause fluid to build up in your neck, which can block your upper airway.
- **Large tonsils and a thick neck**. These features may cause sleep apnea because they narrow your upper airway. Also, having a large tongue and your tongue's position in your mouth can make it easier for your tongue to block your airway while you sleep.
- **Lifestyle habits**. Drinking alcohol and smoking can raise your risk of sleep apnea. Alcohol can make the muscles of your mouth and throat relax, which may close your upper airway. Smoking can cause inflammation in your upper airway, which affects breathing.
- **Obesity**. This condition is a common cause of sleep apnea. People with this condition can have increased fat deposits in their necks that can block the upper airway. Maintaining a healthy weight can help prevent or treat sleep apnea caused by obesity.
- **Sex**. Sleep apnea is more common in men than in women. Men are more likely to have serious sleep apnea and to get sleep apnea at a younger age than women.

## What Raises the Risk of Central Sleep Apnea?

- **Age**. As you get older, normal changes in how your brain controls breathing during sleep may raise your risk of central sleep apnea.
- **Family history and genetics**. Your genes can affect how your brain controls your breathing during sleep. Genetic conditions such as congenital central hypoventilation syndrome (CCHS) can raise your risk.
- **Lifestyle habits**. Drinking alcohol and smoking can affect how your brain controls sleep or the muscles involved in breathing.
- **Opioid use**. Opioid use disorder or long-term use of prescribed opioid-based pain medicines can cause problems with how your brain controls sleep.
- **Health conditions**. Some conditions that affect how your brain controls your airway and chest muscles can raise your risk. These include heart failure, stroke, amyotrophic lateral sclerosis (ALS), and myasthenia gravis. Also, your hormone levels can affect how your brain controls your breathing.
- **Premature birth**. Babies born before 37 weeks of pregnancy have a higher risk of breathing problems during sleep. In most cases, the risk gets lower as the baby gets older.

## Can You Prevent Obstructive Sleep Apnea?

You may be able to prevent OSA by making healthy lifestyle changes, such as eating a heart-healthy diet, aiming for a healthy weight, quitting smoking, and limiting alcohol intake. Your health-care provider may also ask you to sleep on your side and to adopt healthy sleep habits, such as getting the recommended amount of sleep.

## DIAGNOSIS OF SLEEP APNEA

Your health-care provider will ask you about your symptoms, risk factors, and whether you have a family history of sleep apnea. You may need a sleep study to help diagnose sleep apnea.

## Sleep Study

Your health-care provider will ask you to see a sleep specialist or go to a center for a sleep study. Sleep studies can help diagnose which type of sleep apnea you have and how serious it is.

## Sleep Diary

A sleep diary can help you keep track of how long and how well you sleep and how sleepy you feel during the day. These details can help your health-care provider diagnose your condition.

## Ruling Out Other Medical Conditions

Your provider may order other tests to help rule out other medical conditions that can cause sleep apnea.

- Blood tests check the levels of certain hormones to check for endocrine disorders that could contribute to sleep apnea.
  - Thyroid hormone tests can rule out hypothyroidism.
  - Growth hormone tests can rule out acromegaly.
  - Total testosterone and dehydroepiandrosterone sulfate (DHEAS) tests can help rule out polycystic ovary syndrome (PCOS).
- Pelvic ultrasounds examine the ovaries and help detect cysts. This can rule out PCOS.

Your provider will also want to know whether you are using medicines, such as opioids, that could affect your sleep or cause breathing symptoms of sleep apnea. They may want to know whether you have traveled recently to altitudes greater than 6,000 feet because these low-oxygen environments can cause symptoms of sleep apnea for a few weeks after traveling.

## TREATMENT FOR SLEEP APNEA

If a sleep study shows that you have sleep apnea, your health-care provider may talk to you about making lifelong heart-healthy life-style changes. You may also need breathing or oral devices or surgery to help keep your airways open while you sleep.

## Healthy Lifestyle Changes

To help treat your sleep apnea, you may need to adopt lifelong healthy lifestyle changes. These include getting regular physical activity, maintaining healthy sleeping habits and a healthy weight, limiting alcohol, and quitting smoking. Your provider may also ask you to sleep on your side and not on your back. This helps keep your airway open while you sleep.

## Breathing Devices

A breathing device, such as a CPAP machine, is the most common treatment for sleep apnea. A CPAP machine provides constant air pressure in your throat to keep the airway open when you breathe in. Breathing devices work best when you also make healthy lifestyle changes. Side effects of CPAP treatment may include the following:

- congestion
- dry eyes
- dry mouth
- nosebleeds
- runny nose

If you experience stomach discomfort or bloating, you should stop using your CPAP machine and contact your health-care provider. Depending on the type of sleep apnea you have, you may need another type of breathing device, such as an auto-adjusting positive airway pressure (APAP) machine or a bi-level positive airway pressure (BPAP) machine.

## Oral Devices

Oral devices, also called "oral appliances," are custom-fit devices that you typically wear in your mouth while you sleep. There are two types of oral devices that work differently to open the upper airway while you sleep. Some hybrid devices have features of both types.

- Mandibular repositioning mouthpieces are devices that cover the upper and lower teeth and hold the jaw in a position that prevents it from blocking the upper airway.

- Tongue-retaining devices are mouthpieces that hold the tongue in a forward position to prevent it from blocking the upper airway.

A new type of oral device was recently approved by the U.S. Food and Drug Administration (FDA) for use while awake. The device delivers electrical muscle stimulation through a removable mouthpiece that sits around the tongue. You wear the mouthpiece once a day for 20 minutes at a time for six weeks. The device stimulates the tongue muscle while awake to help prevent the tongue from collapsing backward and blocking the airway during sleep.

If you have sleep apnea, your provider may prescribe an oral device if you do not want to use CPAP or cannot tolerate CPAP. They will recommend that you visit a dentist who will custom-make an appliance for you, make sure that it is comfortable, and teach you how to use it to get the best results.

## Therapy for Your Mouth and Facial Muscles

Exercises for your mouth and facial muscles, also called "orofacial therapy," may help treat sleep apnea in children and adults. This therapy helps improve the position of your tongue and strengthens the muscles that control your lips, tongue, upper airway, and face.

## Surgical Procedures

You may need surgery if other treatments do not work for you. Possible surgical procedures include the following:

- adenotonsillectomy to remove your tonsils and adenoids
- surgery to place an implant that monitors your breathing patterns and helps control certain muscles that open your airways during sleep
- surgery to remove some soft tissue from your mouth and throat, which helps make your upper airway bigger
- maxillary or jaw advancement surgery to move your upper jaw (maxilla) and lower jaw (mandible) forward, which helps make your upper airway bigger

## LIVING WITH SLEEP APNEA

If you have been diagnosed with sleep apnea, you will need to schedule regular check-ups to make sure that your treatment is working and whether you have any complications. You may need to repeat your sleep study to monitor your symptoms while using your treatment, especially if you gain or lose a lot of weight. You may also need treatment for other health conditions that cause your sleep apnea or can make it worse.

### How Does Sleep Apnea Affect Your Health?

Undiagnosed or untreated sleep apnea prevents you from getting enough rest, which can cause problems concentrating, remembering things, making decisions, or controlling your behavior, as well as dementia in older adults. In children, sleep apnea can lead to problems with learning and memory, known as "learning disabilities." The daytime sleepiness and fatigue that results from sleep apnea can also impact your child's behavior and desire to be physically active.

Sleep apnea affects many parts of your body. It can cause low oxygen levels in your body during sleep and can prevent you from getting enough good-quality sleep. Also, it takes a lot of effort for you to restart breathing many times during sleep, and this can damage your organs and blood vessels. These factors may raise your risk of the following conditions:

- asthma
- cancers, such as pancreatic, renal, and skin cancers
- chronic kidney disease
- eye problems, such as glaucoma, dry eye, or an eye condition called "keratoconus"
- heart and blood vessel diseases, such as atrial fibrillation, atherosclerosis, difficult-to-control high blood pressure, heart attacks, heart failure, pulmonary hypertension, and stroke
- metabolic syndrome
- pregnancy complications
- type 2 diabetes

## Using and Caring for Your Breathing Device

It is important that you properly use and care for your breathing device.

- Be patient as you learn to use your breathing device. It may take time to adjust to breathing with the help of a CPAP machine.
- Use your breathing device for all sleep, including naps. If you are traveling, be sure to bring your breathing device with you.
- Talk to your health-care provider if the mask of your breathing device is not comfortable, if your mask is not staying on or fitting well, or if it leaks air. Also, tell your provider if you are having difficulty falling or staying asleep if you wake up with a dry mouth, or if you have a stuffy or runny nose. Your provider may ask you to try different masks or nasal pillows or to adjust the machine's pressure timing and settings.
- Clean your mask and wash your face before you put on your mask. This can help make a better seal between the mask and your skin. You may need to try a different breathing device that has a humidifier chamber or provides bi-level or auto-adjusting pressure settings.
- Know how to set up and properly clean all parts of your machine. Be sure to refill prescriptions on time for all of the device's parts that need to be replaced regularly, including the tubes, masks, and air filters.

Your health-care provider, and possibly your insurance provider, may ask to check the data card from your breathing device. This card shows how often you use your device and whether the device is working properly.

## Using and Caring for Your Oral Device

If you are using an oral device, you may need to see your dentist after six months and then every year. Your dentist will check whether your device is working correctly and whether it needs to be adjusted or replaced.

Ask your dentist how to properly care for your oral device. If it does not fit right or your symptoms do not improve, let your dentist know. It is common to feel some discomfort after a device is adjusted until your mouth and facial muscles get used to the new fit.

## Information to Help You Stay Safe

Sleep apnea can raise your risks of complications if you are having surgery, and it can affect how well you drive:

- If you need medicine to make you sleep during surgery or pain medicine after surgery, tell your health-care provider that you have sleep apnea. Your provider may have to take extra steps to make sure that your airway stays open during the surgery and that your pain medicine does not make it harder for your airway to stay open.
- Untreated sleep apnea can make you sleepy during the day and can make it difficult for you to pay attention and make decisions while you drive. This can cause road accidents. Pay attention to your symptoms and do not drive if you feel very tired or sleepy.[1]

## SLEEP APNEA AND WOMEN

Women may be more at risk for sleep apnea during pregnancy or during and after menopause because of hormone changes. Hormone problems in women who have PCOS may also raise the risk of sleep apnea.

## Sleep Apnea Symptoms in Women

Sleep apnea symptoms may be different for women compared with men. Women more often have the following symptoms:

- anxiety
- daytime sleepiness

---

[1] "What Is Sleep Apnea?" National Heart, Lung, and Blood Institute (NHLBI), March 24, 2022. Available online. URL: www.nhlbi.nih.gov/health/sleep-apnea. Accessed March 20, 2023.

- depression
- headaches, especially in the morning
- insomnia
- tiredness
- waking up often during sleep

Because you may not have common sleep apnea symptoms such as snoring, you may not think that you have this condition. It is important that you talk to your health-care provider if you have any of these symptoms or if you have any risk factors for sleep apnea.

## Sleep Apnea and Pregnancy

During pregnancy, changes to a woman's upper airway or to the way the brain controls breathing raise a woman's risk of sleep apnea or make it worse. Sleep apnea is often more serious in the third trimester of pregnancy and may improve after your baby is born. Pregnant women who are older or who have obesity have a higher risk of sleep apnea. In pregnant women, sleep apnea can cause many complications, including the following:

- cesarean sections
- gestational diabetes
- high blood pressure
- low birth weight
- preterm birth

Breathing devices such as CPAP machines are safe for treating sleep apnea during pregnancy. Because pregnancy causes changes to your body, you may need to see a sleep specialist to adjust the settings of your CPAP machine during and after your pregnancy.[2]

---

[2] "Sleep Apnea and Women," National Heart, Lung, and Blood Institute (NHLBI), March 24, 2022. Available online. URL: www.nhlbi.nih.gov/health/sleep-apnea/women. Accessed March 21, 2023.

Section 19.2 | **Obstructive Sleep Apnea**

## WHAT IS OBSTRUCTIVE SLEEP APNEA?

Obstructive sleep apnea (OSA) is a condition in which individuals experience pauses in breathing (apnea) during sleep, which are associated with partial or complete closure of the throat (upper airway; refer to Figure 19.1). Complete closure can lead to apnea, while partial closure allows breathing but decreases the intake of oxygen (hypopnea).

Individuals with OSA may experience interrupted sleep with frequent awakenings and loud snoring. Repeated pauses in breathing lead to episodes of lower-than-normal oxygen levels (hypoxemia) and a buildup of carbon dioxide (hypercapnia) in the bloodstream. Interrupted and poor-quality sleep can lead to daytime sleepiness and fatigue, impaired attention and memory, headaches, depression, and sexual dysfunction. Daytime sleepiness leads to a higher risk of motor vehicle accidents in individuals with OSA. OSA is also associated with an increased risk of developing insulin resistance, which is an inability to regulate blood sugar levels effectively; high blood pressure (hypertension); heart disease; and stroke.

## FREQUENCY OF OBSTRUCTIVE SLEEP APNEA

Obstructive sleep apnea is a common condition. It is estimated to affect 2–4 percent of children and at least 10 percent of adults worldwide. Males are twice as likely as females to have OSA.

## CAUSES OF OBSTRUCTIVE SLEEP APNEA

The causes of OSA are often complex. This condition results from a combination of genetic, health, and lifestyle factors, many of which have not been identified. Studies suggest that variations in multiple genes, each with a small effect, combine to increase the risk of developing the condition. However, it is unclear what contribution each of these genetic changes makes to disease risk. Most of the variations have been identified in single studies, and subsequent research has not verified them.

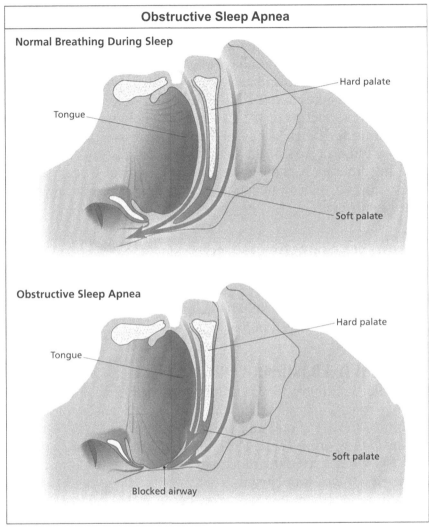

© Infobase

**Figure 19.1.** Obstructive Sleep Apnea

*Infobase*

Genes thought to be associated with the development of OSA are involved in many body processes. These include communication between nerve cells, breathing regulation, control of inflammatory responses by the immune system, development of tissues in the head and face (craniofacial development), the sleep–wake cycle, and appetite control.

Obesity is a major risk factor for OSA, as 60–70 percent of individuals with this condition have obesity. It is thought that excess fatty tissue in the head and neck constricts airways and abdominal fat may prevent the chest and lungs from fully expanding and relaxing. Other risk factors for OSA include alcohol use, frequent nasal congestion, and blockages of the airways, such as enlarged tonsils.

OSA often occurs on its own, without signs and symptoms affecting other parts of the body. However, it can also occur as part of a syndrome, such as mucopolysaccharidosis type I or polycystic ovary syndrome.

## INHERITANCE OF OBSTRUCTIVE SLEEP APNEA

The inheritance pattern of OSA is unclear. Overall, the risk of developing this condition is about 50 percent greater for first-degree relatives (such as siblings or children) of affected individuals than that for the general public.[3]

## TREATMENT FOR OBSTRUCTIVE SLEEP APNEA

There are treatments for OSA that work well. Eric Mann, M.D., Ph.D., deputy director at the Center for Devices and Radiological Health of the U.S. Food and Drug Administration (FDA), says, "Many FDA-approved and FDA-cleared treatments can help people with OSA wake up in the mornings feeling rested and refreshed, improving their overall health."

Getting treatment for OSA is key because OSA not only affects your sleep but also increases your risk of serious health problems and even death. OSA may increase your risk of heart attack, stroke, type 2 diabetes, glaucoma, and some types of cancer, along with other serious health conditions. Lifestyle behavior changes such as losing weight, drinking less alcohol, stopping smoking, and using devices that help you sleep in a certain position may help improve

---

[3] MedlinePlus, "Obstructive Sleep Apnea," National Institutes of Health (NIH), March 1, 2018. Available online. URL: https://medlineplus.gov/genetics/condition/obstructive-sleep-apnea. Accessed March 21, 2023.

OSA but may not make it go away entirely. Taking certain medicines, such as sedatives or sleep aids, that slow or lessen breathing can also contribute to OSA. Talk to your doctor before stopping or starting any medicine.

OSA treatments can work well to manage OSA, but not every treatment is right for everyone. Some treatments work best for people with mild OSA, while others are best for people with more severe OSA. Sometimes, you must try a specific treatment before you can move on to a different treatment. Some treatments involve surgery to correct a narrow airway or a specific part of the airway that may collapse during sleep. Any type of surgery has risks, so talk with your doctor about all of your options before you decide.

The FDA evaluates the safety and effectiveness of certain medical devices before they can be marketed to the public, including the device most often used for OSA. Depending on your health status and the type of OSA you may have, your doctor may prescribe one of these OSA treatments.

## Continuous Positive Airway Pressure Machine

The most common OSA treatment is using a continuous positive airway pressure (CPAP) machine every night during sleep. CPAP machines use mild air pressure to keep your airways open during sleep. The air is delivered through a mask that fits over your nose and mouth or only your nose. CPAP machines are considered the standard treatment for OSA, but you may need to work with a doctor or technician for a few weeks to find the best combination of settings and CPAP accessories for you.

## Nasal Expiratory Positive Airway Pressure

This alternative treatment uses disposable or reusable valves inserted into or over the nostrils during sleep. The valves limit your exhalations which helps maintain pressure to keep your airway open during sleep. Unlike a CPAP machine, expiratory positive airway pressure (EPAP) valves do not need power from an electrical outlet or batteries.

## Oral Appliance

A prescription-only oral appliance is worn during sleep and fits like a sports mouth guard or an orthodontic retainer but is for both the top and bottom teeth. It keeps your jaw positioned forward so that your airway stays open while you sleep. A dentist takes impressions of your teeth, so a custom device can be made and fitted for you.

## Tongue-Retaining Device

This type of oral appliance is worn in the mouth during sleep and includes a part that prevents your tongue from falling back into the airway during sleep.

## Neuromuscular Tongue Muscle Stimulator

A neuromuscular tongue muscle stimulator is a prescription-only device you put in your mouth for 20 minutes a day while you are awake. The device delivers mild electrical currents to your tongue muscle, strengthening it so that it does not relax and block your airway as much during sleep.

## Implantable Nerve Stimulator

The FDA approved a medical device for OSA that can be surgically implanted during an outpatient procedure. A surgeon implants the device, which is similar to a pacemaker, on the upper chest below the collarbone. During surgery, the doctor places wires from the implant near the nerves that control your tongue and nearby muscles. The implant sends mild electrical impulses through the wires to nerves in your tongue muscles during sleep. The nerve stimulation prevents your tongue and the muscles around it from collapsing and blocking your airway during sleep. Most implants have a remote control you use to turn the device on before going to sleep and off after waking up.

## Position Therapy Device

A special pillow or other bed devices may help with mild-to-moderate positional OSA. Positional OSA is caused by lying on your back (face up) during sleep. A special pillow or similar bed device can help you stay sleeping on your side where gravity does not cause your tongue or throat to block your airway. Before purchasing a device, some people try homemade positional methods such as a special pillow or bumpers for the bed.

## Position Monitoring Device/Stimulation

A positional monitoring device can treat mild-to-moderate OSA caused by sleeping on your back. It is worn on the body (usually around the neck or chest) and monitors your sleeping position with a position accelerometer. When you are lying on your back, or face up, during sleep, the device vibrates with increasing intensity until you turn over to sleep on your side.[4]

## Section 19.3 | Central Sleep Apnea

Central sleep apnea (CSA) is a form of sleep disorder characterized by repeated breathing interruptions during sleep due to a communication issue between the brain and the muscles that regulate breathing.

To be diagnosed with CSA, a person must have more than five breathing interruptions per hour of sleep with associated symptoms of disrupted sleep, such as excessive daytime sleepiness.

Unlike obstructive sleep apnea (OSA), which is caused by blocked airways, CSA is the result of insufficient muscle activity that regulates breathing. CSA is less common than OSA and is often tied to an underlying health condition. Identifying whether an individual has CSA, OSA, or both can sometimes be challenging for health-care providers.

If left untreated, CSA can lead to daytime drowsiness and difficulty with thinking, increasing the risk of errors and accidents.

---

[4] "Always Tired? You May Have Sleep Apnea," U.S. Food and Drug Administration (FDA), July 12, 2021. Available online. URL: www.fda.gov/consumers/consumer-updates/always-tired-you-may-have-sleep-apnea. Accessed May 3, 2023.

## CAUSES OF CENTRAL SLEEP APNEA

There are several causes of CSA, including underlying medical conditions such as heart attack, stroke, brain inflammation, and congestive heart failure. Some medications, such as opioid pain-killers, can also cause CSA.

Cheyne-Stokes respiration is another condition that can cause CSA, often affecting people with severe heart failure. This breathing disorder involves cycles of alternating deep, heavy breathing with shallow breathing or even not breathing, especially during sleep.

If the cause of CSA cannot be determined, it is called "idiopathic central sleep apnea."

## SYMPTOMS OF CENTRAL SLEEP APNEA

Many people with CSA may not know they have it because they are asleep when it occurs. However, the most common symptoms of this condition include:

- feeling breathless upon awakening
- shallow breathing instead of complete cessation
- suffering from lack of sleep (insomnia)
- waking up frequently due to a lack of oxygen

If CSA is associated with a nervous system disorder, individuals may also experience daytime sleepiness, chronic fatigue, restless sleep, swallowing difficulties, changes in voice, shortness of breath, and weakness or numbness throughout the body.

## DIAGNOSIS OF CENTRAL SLEEP APNEA

When CSA is suspected, a doctor will inquire about symptoms, obtain the patient's medical history, and perform a physical examination. In addition, other tests such as an echocardiogram, lung function testing, blood tests, and magnetic resonance imaging (MRI) of the brain, spine, or neck may also be performed to diagnose any underlying medical condition. A head or spinal MRI scan can also diagnose CSA by revealing any structural abnormalities in the brain stem or spine.

A doctor may order an overnight sleep study test, the polysomnography, to better diagnose CSA. This test is conducted in a specialized sleep laboratory in a hospital or sleep center. The results of the polysomnography test can aid in identifying the root cause of the patient's apnea, the results of which the doctor, a neurologist, and sometimes a cardiologist will review to devise the appropriate treatment plan.

## TREATMENT FOR CENTRAL SLEEP APNEA

The treatment for CSA primarily depends on the severity of the condition and identifying the root cause. It is essential for individuals to discuss treatment options with their doctor to determine the most effective course of treatment. Treatment approaches for CSA include the following:

- **Treating the underlying medical condition**. The primary approach to treating CSA is to manage the underlying medical condition that causes it. For instance, treating heart failure may alleviate sleep apnea symptoms.
- **Medications**. Medications such as acetazolamide may help stimulate breathing, while others can control heart or nervous system conditions that cause sleep apnea.
- **Oxygen supplementation**. This method is helpful for people who experience low oxygen levels during sleep. A machine can regulate the air pressure to ensure the lungs receive enough oxygen.
- **Continuous positive air pressure (CPAP)**. A CPAP machine supplies constant air pressure into the airways through a mask covering the nose and mouth. Although it is commonly used to treat OSA, it proves beneficial for CSA.
- **Bi-level positive air pressure (BPAP)**. BPAP is similar to CPAP, but the machine adjusts the air pressure based on the inhalation and exhalation levels.
- **Adaptive servo-ventilation (ASV)**. ASV uses a computerized system to regulate breathing by

monitoring the breathing pattern and adjusting the air pressure accordingly.

- **Phrenic nerve stimulation**. This treatment involves implanting a device in the chest that stimulates the diaphragm through the phrenic nerve, which controls the diaphragm. This is more feasible for individuals who do not show positive results from other therapies.
- **Changing or adjusting medication dosage**. If routine medication use, taken for other underlying health conditions, is causing CSA, the health-care provider may recommend changing the medication or adjusting the dosage.

An individual's recovery from CSA depends on addressing the issue that is responsible for the condition. If the cause of CSA is unclear (idiopathic), people generally respond positively to therapy, and their prognosis is typically favorable. However, the effectiveness of treatment may differ based on the specific cause of the condition. If an individual or their family members suspect the possibility of CSA, they should seek medical attention as early as possible. Neglecting to do so could potentially result in the condition worsening over time.

## References

"Central Sleep Apnea," MedlinePlus, July 12, 2021. Available online. URL: https://medlineplus.gov/ency/article/003997.htm. Accessed April 13, 2023.

Eckert, Danny J.; Jordan, Amy S.; Merchia, Pankaj; and Malhotra, Atul. "Central Sleep Apnea," National Center for Biotechnology Information (NCBI), February 2007. Available online. URL: www.ncbi.nlm.nih.gov/pmc/articles/PMC2287191. Accessed April 13, 2023.

Roth, Erica. "Central Sleep Apnea," Healthline Media, April 2, 2019. Available online. URL: www.healthline.com/health/sleep/central-sleep-apnea. Accessed April 13, 2023.

Singh, Jaspal. "Basics of Central Sleep Apnea," American College of Cardiology Foundation (ACC), January 8,

2013. Available online. URL: www.acc.org/latest-in-cardiology/articles/2014/07/22/08/25/basics-of-central-sleep-apnea. Accessed April 13, 2023.

Suni, Eric. "Central Sleep Apnea," Sleep Foundation, March 29, 2023. Available online. URL: www.sleepfoundation.org/sleep-apnea/central-sleep-apnea. Accessed April 13, 2023.

## Section 19.4 | Snoring

Snoring is the sound you make when your breathing is blocked while you are asleep. The sound is caused by tissues at the top of your airway that strike each other and vibrate. Snoring is common, especially among older people and people who are overweight.

When severe, snoring can cause frequent awakenings at night and daytime sleepiness. It can disrupt your bed partner's sleep. Snoring can also be a sign of a serious sleep disorder called "sleep apnea." You should see your health-care provider if you are often tired during the day, do not feel that you sleep well, or wake up gasping.

To reduce snoring, do the following:

- Lose weight if you are overweight, as it may help, but thin people can snore, too.
- Cut down or avoid alcohol and other sedatives at bedtime.
- Do not sleep flat on your back.[5]

## IS SNORING A PROBLEM?

Long the material for jokes, snoring is generally accepted as common and annoying in adults but as nothing to worry about. However, snoring is no laughing matter. Frequent, loud snoring is

---

[5] MedlinePlus, "Snoring," National Institutes of Health (NIH), August 4, 2016. Available online. URL: https://medlineplus.gov/snoring.html. Accessed March 21, 2023.

often a sign of sleep apnea and may increase your risk of developing cardiovascular disease (CVD) and diabetes. Snoring may also lead to daytime sleepiness and impaired performance.

Snoring is caused by a narrowing or partial blockage of the airways at the back of your mouth, throat, or nose. This obstruction results in increased air turbulence when breathing in, causing the soft tissues in your upper airways to vibrate. The end result is a noisy snore that can disrupt the sleep of your bed partner. This narrowing of the airways is typically caused by the soft palate, tongue, and throat relaxing while you sleep, but allergies or sinus problems can also contribute to a narrowing of the airways, as can being overweight and having extra soft tissue around your upper airways.

The larger the tissues in your soft palate (the roof of your mouth in the back of your throat), the more likely you are to snore while sleeping. Alcohol or sedatives taken shortly before sleep also promote snoring. These drugs cause greater relaxation of the tissues in your throat and mouth. Surveys reveal that about one-half of all adults snore and 50 percent of these adults do so loudly and frequently. African Americans, Asians, and Hispanics are more likely to snore loudly and frequently than Caucasians, and snoring problems increase with age.

Not everyone who snores has sleep apnea, but people who have sleep apnea typically do snore loudly and frequently. Sleep apnea is a serious sleep disorder, and its hallmark is loud, frequent snoring with pauses in breathing or shallow breaths while sleeping. Even if you do not experience these breathing pauses, snoring can still be a problem for you as well as for your bed partner. Snoring adds extra effort to your breathing, which can reduce the quality of your sleep and lead to many of the same health consequences as sleep apnea.

One study found that older adults who did not have sleep apnea, but who snored six to seven nights a week, were more than twice as likely to report being extremely sleepy during the day than those who never snored. The more people snored, the more daytime fatigue they reported. Sleepiness may help explain why snorers are more likely to be in car crashes than people who do not snore. Loud snoring can also disrupt the sleep of bed partners and strain marital relations, especially if snoring causes the spouses to sleep in separate bedrooms.

In addition, snoring increases the risk of developing diabetes and heart disease. One study found that women who snored regularly were twice as likely as those who did not snore to develop diabetes, even if they were not overweight (another risk factor for diabetes). Other studies suggest that regular snoring may raise the lifetime risk of developing high blood pressure, heart failure, and stroke.

About one-third of all pregnant women begin snoring for the first time during their second trimester. If you are snoring while pregnant, let your doctor know. Snoring during pregnancy can be associated with high blood pressure and can have a negative effect on your baby's growth and development. Your doctor will keep a close eye on your blood pressure throughout your pregnancy and can let you know if any additional evaluations for snoring might be useful. In most cases, snoring and any related high blood pressure will go away shortly after delivery. Snoring can also be a problem in children. As many as 10–15 percent of young children, who typically have enlarged adenoids and tonsils (both tissues in the throat), snore on a regular basis. Several studies show that children who snore (with or without sleep apnea) are more likely than those who do not snore to score lower on tests that measure intelligence, memory, and attention span. These children also have more problematic behavior, including hyperactivity. The end result is that children who snore do not perform as well in school as those who do not snore. Strikingly, snoring was linked to a greater drop in intelligence quotient (IQ) than that seen in children who had elevated levels of lead in their blood. Although the behavior of children improves after they stop snoring, studies suggest they may continue to get poorer grades in school, perhaps because of the lasting effects on the brain linked to snoring. You should have your child evaluated by your doctor if the child snores loudly and frequently—three to four times a week—especially if you note brief pauses in breathing while asleep and if there are signs of hyperactivity or daytime sleepiness, inadequate school achievement, or slower than expected development.

Surgery to remove the adenoids and tonsils of children can often cure their snoring and any associated sleep apnea. Such surgery has been linked to a reduction in hyperactivity and improved ability to pay attention, even in children who showed no signs of sleep apnea before surgery.

Snoring in older children and adults may be relieved by less invasive measures, however. These measures include losing weight, refraining from the use of tobacco, sleeping on the side rather than on the back, or elevating the head while sleeping. Treating chronic congestion and refraining from alcohol or sedatives before sleeping may also decrease snoring. In some adults, snoring can be relieved by dental appliances that reposition the soft tissues in the mouth. Although numerous over-the-counter (OTC) nasal strips and sprays claim to relieve snoring, no scientific evidence supports those claims.[6]

## Section 19.5 | Congenital Central Hypoventilation Syndrome

## WHAT IS CONGENITAL CENTRAL HYPOVENTILATION SYNDROME?

Congenital central hypoventilation syndrome (CCHS) is a disorder that affects normal breathing. People with this disorder take shallow breaths (hypoventilate), especially during sleep, resulting in a shortage of oxygen and a buildup of carbon dioxide in the blood. Ordinarily, the part of the nervous system that controls involuntary body processes (autonomic nervous system) would react to such an imbalance by stimulating the individual to breathe more deeply or wake up. This nervous system reaction is impaired in people with CCHS. They must be supported by a machine to help them breathe (mechanical ventilation) or a device that stimulates a normal breathing pattern (diaphragm pacemaker). Some affected individuals need this support 24 hours a day, while others need it only at night.

---

[6] "Your Guide to Healthy Sleep," National Heart, Lung, and Blood Institute (NHLBI), August 2011. Available online. URL: www.nhlbi.nih.gov/files/docs/public/sleep/healthy_sleep.pdf. Accessed March 21, 2023.

## SYMPTOMS OF CONGENITAL CENTRAL HYPOVENTILATION SYNDROME

Symptoms of CCHS usually become apparent shortly after birth when affected infants hypoventilate upon falling asleep. In these infants, a lack of oxygen in the blood often causes a bluish appearance of the skin or lips (cyanosis). In some milder cases, CCHS may not become apparent until later in life. In addition to the breathing problem, people with CCHS may have difficulty regulating their heart rate and blood pressure, for example, in response to exercise or changes in body position. They also have decreased perception of pain, low body temperature, and occasional episodes of heavy sweating.

People with CCHS may have additional problems affecting the nervous system. About 20 percent of people with CCHS have abnormalities in the nerves that control the digestive tract (Hirschsprung disease), resulting in severe constipation, intestinal blockage, and enlargement of the colon. (Some researchers refer to the combination of CCHS and Hirschsprung disease as Haddad syndrome.) Some affected individuals develop learning difficulties or other neurological problems. People with CCHS are also at increased risk of developing certain tumors of the nervous system called "neuroblastomas," "ganglioneuromas," and "ganglioneuroblastomas."

Additionally, individuals with CCHS usually have eye abnormalities, including a decreased response of the pupils to light. People with CCHS, especially children, may have a characteristic appearance with a short, wide, somewhat flattened face often described as "box-shaped."

In CCHS, life expectancy and the extent of any intellectual disabilities depend on the severity of the disorder, the timing of the diagnosis, and the success of treatment.

## FREQUENCY OF CONGENITAL CENTRAL HYPOVENTILATION SYNDROME

Congenital central hypoventilation syndrome is a relatively rare disorder. More than 1,000 individuals with this condition have been identified. Researchers believe that some cases of sudden infant death syndrome (SIDS) or sudden unexplained death in children may be caused by undiagnosed CCHS.

## CAUSES OF CONGENITAL CENTRAL HYPOVENTILATION SYNDROME

Mutations in a gene called "*PHOX2B*" cause CCHS. The *PHOX2B* gene provides instructions for making a protein that is important during development before birth. The PHOX2B protein helps support the formation of nerve cells (neurons) and regulates the process by which the neurons mature to carry out specific functions (differentiation). The protein is active in the neural crest, which is a group of cells in the early embryo that give rise to many tissues and organs. Neural crest cells migrate to form parts of the autonomic nervous system, many tissues in the face and skull, and other tissue and cell types.

*PHOX2B* gene mutations that cause CCHS are believed to interfere with the PHOX2B protein's role in supporting neuron formation and differentiation, especially in the autonomic nervous system. As a result, bodily functions that are controlled by this system, including regulation of breathing, heart rate, blood pressure, and body temperature, are inconsistent in CCHS.

## INHERITANCE OF CONGENITAL CENTRAL HYPOVENTILATION SYNDROME

This condition is inherited in an autosomal dominant pattern, which means one copy of the altered gene in each cell is sufficient to cause the disorder.

More than 90 percent of cases of CCHS result from new mutations in the *PHOX2B* gene. These cases occur in people with no history of the disorder in their family. Occasionally, an affected person inherits the mutation from one affected parent. The number of such cases has been increasing as better treatment has allowed more affected individuals to live into adulthood and start families.

About 5–10 percent of affected individuals inherit the altered gene from an unaffected parent who has a *PHOX2B* gene mutation only in their sperm or egg cells. This phenomenon is called "germline mosaicism." A parent with mosaicism for a *PHOX2B* gene mutation may not show any signs or symptoms of CCHS.[7]

[7] MedlinePlus, "Congenital Central Hypoventilation Syndrome," National Institutes of Health (NIH), September 1, 2019. Available online. URL: https://medlineplus.gov/genetics/condition/congenital-central-hy-poventilation-syn-drome. Accessed March 21, 2023.

# Chapter 20 | **Circadian Rhythm Disorders**

## WHAT ARE CIRCADIAN RHYTHM DISORDERS?

Circadian rhythm disorders, also known as "sleep–wake cycle disorders," are problems that occur when your body's internal clock, which tells you when it is time to sleep or wake, is out of sync with your environment. Your internal clock, called a "circadian clock," cycles about every 24 hours. These repeating 24-hour cycles are called the "circadian rhythm."

Your body tries to align your sleep–wake cycle to cues from the environment, such as when it gets light or dark outside when you eat, and when you are physically active. When your sleep–wake cycle is out of sync with your environment, you may have difficulty sleeping, and the quality of your sleep may be poor. Disruptions of your sleep–wake cycle that interfere with daily activities may mean that you have a circadian rhythm disorder.

Disruptions in your sleep patterns can be temporary and caused by your sleep habits, job, or travel. Or a circadian rhythm disorder can be long-term and caused by aging, your genes, or a medical condition. You may have symptoms such as extreme daytime sleepiness, decreased alertness, and problems with memory and decision-making.

To diagnose a circadian rhythm disorder, your doctor may ask about your sleep habits and may suggest a sleep study and some other diagnostic tests. Your treatment plan will depend on the type and cause of your circadian rhythm disorder. You can take steps to prevent circadian rhythm disorders by making healthy lifestyle changes to improve your sleep habits. If left untreated, circadian rhythm disorders may increase the risk of certain health problems or lead to workplace and road accidents.

## TYPES OF CIRCADIAN RHYTHM DISORDERS

The types of circadian rhythm disorders are advanced sleep–wake phase disorder (ASWPD) or delayed sleep–wake phase disorder (DSWPD), irregular or non-24-hour sleep–wake rhythm disorder, and shift work or jet lag disorder. The type you may have is based on your pattern of sleep and wakefulness.

### Advanced Sleep–Wake Phase Disorder

If you have ASWPD, you may find it very difficult to stay awake in the early evening and, as a result, wake up too early in the morning. This can interfere with work, school, or social responsibilities.

### Delayed Sleep–Wake Phase Disorder

This is one of the most common circadian rhythm disorders. If you have DSWPD, you may fall asleep later than you would like and then find it difficult to wake up on time in the morning. DSWPD often interferes with work, school, or social responsibilities. You may get too little sleep, which can lead to daytime tiredness or anxiety.

### Irregular Sleep–Wake Rhythm Disorder

If you have irregular sleep–wake rhythm disorder (ISWRD), you may have several short periods of sleep and wakefulness. You may be unable to sleep during the night and take multiple naps during the day due to excessive sleepiness. You may not feel rested after sleep.

### Jet Lag Disorder

This is often a temporary disorder that may affect you if you travel across at least two time zones in a short period. Your sleep–wake rhythm falls out of sync with the local time at your destination, so you may feel sleepy or alert at the wrong time of day or night.

The jet lag disorder is often more severe when you travel east than when you travel west.

Some people experience social jet lag, which can occur when you go to activities on weekends or days off at much later times than you do on weekdays or workdays. This is not considered a disorder.

## Non-24-Hour Sleep–Wake Rhythm Disorder

This type of circadian rhythm disorder occurs when your sleep–wake rhythm is not in sync with the 24-hour day. When this happens, your sleep times may gradually become more delayed. For example, your sleep time may be delayed to the point that you are going to sleep at noon instead of at night. This often occurs when light exposure is very limited, and it is common in people who are completely blind. You may have periods of insomnia and daytime sleepiness, followed by periods with no symptoms, when your circadian rhythms happen to align with your environment.

## Shift Work Disorder

Shift work disorder affects those who work during the night or on a rotating schedule. Because of your work schedule, you may not be able to get uninterrupted quality sleep when your body needs it. Shift work disorder can cause insomnia, extreme tiredness, and sleepiness while working at night.

## SYMPTOMS OF CIRCADIAN RHYTHM DISORDER

Symptoms of circadian rhythm disorders can vary depending on the type of circadian rhythm disorder you have and how severe your condition is. Many of the symptoms of circadian rhythm disorders occur because you are not getting enough good-quality sleep when your body needs it. Undiagnosed and untreated circadian rhythm disorders may increase your risk of certain health conditions or cause workplace or road accidents. Speak with your healthcare provider to learn more about diagnosis and treatment options.

The following are some of the symptoms of rhythm disorder:
- difficulty falling asleep, staying asleep, or both
- excessive daytime sleepiness or sleepiness during shift work

- extreme tiredness and exhaustion
- lethargy
- decreased alertness and difficulty concentrating
- impaired judgment in risky situations, such as while driving, and trouble controlling mood and emotions
- aches and pains, including headaches
- stomach problems in people who have jet lag disorder

## How Do Circadian Rhythm Disorders Affect Judgment?

Circadian rhythm disorders often cause sleep deprivation, a condition that occurs when you do not get the recommended amount of uninterrupted quality sleep (seven to nine hours for adults). Sleep deprivation can change how well your brain judges risky situations and behaviors. When you do not get enough sleep, you may underestimate the risks and overestimate the rewards of certain situations. This may lead you to make riskier choices than you would have made if you were well-rested. Not getting enough sleep when you need it can also increase your risk for accidents, such as those caused by drowsy driving after working a night shift.

## CAUSES AND RISK FACTORS OF CIRCADIAN RHYTHM DISORDER

Circadian rhythm disorders occur when your sleep–wake cycle is out of sync with your environment. Many factors, both internal and external, can cause you to have problems sleeping and raise your risk for a circadian rhythm disorder.

## What Causes Circadian Rhythm Disorders?

Genetic conditions that affect your brain or hormone can cause circadian rhythm disorders. For example, Smith-Magenis syndrome is a genetic condition that may affect how much or how often your body makes the hormone melatonin, which helps you sleep. Sleep patterns may be completely reversed, causing daytime sleepiness and wakeful nights.

Did you know that your sleep–wake cycle and your risk for circadian rhythm disorders may be different from that of someone else? This is controlled by the genes in your deoxyribonucleic acid (DNA). Some people naturally wake early, while others naturally stay up late. Some people can more easily adjust their circadian rhythm to match their environment. If you are one of these people, you may be less likely to develop jet lag disorder and shift work disorder. You may develop circadian rhythm disorders if your patterns do not align with your work, school, or social responsibilities. Talk to your doctor about your symptoms.

## What Raises Your Risk of Circadian Rhythm Disorders?

Many things can lead to a circadian rhythm disorder. Some you cannot change, such as your age, family history, or sex. Some you can manage, such as your lifestyle or occupation.

## Age

The rhythm and timing of your sleep–wake cycle can change with age because of changes in your brain. Teens may naturally have a later bedtime than adults, which raises their risk for DSWPD. Older adults usually go to sleep and wake up early. This raises their risk for ASWPD. Older adults are also at higher risk for shift work disorder and jet lag disorder.

## Environment or Occupation

People who work during the night have a higher risk for shift work disorder. Jet lag disorder is more common in pilots, flight attendants, athletes, and people who often travel for business.

## Family History or Genetics

Your genetic preference for an early or late bedtime can raise your risk for ASWPD or DSWPDr if your rhythm is out of sync with your environment or social responsibilities. Changes in the genes that control your circadian rhythm, called "circadian clock genes," can also raise your risk.

## Lifestyle Habits

Lifestyle habits can raise your risk for circadian rhythm disorders. These include:
- alcohol use
- chronic caffeine use
- frequent air travel
- illegal drug use
- lack of exposure to natural light during the day
- unhealthy sleep habits, such as regularly staying up late and being exposed at nighttime to artificial light, such as from a TV screen, smartphone, or very bright alarm clock

## Other Medical Conditions

Several medical conditions can increase your risk for circadian rhythm disorders, including:
- autism spectrum disorders
- certain genetic conditions, such as Smith-Magenis syndrome, Angelman syndrome, and Huntington disease
- conditions that affect eyesight, such as blindness and macular degeneration, which raise the risk for a non-24-hour sleep–wake rhythm disorder
- conditions that cause damage to the brain, such as traumatic brain injuries, strokes, and brain tumors
- mental health conditions, such as bipolar disorder, major depression, obsessive-compulsive disorder, and schizophrenia, which raise the risk of DSWPD
- neurodegenerative diseases, such as Alzheimer disease (AD), dementia, and Parkinson disease (PD), which are more common in older adults and can increase the risk for irregular sleep–wake phase disorder

## Sex

Men are more likely to have ASWPD than women. Women may be likely to experience circadian rhythm disorders at certain stages of life.
- Hormonal changes that happen during pregnancy, after childbirth, and at menopause can cause problems with sleep.

- Discomfort during pregnancy may also prevent good-quality sleep.
- After childbirth, sleep interruptions and nighttime exposure to light while caring for a newborn can increase your risk for circadian rhythm disorders.

## Can Circadian Rhythm Disorders Be Prevented?

If you are at risk for circadian rhythm disorders, your doctor may recommend certain lifestyle changes to help prevent a circadian rhythm disorder. For example, your doctor may talk to you about avoiding bright light and caffeine close to your bedtime.

Other preventive steps may help depending on your stage of life or work.

### FOR NEW PARENTS

While caring for a newborn at night, keep the lights as dim as possible.

### FOR SHIFT WORKERS

The following steps may help prevent shift work disorder:
- Take a short nap before your night shift to help prevent sleepiness at work.
- Adopt a sleep schedule on your days off that overlaps with your sleep time on workdays.
- Avoid multiple schedule switches between day and night shifts, if possible.

### FOR LONG-DISTANCE TRAVEL

The following steps may help prevent jet lag disorder:
- A few days before traveling, begin adjusting your sleep–wake cycle to match the time at your destination. You may gradually change your sleep schedule and use a bright light to help advance or delay your waking time.
- If you can, arrive at your destination a few days before an important event to help you gradually adjust to the local time. Your body adjusts to 11.5 changes in time zones per day.

- Spend plenty of time outside at your destination. Outdoor light may shorten symptoms of jet lag.

## DIAGNOSIS OF CIRCADIAN RHYTHM DISORDER

To diagnose a circadian rhythm disorder, your doctor may review your medical history; ask about your symptoms, sleep patterns, and environment; do a physical exam; and order diagnostic tests.

### Medical History and Physical Exam

Your doctor will want to learn about your symptoms and risk factors to help diagnose a circadian rhythm disorder. To do this, your doctor may ask the following questions:

- **When, how long, and how well you sleep**. If you do not know for sure, your doctor may ask you to keep a sleep diary to help you keep track.
- **Your symptoms and when they began**. Symptoms that have lasted for three months or more may indicate a circadian rhythm disorder.
- **Your personal and family history of health conditions**. These may be risk factors for a circadian rhythm disorder.
- **Your use of caffeine or drugs and exposure to artificial light**. These lifestyle habits may cause insomnia or tiredness.
- **Whether you are pregnant or undergoing menopause**. Changing hormone levels during menopause or pregnancy can affect the quality of women's sleep.

Your doctor may also examine you. A physical exam can help your doctor rule out other medical conditions that may prevent good-quality sleep, such as chronic pain, heart or lung diseases, or large tonsils or small airways that may be a sign of sleep apnea.

## Diagnostic Tests

Your doctor may recommend one or more of the following tests:
- Actigraphy involves wearing a small motion sensor for 3–14 days to measure your sleep–wake cycles.
- Sleep studies measure how well you sleep and how your body responds to sleep problems.

Your doctor may do other studies to look at your natural patterns of sleep and wakefulness. Your doctor may repeatedly measure your body temperature and the levels of melatonin and cortisol in your blood or saliva. The way these rise and fall over time can help determine the type of circadian rhythm disorder you may have.

## TREATMENT FOR CIRCADIAN RHYTHM DISORDERS

Treatments for circadian rhythm disorders aim to reset your sleep–wake rhythm to align with your environment. Your treatment plan will depend on the type and severity of your circadian rhythm disorder. The most common treatments are healthy lifestyle changes, bright light therapy, and melatonin. Often, your doctor will recommend a combination of these treatments.

## Healthy Lifestyle Changes

To help reset your sleep–wake cycle, your doctor may recommend that you establish a daily routine with set activities that happen during the day and another set of activities that happen at night. This may help manage the symptoms of circadian rhythm disorders.
- Keep a regular meal schedule, especially if you are a shift worker or sleep at irregular times of the day or night.
- Start a regular bedtime routine. Sleep in a cool, quiet place and follow a relaxing bedtime routine that limits stress. These practices, along with regular sleep and

waking times, can help you fall asleep faster and stay asleep longer.

- Avoid daytime naps, especially in the afternoon. However, shift workers may benefit from a short nap before the start of their shift.
- Get regular physical activity. Your doctor may recommend getting regular physical activity during the daytime and avoiding exercising close to bedtime, which may make it hard to fall asleep.
- Limit caffeine, alcohol, nicotine, and some medicines, especially close to bedtime.
- Manage your exposure to light. Light is the strongest signal in the environment to help reset your sleep–wake cycle. You may need more sunlight during the day and less artificial light at night from TV screens and electronic devices. Artificial light can lower your melatonin levels, making it harder to fall asleep. Light-blocking glasses, screen filters, or smartphone apps can help dim the light from your electronic devices. Dim lighting for a period before bed may also help reduce the symptoms of a circadian rhythm disorder. For shift workers, wearing light-blocking glasses when you are outside during the day may help.

## Light Therapy

Your doctor may suggest that you try light therapy to treat some types of circadian rhythm disorders. With this approach, you plan time each day to sit in front of a light box, which produces bright light similar to sunlight. Light visors and light glasses may also be effective. Light therapy may help adjust how much melatonin your body makes to reset your sleep–wake cycle.

- To move your sleep and wake times earlier, use the lightbox when you wake up in the morning. This may also help reduce daytime sleepiness. This method may be used to help treat delayed sleep–wake phase disorder, irregular sleep–wake rhythm disorder, and jet lag disorder when you travel east.

- To move your sleep and wake times later, use the lightbox late in the afternoon or early in the evening. This method may be used to help treat advanced sleep–wake phase disorder, shift work disorder, and jet lag disorder when you travel west.

Side effects of light therapy may include agitation, eye strain, headaches, migraines, and nausea. Ask your doctor before using light therapy if you have an eye condition or use medicines that make you sensitive to light.

## Medicines or Supplements

Your doctor may recommend melatonin medicines or supplements to help align your sleep–wake cycle with your environment.

- Melatonin medicine, called "melatonin receptor agonists," can help treat non-24-hour sleep–wake rhythm disorder. Side effects can include dizziness and fatigue.
- Melatonin supplements are lab-made versions of the sleep hormone that your doctor may recommend for DSWPD, irregular sleep–wake rhythm disorder, and non-24-hour sleep–wake rhythm disorder. These supplements are not regulated by the U.S. Food and Drug Administration (FDA). Because of this, the dose and purity of these supplements can vary between brands. Talk with your doctor about how to find safe, effective melatonin supplements, as well as any possible side effects or medicine interactions, especially if you are pregnant or trying to become pregnant. Side effects of melatonin may include excess sleepiness, headaches, high blood pressure, low blood pressure, stomach upsets, and worsening symptoms of depression.

Your doctor may talk to you about other ways to treat the symptoms of circadian rhythm disorders:

- Caffeine may help prevent daytime sleepiness. Your doctor may recommend that you avoid caffeine within eight hours of your desired bedtime.
- Sleep-promoting medicines, such as benzodiazepines and zolpidem, can help you fall asleep faster and stay asleep longer. These medicines may cause side effects and complications, such as muscle weakness and confusion, that may be more severe in older adults and people who have dementia.
- Wake-promoting medicines, such as modafinil and armodafinil, can help you stay alert and improve performance during shift work. The effects of these medicines may last only for a short time, and you may still experience some sleepiness.

## LIVING WITH A CIRCADIAN RHYTHM DISORDER

If you have been diagnosed with a circadian rhythm disorder, it is important that you continue your treatment. Follow-up care can vary depending on your response to treatment and what causes your sleep problems.

### Tips for Managing Your Condition at Home

- **Follow your treatment plan**. It is important that you follow your doctor's instructions to help avoid the symptoms and complications of circadian rhythm disorders.
- **Get regular follow-up care**. Talk with your doctor about how often to schedule office visits and medical tests. You may need more sleep studies or regular tests to monitor your melatonin levels. Between visits, tell your doctor if you have any new symptoms, if your symptoms worsen, or if you have any complications because of your medicines.
- **Keep a sleep diary**. To monitor improvements in your pattern of sleep and wakefulness and in your quality of sleep.

## Learn Precautions to Help You Stay Safe

To avoid accidents caused by fatigue and daytime sleepiness, it is important to identify when you are too tired to drive, operate heavy machinery, or work. Consider using public transportation if you are too tired to drive.

## How Can Circadian Rhythm Disorders Affect Your Health?

Left untreated, circadian rhythm disorders can increase your risk for the following health conditions:

- **Weakened immune system**. It can lead to infections and poor recovery from illnesses.
- **Cardiovascular diseases and cognitive and behavioral disorders**. Atherosclerosis or stroke (cardiovascular diseases) and decreases in attention, vigilance, concentration, motor skills, and memory (cognitive and behavioral disorders) can lead to reduced productivity, workplace mistakes, or road accidents. In teens and young adults, circadian rhythm disorders can cause risky behavior and problems with concentrating at school, controlling emotions, and coping with stress.
- **Digestive disorders**. They include stomach ulcers, gastroesophageal reflux disease (GERD), and irritable bowel syndrome (IBS). Circadian rhythm disorders may influence the signaling from the brain to the gastrointestinal tract. They may also increase inflammation in the bowel, which can lead to digestive symptoms.
- **Fertility problems**. Circadian rhythm disorders may disrupt the hormone cycle that controls fertility and reproduction.
- **Metabolism disorders**. These disorders can lead to diabetes, metabolic syndrome, and overweight and obesity.
- **Mood disorders**. Irritability, anxiety, and depression are a few examples of these disorders that may be aggravated by circadian rhythm disorders.

- **Worsening of other sleep disorders**. Circadian rhythm disorders can increase your risk of sleep disorders, such as sleep apnea.[1]

---

[1] "What Are Circadian Rhythm Disorders?" National Heart, Lung, and Blood Institute (NHLBI), March 24, 2022. Available online. URL: www.nhlbi.nih.gov/health/circadian-rhythm-disorders. Accessed March 21, 2023.

# Chapter 21 | Insomnia

## Chapter Contents

## Section 21.1 | Understanding Insomnia

Insomnia is one of the most commonly reported sleep problems. One in four women has some insomnia symptoms, such as trouble falling asleep, trouble staying asleep, or both. About one in seven adults has chronic (long-term) insomnia. Chronic insomnia can affect your ability to do daily tasks such as working, going to school, or caring for yourself. Insomnia is more common in women, especially older women, than men.

## WHAT IS INSOMNIA?

Insomnia is a common sleep disorder. It is defined as an inability to go to sleep, waking up too early, or feeling unrested after sleep for at least three nights a week for at least three months. Most adult women need to get seven or more hours of sleep a night to feel rested.

Chronic or long-term insomnia makes it difficult to accomplish routine tasks such as going to work or school and taking care of yourself. Insomnia can lead to or contribute to the development of other health problems, such as depression, heart disease, and stroke.

## WHAT ARE THE DIFFERENT TYPES OF INSOMNIA?

The following are the two types of insomnia:
- **Primary insomnia**. Primary insomnia is a disorder. It is not a symptom or a side effect of another medical condition. Your doctor may diagnose your sleeplessness as primary insomnia after ruling out other medical conditions as a cause.
- **Secondary insomnia**. Secondary insomnia is caused by or happens alongside other health conditions or as a side effect of prescribed medicines. It can be acute (short-term) or chronic (long-term). Most people with chronic insomnia have secondary insomnia.

## WHAT CAUSES PRIMARY INSOMNIA?

The exact cause of primary insomnia is unknown. It may be life-long, or it can happen because of changes in your routine during travel or stressful life events.

## WHAT CAUSES SECONDARY INSOMNIA?

Conditions that may trigger or happen at the same time as secondary insomnia include the following:

- mental health conditions, such as depression, anxiety, or posttraumatic stress disorder (PTSD)
- traumatic brain injury (TBI)
- neurological (brain) disorders, such as Alzheimer disease (AD) or Parkinson disease (PD)
- conditions that cause chronic pain, such as arthritis
- conditions that make it hard to breathe, such as asthma and sleep apnea
- trouble with hormones, including thyroid problems
- gastrointestinal disorders, such as heartburn
- stroke
- other sleep disorders, such as restless legs syndrome (RLS)
- menopause symptoms, such as hot flashes
- cancer
- side effects of medicines, such as those to treat cancer, asthma, heart disease, allergies, and colds

Talk to your doctor or nurse if you think another health problem could be causing insomnia.

Other things that can keep you from getting enough sleep include the following:

- **Caffeine, tobacco, and alcohol.** Caffeine and nicotine in tobacco products can disrupt sleep, especially if taken within several hours of going to bed. Alcohol may make it easier to fall asleep at first, but it can cause you to wake up too early and not be able to fall back asleep.
- **A traumatic event.** People who witness or experience a traumatic event, such as an accident, natural disaster,

physical attack, or war, can have trouble falling and staying asleep. Getting treatment for symptoms of anxiety or PTSD as a result of the trauma can help insomnia get better.

- **A bad sleep environment**. Having a bed or place to sleep that is uncomfortable, unsafe, noisy, or too bright can make it difficult to fall asleep.
- **A partner with sleep problems**. If you sleep with a partner who snores or has sleep apnea, your sleep may be more restless and interrupted. Snoring and sleep apnea can be treated.
- **Pregnancy**. During pregnancy, especially in the third trimester, you may wake up more often than usual because of discomfort, leg cramps, or needing to use the bathroom.
- **Having a new baby**. Changing hormone levels after childbirth can disrupt your sleep. Very young babies do not usually sleep longer than a few hours at a time and need to be fed every few hours.

## WHO GETS INSOMNIA?

Anyone can get insomnia, but it affects more women than men. More than one in four women in the United States experience insomnia, compared with fewer than one in five men. In one study, women of all ages reported worse sleep quality than men, including taking longer to fall asleep, sleeping for shorter periods of time, and feeling sleepier when awake.

Older women are at a higher risk of insomnia. Other people at risk for insomnia include those who:

- have a lot of stress
- have depression or other mental health conditions
- work nights or have an irregular sleep schedule, such as shift workers
- travel long distances with time changes, such as air travelers
- have certain medical conditions, such as sleep apnea, asthma, and fibromyalgia

## WHY DO MORE WOMEN THAN MEN HAVE INSOMNIA?

Women may be more likely to have insomnia than men because women experience unique hormonal changes that can cause insomnia symptoms. These include hormonal changes during:

- the menstrual cycle, especially in the days leading up to their period when many women report problems going to sleep and staying asleep, which is especially common in women who have premenstrual dysphoric disorder (PMDD), a more severe type of premenstrual syndrome (PMS)
- pregnancy, especially in the third trimester, when women may wake up often because of discomfort, leg cramps, or needing to use the bathroom
- perimenopause and menopause when hot flashes and night sweats can disturb sleep

Also, some health problems that can cause secondary insomnia are more common in women than in men. These include the following:

- **Depression and anxiety**. People with insomnia are 10 times more likely to have depression and 17 times more likely to have anxiety. Researchers are not sure if mental health conditions lead to insomnia or if insomnia leads to mental health conditions. But not getting enough sleep may make mental health conditions worse.
- **Fibromyalgia**. The pain experienced with fibromyalgia can make it difficult to fall asleep and stay asleep.

## HOW LONG DOES INSOMNIA LAST?

It depends. Insomnia can be acute (short-term) or chronic (long-term). While acute insomnia may last for only a few days or weeks, chronic insomnia can last for three months or more.

## WHAT ARE THE SYMPTOMS OF INSOMNIA?

The most common symptom of insomnia is difficulty sleeping—either going to sleep, staying asleep, or waking up too early. If you have insomnia, you may:

- lie awake for a long time without going to sleep
- wake up during the night and find it difficult to go back to sleep
- not feel rested when you wake up

Lack of sleep may cause other symptoms during the daytime. For example, you may wake up feeling tired, and you may have low energy during the day. It can also cause you to feel anxious, depressed, or irritable, and you may have a hard time concentrating or remembering things.

## HOW DOES INSOMNIA AFFECT WOMEN'S HEALTH?

Insomnia can cause you to feel tired, anxious, or irritable in the short term. Over time, lack of sleep may increase your risk for more serious problems, including the following:

- accidents
- health problems, including diabetes and high blood pressure
- increased risk for falls, especially in older women

Women who have long-term insomnia may be more at risk than men with long-term insomnia for mood problems, heart disease and stroke, and obesity.[1]

---

[1] Office on Women's Health (OWH), "Insomnia," U.S. Department of Health and Human Services (HHS), February 22, 2021. Available online. URL: www.womenshealth.gov/a-z-topics/insomnia. Accessed March 21, 2023.

## Section 21.2 | **Fatal Familial Insomnia**

### WHAT IS FATAL FAMILIAL INSOMNIA?

Fatal familial insomnia (FFI) affects the thalamus, the part of the brain that controls the sleep–wake cycle. Symptoms typically begin between the ages of 40 and 60 years. The most common symptoms are sleep disturbance, psychiatric problems, weight loss, and balance problems. Other symptoms include high blood pressure, excess sweating, and difficulty controlling body temperature. These symptoms tend to get worse over time. FFI is usually fatal in 6–36 months. Almost all cases of FFI occur due to a specific variant in the *PRNP* gene and are inherited in an autosomal dominant pattern. Diagnosis is based on the symptoms, clinical exam, sleep study, and imaging studies. The results of genetic testing can help confirm the diagnosis. Treatment for FFI is focused on managing the symptoms.

### SYMPTOMS OF FATAL FAMILIAL INSOMNIA

The following list includes the most common signs and symptoms in people with FFI. These features may be different from person to person. Some people may have more symptoms than others, and they can range from mild to severe. This list does not include every symptom that has been described in the condition.

Symptoms of FFI may include the following:
- inability to fall asleep or stay asleep (insomnia)
- difficulty thinking and concentrating (cognitive impairment)
- short-term memory loss
- weight loss
- difficulty coordinating movements
- high blood pressure
- inability to maintain body temperature
- excessive sweating and tearing

The first symptoms of FFI usually begin between the ages of 40 and 60 years. Initial symptoms usually include difficulty sleeping and problems with thinking and concentration. Insomnia gets worse over time, leading to high blood pressure, rapid heart rate, weight loss, and trouble controlling body temperature. Other symptoms that may develop include uncoordinated movements (ataxia), hallucinations, severe confusion (delirium), and difficulty swallowing. Death usually occurs within 6–36 months after symptoms begin. Death is usually due to heart problems or infections.

## CAUSES OF FATAL FAMILIAL INSOMNIA

Fatal familial insomnia occurs when the *PRNP* gene is not working correctly. Deoxyribonucleic acid (DNA) changes known as "pathogenic variants" are responsible for making genes work incorrectly or, sometimes, not at all. In almost every case, FFI is caused by a very specific variant in the *PRNP* gene.

## INHERITANCE OF FATAL FAMILIAL INSOMNIA

Fatal familial insomnia is inherited in an autosomal dominant pattern. All individuals inherit two copies of each gene. Autosomal means the gene is found on one of the numbered chromosomes found in both sexes. Dominant means that only one altered copy of a gene is necessary to have the condition. The variant can be inherited from either parent. Sometimes, an autosomal dominant condition occurs because of a new genetic variant (de novo), and there is no history of this condition in the family.

Each child of an individual with an autosomal dominant condition has a 50 percent or one in two chance of inheriting the variant and the condition. Typically, children who inherit a dominant variant will have the condition, but they may be more or less severely affected than their parents. Sometimes, a person may have a gene variant for an autosomal dominant condition and show no signs or symptoms of the condition.

## DIAGNOSIS OF FATAL FAMILIAL INSOMNIA

Fatal familial insomnia is diagnosed based on the symptoms, clinical exam, a sleep study (polysomnography), and imaging tests.

The results of genetic testing may be helpful to help confirm the diagnosis. A list of features for diagnosing FFI (diagnostic criteria) has been published.

## TREATMENT FOR FATAL FAMILIAL INSOMNIA

Treatment for FFI is focused on managing the symptoms and providing comfort for the person with FFI.

Specialists involved in the care of someone with FFI may include the following:
- neurologist
- medical geneticist
- social worker[2]

[2] Genetic and Rare Diseases Information Center (GARD), "Fatal Familial Insomnia," National Center for Advancing Translational Sciences (NCATS), November 11, 2020. Available online. URL: https://rarediseases.info.nih.gov/diseases/6429/fatal-familial-insomnia. Accessed March 24, 2023.

# Chapter 22 | Excessive Sleeping

## Chapter Contents

## Section 22.1 | **Hypersomnia**

## WHAT IS HYPERSOMNIA?

Hypersomnia refers to medical conditions in which you repeatedly feel excessively tired during the day (called "excessive daytime sleepiness") or sleep longer than usual at night. It is different from feeling tired due to lack of or interrupted sleep at night. If you have hypersomnia, you might fall asleep repeatedly during the day, often at inappropriate times such as at work or during a meal. These daytime naps usually provide no relief from symptoms. Hypersomnia can occur on its own or be caused by:

- another sleep disorder (such as insomnia or sleep apnea)
- another medical condition (including multiple sclerosis, depression, encephalitis, epilepsy, or obesity)
- drug or alcohol abuse
- dysfunction of part of the nervous system

It can also result from a physical problem, such as a tumor, head trauma, or injury to the central nervous system (CNS). Symptoms include the following:

- difficulty waking from a long sleep
- slow thinking
- slow speech
- memory difficulty
- anxiety
- increased irritation
- decreased energy
- hallucinations

Medications are available to treat one form of hypersomnia. Other medicines may be used to treat symptoms. Lifestyle changes can include avoiding caffeine or alcohol, avoiding night work and social activities that delay bedtime, and going to bed at a regular time. Counseling and support groups can also help you learn to cope with hypersomnia.

## HOW CAN YOU OR YOUR LOVED ONE HELP IMPROVE CARE FOR PEOPLE WITH HYPERSOMNIA?

Consider participating in a clinical trial (www.ninds.nih.gov/health-information/clinical-trials), so clinicians and scientists can learn more about hypersomnia and related disorders. Clinical research uses human volunteers to help researchers learn more about a disorder and perhaps find better ways to safely detect, treat, or prevent disease.

All types of volunteers are needed—those who are healthy or may have an illness or disease—of all different ages, sexes, races, and ethnicities to ensure that study results apply to as many people as possible and that treatments will be safe and effective for everyone who will use them.[1]

## WHAT IS IDIOPATHIC HYPERSOMNIA?

Idiopathic hypersomnia (IH) is a neurological sleep disorder that can affect many aspects of a person's life. Symptoms often begin between adolescence and young adulthood and develop over weeks to months. People with IH have a hard time staying awake and alert during the day (chronic excessive daytime sleepiness). They may fall asleep unintentionally or at inappropriate times, interfering with daily functioning. They may also have difficulty waking up from nighttime sleep or daytime naps. Sleeping longer at night does not appear to improve daytime sleepiness. The cause of IH is not known. Some people with IH have other family members with a sleep disorder such as IH or narcolepsy.

## WHEN DO SYMPTOMS OF IDIOPATHIC HYPERSOMNIA BEGIN?

Symptoms of this disease may start to appear at any time in life. The age symptoms may begin to appear between diseases. Symptoms may begin in a single age range or during several age ranges. The symptoms of some diseases may begin at any age. Knowing when symptoms begin to appear can help medical providers find the correct diagnosis.

---

[1] "Hypersomnia," National Institute of Neurological Disorders and Stroke (NINDS), February 7, 2023. Available online. URL: www.ninds.nih.gov/health-information/disorders/hypersomnia. Accessed March 28, 2023.

## SYMPTOMS OF IDIOPATHIC HYPERSOMNIA

The number and severity of symptoms experienced may differ among people with this disease. Your experience may be different from others, and you should consult your primary care provider for more information.[2]

## Section 22.2 | Kleine-Levin Syndrome

## WHAT IS KLEINE-LEVIN SYNDROME?

Kleine-Levin syndrome is a rare disorder that primarily affects teenage males. Approximately 70 percent of people living with Kleine-Levin syndrome are male.

Symptoms include repeated but reversible periods of excessive sleep (up to 20 hours per day). Symptoms happen as "episodes," which typically last a few days to a few weeks, and may be related to malfunction of the parts of the brain that are in charge of appetite (hypothalamus) and sleep (thalamus).

Episodes often start suddenly and may include the following:

- flu-like symptoms
- overeating
- irritability
- childishness
- disorientation (not being sure where you are or what is happening)
- hallucinations (seeing or hearing things that are not there)
- an abnormally unlimited sex drive

A person's mood can be depressed as a result of Kleine-Levin syndrome, but the mood does not cause the disorder. People with the disorder are completely "normal" between episodes, but they

---

[2] Genetic and Rare Diseases Information Center (GARD), "Idiopathic Hypersomnia," National Center for Advancing Translational Sciences (NCATS), February 2023. Available online. URL: https://rarediseases.info.nih.gov/diseases/8737/idiopathic-hypersomnia. Accessed March 28, 2023.

may not be able to remember everything that happened in the episodes. It may be weeks or more before symptoms come back.

There is no sure treatment for Kleine-Levin syndrome. People with the disorder are often advised to carefully keep track of their symptoms (an approach called "watchful waiting") at home instead of treating the disorder with medicines. Stimulant pills, including amphetamines, methylphenidate, and modafinil, are used to treat sleepiness—but they may increase irritability and will not improve the person's ability to think and reason normally.

Because of similarities between Kleine-Levin syndrome and certain mood disorders, doctors may prescribe lithium and carbamazepine. In some cases, these drugs have prevented further episodes of the disorder.

Kleine-Levin syndrome is different from having repeated cycles of sleepiness during the premenstrual period in teenage girls. Those cycles may be controlled with birth control pills. The disorder is also different from encephalopathy (brain damage or brain disease), repeated depression, or psychosis (losing touch with reality).[3]

## WHEN DO SYMPTOMS OF KLEINE-LEVIN SYNDROME BEGIN?

Symptoms of this disease may start to appear from childhood to adulthood. The age symptoms may begin to appear between diseases. Symptoms may begin in a single age range or during several age ranges. The symptoms of some diseases may begin at any age. Knowing when symptoms began to appear can help medical providers find the correct diagnosis.[4]

---

[3] "Kleine-Levin Syndrome," National Institute of Neurological Disorders and Stroke (NINDS), January 20, 2023. Available online. URL: www.ninds.nih.gov/health-information/disorders/kleine-levin-syndrome. Accessed March 28, 2023.
[4] Genetic and Rare Diseases Information Center (GARD), "Kleine Levin Syndrome," National Center for Advancing Translational Sciences (NCATS), February 2023. Available online. URL: https://rarediseases.info.nih.gov/diseases/3117/kleine-levin-syndrome. Accessed March 28, 2023.

## HOW CAN YOU OR YOUR LOVED ONE HELP IMPROVE CARE FOR PEOPLE WITH KLEINE-LEVIN SYNDROME?

Consider participating in a clinical trial, so clinicians and scientists can learn more about Kleine-Levin syndrome and related disorders. Clinical research uses human volunteers to help researchers learn more about a disorder and perhaps find better ways to safely detect, treat, or prevent disease.

All types of volunteers are needed—those who are healthy or may have an illness or disease—of all different ages, sexes, races, and ethnicities to ensure that study results apply to as many people as possible and that treatments will be safe and effective for everyone who will use them.[5]

---

[5] See footnote [3].

# Chapter 23 | **Narcolepsy**

## Chapter Contents

## Section 23.1 | **Narcolepsy: An Overview**

## WHAT IS NARCOLEPSY?

Narcolepsy is a chronic neurological disorder that affects the brain's ability to control sleep–wake cycles. People with narcolepsy may feel rested after waking but then feel very sleepy throughout much of the day. Many individuals with narcolepsy also experience uneven and interrupted sleep that can involve waking up frequently during the night.

Narcolepsy can greatly affect daily activities. People may unwillingly fall asleep even if they are in the middle of an activity, such as driving, eating, or talking. Other symptoms may include sudden muscle weakness while awake that makes a person go limp or unable to move (cataplexy), vivid dream-like images or hallucinations, and total paralysis just before falling asleep or just after waking up (sleep paralysis).

In a normal sleep cycle, a person enters rapid eye movement (REM) sleep after about 60–90 minutes. Dreams occur during REM sleep, and the brain keeps muscles limp during this sleep stage, which prevents people from acting out their dreams. People with narcolepsy frequently enter REM sleep rapidly within 15 minutes of falling asleep. Also, muscle weakness or dream activity of REM sleep can occur during wakefulness or be absent during sleep. This helps explain some symptoms of narcolepsy.

If left undiagnosed or untreated, narcolepsy can interfere with psychological, social, and cognitive function and development and can inhibit academic, work, and social activities.

Narcolepsy is a lifelong problem, but it does not usually worsen as the person ages. Symptoms can partially improve over time, but they will never disappear completely. The most typical symptoms are as follows:

- **Excessive daytime sleepiness (EDS).** All individuals with narcolepsy have EDS, and it is often the most obvious symptom. EDS is characterized by persistent sleepiness, regardless of how much sleep an individual gets at night. However, sleepiness in narcolepsy is more like a "sleep attack," where an overwhelming sense of sleepiness comes on quickly. In between sleep attacks, individuals have normal levels of alertness, particularly if doing activities that keep their attention.

- **Cataplexy**. This sudden loss of muscle tone while a person is awake leads to weakness and a loss of voluntary muscle control. It is often triggered by sudden, strong emotions such as laughter, fear, anger, stress, or excitement. The symptoms of cataplexy may appear weeks or even years after the onset of EDS. Some people may only have one or two attacks in a lifetime, while others may experience many attacks a day. In about 10 percent of cases of narcolepsy, cataplexy is the first symptom to appear and can be misdiagnosed as a seizure disorder. Attacks may be mild and involve only a momentary sense of minor weakness in a limited number of muscles, such as a slight drooping of the eyelids. The most severe attacks result in a total body collapse during which individuals are unable to move, speak, or keep their eyes open. But, even during the most severe episodes, people remain fully conscious, a characteristic that distinguishes cataplexy from fainting or seizure disorders. The loss of muscle tone during cataplexy resembles paralysis of muscle activity that naturally occurs during REM sleep. Episodes last a few minutes at most and resolve almost instantly on their own. While scary, the episodes are not dangerous as long as the individual finds a safe place in which to collapse.
- **Sleep paralysis**. The temporary inability to move or speak while falling asleep or waking up usually lasts only a few seconds or minutes and is similar to REM-induced inhibitions of voluntary muscle activity. Sleep paralysis resembles cataplexy, except it occurs at the edges of sleep. As with cataplexy, people remain fully conscious. Even when severe, cataplexy and sleep paralysis do not result in permanent dysfunction—after episodes end, people rapidly recover their full capacity to move and speak.

- **Hallucinations**. Very vivid and sometimes frightening images can accompany sleep paralysis and usually occur when people are falling asleep or waking up. Most often, the content is primarily visual, but any of the other senses can be involved.

Additional symptoms include the following:
- **Fragmented sleep and insomnia**. While individuals with narcolepsy are very sleepy during the day, they usually also experience difficulties staying asleep at night. Sleep may be disrupted by insomnia, vivid dreaming, sleep apnea, acting out while dreaming, and periodic leg movements.
- **Automatic behaviors**. Individuals with narcolepsy may experience temporary sleep episodes that can be very brief, lasting no more than seconds at a time. A person falls asleep during an activity (e.g., eating, talking) and automatically continues the activity for a few seconds or minutes without conscious awareness of what they are doing. This happens most often while people are engaged in habitual activities such as typing or driving. They cannot recall their actions, and their performance is almost always impaired. Their handwriting may, for example, degenerate into an illegible scrawl, or they may store items in bizarre locations and then forget where they placed them. If an episode occurs while driving, individuals may get lost or have an accident. People tend to awaken from these episodes feeling refreshed, finding that their drowsiness and fatigue have temporarily subsided.

The following are the two major types of narcolepsy:
- **Type 1 narcolepsy**. It was previously known as "narcolepsy with cataplexy." This diagnosis is based on the individual either having low levels of a brain hormone (hypocretin) or reporting cataplexy and having excessive daytime sleepiness on a special nap test.

- **Type 2 narcolepsy**. It was previously known as "narcolepsy without cataplexy." People with this condition experience excessive daytime sleepiness but usually do not have muscle weakness triggered by emotions. They usually also have less severe symptoms and have normal levels of the brain hormone hypocretin.

A condition known as "secondary narcolepsy" can result from an injury to the hypothalamus, a region deep in the brain that helps regulate sleep. In addition to experiencing the typical symptoms of narcolepsy, individuals may also have severe neurological problems and sleep for long periods (more than 10 hours) each night.

## WHO IS MORE LIKELY TO GET NARCOLEPSY?

Narcolepsy affects both females and males equally. Symptoms often start in childhood, adolescence, or young adulthood (aged 7–25) but can occur at any time in life. Since people with narcolepsy are often misdiagnosed with other conditions, such as psychiatric disorders or emotional problems, it can take years for someone to get the proper diagnosis.

Narcolepsy may have several causes. Nearly all people with narcolepsy who have cataplexy have extremely low levels of the naturally occurring chemical hypocretin, which promotes wakefulness and regulates REM sleep. Hypocretin levels are usually normal in people who have narcolepsy without cataplexy.

Although the cause of narcolepsy is not completely understood, current research suggests that narcolepsy may be the result of a combination of factors working together to cause a lack of hypocretin. These factors include the following:

- **Autoimmune disorders**. When cataplexy is present, the cause is most often the loss of brain cells that produce hypocretin. Although the reason for this cell loss is unknown, it appears to be linked to abnormalities in the immune system. Autoimmune disorders occur when the body's immune system turns against itself and mistakenly attacks healthy cells or tissue. Researchers believe that in individuals with narcolepsy, the body's immune system selectively attacks the hypocretin-containing brain cells because of a combination of genetic and environmental factors.

- **Family history**. Most cases of narcolepsy are sporadic, meaning the disorder occurs in individuals with no known family history. However, clusters in families sometimes occur. Up to 10 percent of individuals diagnosed with narcolepsy with cataplexy report having a close relative with similar symptoms.
- **Brain injuries**. Rarely, narcolepsy results from traumatic injury to parts of the brain that regulate wakefulness and REM sleep or from tumors and other diseases in the same regions.

In the past few decades, scientists have made considerable progress in understanding narcolepsy and identifying genes strongly associated with the disorder. Groups of neurons in several parts of the brain interact to control sleep, and the activity of these neurons is controlled by a large number of genes. The loss of hypocretin-producing neurons in the hypothalamus is the primary cause of type 1 narcolepsy. These neurons are important for stabilizing sleep and wake states.

The human leukocyte antigen (*HLA*) system of genes plays an important role in regulating the immune system. This gene family provides instructions for making a group of related proteins called the "HLA complex," which helps the immune system distinguish between good proteins from an individual's own body and bad ones made by foreign invaders such as viruses and bacteria.

One of the genes in this family is *HLA-DQB1*. A variation in this gene, called "*HLA-DQB1*06:02*," increases the chance of developing narcolepsy, particularly the type of narcolepsy with cataplexy and a loss of hypocretins (also known as "orexins"). *HLA-DQB1*06:02* and other *HLA* gene variations may increase susceptibility to an immune attack on hypocretin neurons, causing these cells to die. Most people with narcolepsy have this gene variation and may also have specific versions of closely related *HLA* genes.

However, it is important to note that these gene variations are common in the general population and only a small portion of the people with the *HLA-DQB1\*06:02* variation will develop narcolepsy. This indicates that other genetic and environmental factors are important in determining if an individual will develop the disorder.

Narcolepsy follows a seasonal pattern and is more likely to develop in the spring and early summer after the winter season, a time when people are more likely to get sick. By studying people soon after they develop the disorder, scientists have discovered that individuals with narcolepsy have high levels of antistreptolysin O antibodies, indicating an immune response to a recent bacterial infection such as strep throat. Also, the H1N1 influenza epidemic in 2009 resulted in a large increase in the number of new cases of narcolepsy. Together, this suggests that individuals with the *HLA-DQB1\*06:02* variation are at risk for developing narcolepsy after they are exposed to a specific trigger, such as certain infections that trick the immune system into attacking the body.

## HOW IS NARCOLEPSY DIAGNOSED AND TREATED?
### Diagnosing Narcolepsy
A clinical examination and detailed medical history are essential for the diagnosis and treatment of narcolepsy. Individuals may be asked by their doctor to keep a sleep journal noting the times of sleep and symptoms over a one- to two-week period. A physical exam can rule out or identify other neurological conditions that may be causing the symptoms.

Two specialized tests, which can be performed in a sleep disorders clinic, are required to establish a diagnosis of narcolepsy:

- **Polysomnogram (PSG or sleep study).** The PSG is an overnight recording of brain and muscle activity, breathing, and eye movements. A PSG can help reveal whether REM sleep occurs early in the sleep cycle and if an individual's symptoms result from another condition, such as sleep apnea.
- **Multiple sleep latency test (MSLT).** The MSLT assesses daytime sleepiness by measuring how quickly a person falls asleep and whether they enter REM sleep.

Occasionally, it may be helpful to measure the level of hypocretin in the fluid that surrounds the brain and spinal cord. To perform this test, a doctor will withdraw a sample of the cerebrospinal fluid using a lumbar puncture (also called a "spinal tap") and measure the level of hypocretin-1.

## Treating Narcolepsy

Although there is no cure for narcolepsy, some of the symptoms can be treated with medicines and lifestyle changes.

## MEDICATIONS

- **Modafinil**. The initial line of treatment is usually a central nervous system (CNS) stimulant such as modafinil. Modafinil is usually prescribed first because it is less addictive and has fewer side effects than older stimulants. For most people, these drugs are generally effective at reducing daytime drowsiness and improving alertness.
- **Amphetamine-like stimulants**. In cases where modafinil is not effective, doctors may prescribe amphetamine-like stimulants such as methylphenidate to alleviate EDS. However, these medications must be carefully monitored because they can have side effects.
- **Antidepressants**. Two classes of antidepressant drugs have proven effective in controlling cataplexy in many individuals: tricyclics (including imipramine, desipramine, clomipramine, and protriptyline) and selective serotonin and noradrenergic reuptake inhibitors (including venlafaxine, fluoxetine, and atomoxetine).
- **Sodium oxybate**. It (also known as "gamma-hydroxybutyrate" or "GHB") has been approved by the U.S. Food and Drug Administration (FDA) to treat cataplexy and excessive daytime sleepiness in individuals with narcolepsy. Due to safety concerns associated with the use of this drug, the distribution of sodium oxybate is tightly restricted.

- **Histamine 3 receptor antagonist/inverse agonist.**
  Pitolisant was recently approved by the FDA as the only
  nonscheduled product for treating excessive daytime
  sleepiness or cataplexy in adults with narcolepsy.
  Pitolisant, which has been commercially available in the
  United States since 2019, is thought to increase histamine
  levels in the brain. The most common adverse reactions to
  pitolisant are insomnia, nausea, and anxiety.

## LIFESTYLE CHANGES

Drug therapy should accompany various lifestyle changes.
Remembering the following seven tips may be helpful:

- **Take short naps.** Many individuals take short, regularly
  scheduled naps at times when they tend to feel
  sleepiest.
- **Maintain a regular sleep schedule.** Going to bed and
  waking up at the same time every day, even on the
  weekends, can help people sleep better.
- **Avoid caffeine or alcohol before bed.** Individuals
  should avoid alcohol and caffeine for several hours
  before bedtime.
- **Avoid smoking, especially at night.** Smoking at
  night should be avoided as it can even cause sleeping
  conditions, such as sleep apnea.
- **Exercise daily.** Exercising for at least 20 minutes
  per day at least four or five hours before bedtime
  also improves sleep quality and can help people with
  narcolepsy avoid gaining excess weight.
- **Avoid large, heavy meals right before bedtime.** Eating
  very close to bedtime can make it harder to sleep.
- **Relax before bed.** Relaxing activities such as a
  warm bath before bedtime can help promote
  sleepiness. Also, make sure the sleep space is cool and
  comfortable.

Safety precautions, particularly when driving, are important
for everyone with narcolepsy. Suddenly falling asleep or losing

muscle control can transform actions that are ordinarily safe, such as walking down a long flight of stairs, into hazards.

The Americans with Disabilities Act (ADA) requires employers to provide reasonable accommodations for all employees with disabilities. Adults with narcolepsy can often negotiate with employers to modify their work schedules, so they can take naps when necessary and perform their most demanding tasks when they are most alert.

Similarly, children and adolescents with narcolepsy may be able to work with school administrators to accommodate special needs, such as taking medications during the school day, modifying class schedules to fit in a nap, and other strategies. Additionally, support groups can be extremely beneficial for people with narcolepsy.

## WHAT ARE THE LATEST UPDATES ON NARCOLEPSY?

The mission of the National Institute of Neurological Disorders and Stroke (NINDS) is to seek fundamental knowledge about the brain and nervous system and to use that knowledge to reduce the burden of neurological disease. The NINDS, a component of the National Institutes of Health (NIH), along with several other NIH institutes and centers, supports research on narcolepsy and other sleep disorders through grants to medical institutions across the country.

Additionally, the National Heart, Lung, and Blood Institute (NHLBI) manages the National Center on Sleep Disorders Research (NCSDR), which coordinates federal government sleep research activities, promotes doctoral and postdoctoral training programs, and educates the public and health-care professionals about sleep disorders.

### Genetics and Biochemicals

The NINDS-sponsored researchers are conducting studies devoted to further clarifying the wide range of genetic—both *HLA* genes and non-*HLA* genes—and environmental factors that may cause narcolepsy. Other investigators are using animal models to better understand hypocretin and other chemicals, such as glutamate, that may play a key role in regulating sleep and wakefulness. Researchers are also investigating wake-promoting compounds to widen the range of available therapeutic options and create treatment options that reduce undesired side effects and decrease the potential for abuse. A greater understanding of the complex genetic and biochemical bases of narcolepsy will eventually lead to new therapies to control symptoms and may lead to a cure.

## Immune System

Abnormalities in the immune system may play an important role in the development of narcolepsy. NINDS-sponsored scientists have demonstrated the presence of unusual immune system activity in people with narcolepsy. Furthermore, strep throat and certain varieties of influenza are now thought to be triggers in some at-risk individuals. Other NINDS researchers are also working to understand why the immune system destroys hypocretin neurons in narcolepsy in the hopes of finding a way to prevent or cure the disorder.

## Sleep Biology

The NINDS continues to support investigations into the basic biology of sleep, such as examining the brain mechanisms involved in generating and regulating REM sleep and other sleep behaviors. Since sleep and circadian rhythms are controlled by networks of neurons in the brain, NINDS researchers are also examining how neuronal circuits function in the body and contribute to sleep disorders such as narcolepsy. A more comprehensive understanding of the complex biology of sleep will give scientists a better understanding of the processes that underlie narcolepsy and other sleep disorders.

## HOW CAN YOU OR YOUR LOVED ONE HELP IMPROVE CARE FOR PEOPLE WITH NARCOLEPSY?

The NeuroBioBank serves as a central point of access to collections that span neurological, neuropsychiatric, and neurodevelopmental diseases and disorders. Tissue from individuals with narcolepsy is needed to enable scientists to study this disorder more intensely. Participating groups include brain and tissue repositories, researchers, NIH program staff, information technology experts, disease advocacy groups, and, most importantly, individuals seeking information about opportunities to donate.

Additionally, the NINDS supports genetic and immunological research in narcolepsy at the Stanford University Center for Narcolepsy. Blood samples from individuals with narcolepsy can be sent by mail and are needed to enable scientists to study this disorder more intensely.

Consider participating in a clinical trial, so clinicians and scientists can learn more about narcolepsy and related disorders. Clinical research uses human volunteers to help researchers learn more about a disorder and perhaps find better ways to detect, treat, or prevent disease safely.

All types of volunteers are needed—those who are healthy or may have an illness or disease—of all different ages, sexes, races, and ethnicities to ensure that study results apply to as many people as possible and that treatments will be safe and effective for everyone who will use them.[1]

## Section 23.2 | Immune System's Role in Narcolepsy

Scientists funded by the National Institutes of Health (NIH) have identified a gene associated with narcolepsy, a disorder that causes disabling daytime sleepiness, sleep attacks, irresistible bouts of sleep that can strike at any time, and disturbed sleep at night. The gene has a known role in the immune system, which strongly suggests that autoimmunity, in which the immune system turns against the body's own tissues, plays an important role in the disorder.

---

[1] "Narcolepsy," National Institute of Neurological Disorders and Stroke (NINDS), January 20, 2023. Available online. URL: www.ninds.nih.gov/health-information/disorders/narcolepsy. Accessed March 29, 2023.

"The link between narcolepsy and autoimmunity was proposed decades ago, but efforts to verify it have failed repeatedly. Current findings leave little doubt that autoimmunity plays a role," says Merrill Mitler, Ph.D., a program director with the National Institute of Neurological Disorders and Stroke (NINDS). The study was funded principally by the NINDS, with additional support from the National Institute of Mental Health (NIMH), the National Heart, Lung, and Blood Institute (NHLBI), and the National Institute of Allergy and Infectious Diseases (NIAID), all components of the NIH.

The new study, which appears today in *Nature Genetics*, focused on narcolepsy with cataplexy—a sudden loss of muscle tone that can cause a person to collapse, with or without falling asleep. About 1 in 2,000 Americans has narcolepsy–cataplexy. The symptoms of narcolepsy–cataplexy have been shown to result from the death of a small group of brain cells that normally regulate the sleep–wake cycle by releasing chemicals called "hypocretins."

Genetic and environmental factors both clearly play a role in narcolepsy–cataplexy. Until now, the best evidence for autoimmunity as a cause of the disorder was the discovery that nearly everyone with the disorder has unique variants of a gene called "*HLA-DQB1\*0602*." This is one of the genes that encodes HLA proteins, which dot the surface of the body's cells and help the immune system identify foreign proteins. Some researchers theorize that the HLA variants found in people with narcolepsy–cataplexy predispose them to an autoimmune reaction that destroys their hypocretin-producing cells.

There are gaps in that theory, however, says Emmanuel Mignot, M.D., Ph.D., director of the Center for Narcolepsy at Stanford University School of Medicine in Palo Alto, California, and a Howard Hughes Medical Institute investigator. Dr. Mignot discovered the link between narcolepsy and the hypocretins and helped establish the link to the HLA system. HLA proteins are found in many tissues, including the brain, where they may affect brain development, he says.

HLA variations, however, do not fully account for narcolepsy–cataplexy. Dr. Mignot led a genome-wide association study to search for other genes associated with narcolepsy–cataplexy. These studies involve scanning the genome—the entire set of deoxyribonucleic acid (DNA)—for small differences between people who have a disorder and people who do not. Dr. Mignot's study included more than 4,000 individuals, all of whom had the HLA variants that predispose to narcolepsy–cataplexy, but only about half of whom had the disorder. Participants were recruited so that many genetic groups were represented. Subjects were from the United States and eight countries in Europe and Asia; hundreds were African American, Korean, and Japanese, groups known to have a high incidence of the disorder.

The researchers discovered that in addition to unique HLA variants, people with narcolepsy–cataplexy are also likely to have unique variants of the *TCRA* gene, which encodes a receptor protein on the surface of T cells. T cells are the mobile infantry of the immune system. In concert with the HLA proteins, the T cell receptor enables T cells to recognize and attack foreign invaders, such as bacteria and viruses. Changes to the T cell receptor could increase the likelihood that the cells will direct their attack against the body.

The findings of Dr. Mignot's group indicate that narcolepsy–cataplexy is linked to autoimmunity and involves T cells. The research could lead to new approaches to prevention and treatment. One possibility may be preventing the disorder by stopping the effects of the autoimmune process. "If we can define the changes in the T cell receptor associated with narcolepsy–cataplexy, we might be able to develop drugs that block the protein's abnormal activity and prevent the onset of the disorder," says Dr. Mignot. Current treatments, such as stimulant drugs for combating daytime sleepiness and antidepressants for cataplexy, are only able to control symptoms and do not address the underlying loss of hypocretin cells.

It is important to note that this study, like most genome-wide association studies, did not identify genetic variants that directly cause narcolepsy–cataplexy. Instead, it identifies groups that are more likely to show narcolepsy–cataplexy and groups that are less likely to show the disorder. In people with the HLA variants that predispose to narcolepsy–cataplexy, there is about a 20-fold higher frequency of the disorder if variants in the *TCRA* gene are present. It is yet to be known which people with the genetic variants will go on to develop narcolepsy–cataplexy.

Other risk factors for narcolepsy–cataplexy remain to be discovered, and Dr. Mignot's findings could provide clues to their identity. For example, further studies to characterize the T cells in people with narcolepsy–cataplexy could help reveal whether specific environmental factors—such as infections—contribute to the disorder. Dr. Mignot's findings could also lead to a better understanding of other autoimmune diseases where *HLA* genes are known to play a role, such as multiple sclerosis and type 1 diabetes.[2]

---

[2] "Genetic Study Confirms the Immune System's Role in Narcolepsy," National Institutes of Health (NIH), May 3, 2009. Available online. URL: https://nih.gov/news-events/news-releases/genetic-study-confirms-immune-systems-role-narcolepsy. Accessed March 24, 2023.

# Chapter 24 | **Nocturnal Sleep-Related Eating Disorder**

About 1–3 percent of the general population appears to be affected by sleep-related eating disorders (SREDs). Both women and men can have these disorders, but these are more common among women. Sleep eating is also known to run in the family. The onset of this disease is typically between the ages of 20 and 40. SREDs can also be triggered by other sleep disorders or medical conditions.

## WHAT IS NOCTURNAL SLEEP-RELATED EATING DISORDER?
Sleep eating is a disorder in which the patient is hungry and eats at night. Patients diet during the day and are vulnerable to eating at night but have no memory of doing so. In most cases, people with SREDs have a history of alcoholism, drug abuse, and other sleep disorders. They often eat different types of food at odd hours and may even eat inedible substances. They lose their appetite for food, which often results in anxiety, stress, or depression.

More than 50 percent of these individuals gain weight from consuming food during sleeping hours. They also feel drowsy and experience extreme emotions. Sometimes, low blood sugar (hypoglycemia) can also cause SREDs. Dyssomnia is a conscious behavior, while parasomnia is an unconscious behavior. People with SREDs usually:

- become ill from inadequately cooked food or ingesting toxic substances

- develop metabolic conditions (type 2 diabetes or elevated cholesterol)
- develop cavities or tooth decay from eating sugary foods
- have unrefreshing sleep and feel sleepy or tired during the day
- injure themselves preparing food (lacerations, burns)
- gain weight

Sleep eating is an arousal disorder in which:
- the patient indulges in abnormal behavior during arousal from slow-wave sleep
- the patient indulges in repetitive and automatic motor activity
- the patient is unaware of the entire episode as it is occurring
- the patient finds it difficult to wake up despite vigorous attempts

## SYMPTOMS OF NOCTURNAL SLEEP-RELATED EATING DISORDERS

People with SREDs often eat toxic substances and often in strange combinations. Continuous episodes of binge eating only occur when the patients are partially awake. The following conditions are seen in people with SRED:
- doing something dangerous while getting or cooking food
- continuous episodes of binge eating and drinking during the time when they sleep
- having eating episodes that disturb their sleep and cause insomnia, resulting in unrefreshing sleep
- decline in health from eating foods that are high in calories
- having a loss of appetite in the morning

If something else is causing the problem, it may be one of the following reasons:
- a mental health disorder
- a medical condition

- another sleep disorder
- substance abuse
- medication use

## RISK FACTORS OF NOCTURNAL SLEEP-RELATED EATING DISORDER

About 65–80 percent of SRED patients are females between the ages of 22 and 29. SREDs can also occur from the use of certain medicines that are used to treat depression and other sleep problems. Sleep disorder is an ongoing problem, and most people with SRED were sleepwalkers as children. Sleep-related disorders include the following:

- restless legs syndrome (RLS)
- periodic limb movement disorder (PLMD)
- obstructive sleep apnea (OSA)
- irregular sleep–wake rhythm disorder (ISWRD)
- sleep-related dissociative disorders

The following are the factors that may lead to the development of SRED:

- dieting during the day
- daytime eating disorders
- ending the abuse of alcohol or drugs
- use of certain medications
- quitting smoking

SRED may result in:

- encephalitis (brain swelling)
- hepatitis (liver infection)
- narcolepsy
- stress

## DIAGNOSIS OF NOCTURNAL SLEEP-RELATED EATING DISORDER

It is important for patients to inform their doctor when this eating disorder begins. Keep your doctor informed about your complete medical history. Make sure to inform the doctor of any medication that you have been taking. Maintain a sleep diary to help the doctor understand your sleeping patterns. The doctor will do an overnight sleep study called a "polysomnogram." The polysomnogram will chart your brain waves, heartbeat, and breathing as you sleep. The unusual behaviors that occur during the night will be recorded on a video, which will help your doctor determine the patterns of your SRED.

## TREATMENT FOR NOCTURNAL SLEEP-RELATED EATING DISORDER

Treatment for SREDs involves stress management classes, counseling, clinical interview, and limited intake or avoidance of alcohol and caffeine. The physician may change some of your medicines to make it easier for you to treat SREDs. Plenty of sleep is required on a daily basis. It is important to consult a sleep specialist to check for signs of sleep disorders.

Consulting a psychotherapist may help reduce stress and anxiety. The physician may recommend medicines such as benzodiazepine to treat your sleep-related disorder. Mirapex and Sinemet are effective dopaminergic agents for sleep eaters.

### References

"Sleep Eating Disorder—Overview and Facts," American Academy of Sleep Medicine, September 2020. Available online. URL: www.sleepeducation.org/sleep-disorders-by-category/parasomnias/sleep-eating-disorder/overview-facts. Accessed May 8, 2023.

"Sleep-Related Eating Disorders," The Cleveland Clinic Foundation, April 22, 2017. Available online. URL: https://my.clevelandclinic.org/health/articles/12123-sleep-related-eating-disorders. Accessed May 8, 2023.

"Sleep-Related Eating Disorders," National Center for Biotechnology Information (NCBI), November 2006. Available online. URL: www.ncbi.nlm.nih.gov/pmc/articles/PMC2945843. Accessed May 8, 2023.

# Chapter 25 | **Parasomnias**

## WHAT ARE PARASOMNIAS?

Parasomnias are "odd" actions that we do or unpleasant events that we experience while asleep or while partially asleep. Almost everyone has a nightmare. A nightmare is considered a parasomnia since it is an unpleasant event that occurs while we are asleep.

The term "parasomnia" is much broader than just nightmares, however. Other common parasomnia events include:
- rapid eye movement (REM) behavior disorder (RBD)
- sleep paralysis
- sleepwalking
- confusional arousals

## WHAT ARE COMMON PARASOMNIAS?

Parasomnias are typically classified by whether they occur during REM sleep or non-REM sleep. The REM sleep parasomnias tend to present as traits of wakefulness while in REM sleep or as traits of REM sleep while awake. The non-REM sleep parasomnias tend to present as a middle ground where the patient is doing activities but is not fully awake.

### Rapid Eye Movement Behavior Disorder

Most dreaming occurs in REM sleep. Normally, in REM sleep, most of our body muscles are paralyzed to prevent us from acting out our dreams. In REM behavior disorder, a person does not have this protective paralysis during REM sleep. A person, therefore, might "act out" their dream. Since dreams may involve violence and protecting oneself, a person acting out their dream may injure themselves or their bed partner. The person will usually recall the dream but not realize that they were moving in real life.

## Sleep Paralysis and Sleep Hallucinations

REM sleep is usually associated with dreams, and the body paralyzes most of the muscles, so dreams do not get acted out. Sometimes, REM-related paralysis or dream images can occur when falling asleep or when waking up from sleep. Sleep paralysis and sleep hallucinations can occur together or alone. The person is fully aware of what is happening. Events can be very scary. An event will usually last seconds to minutes and fortunately end on its own.

## Sleepwalking

In sleepwalking, the person is just awake enough to be active but is still asleep and unaware of the activities. Sometimes, disorders such as sleepwalking are called "disorders of arousal" since the person is in a mixed state of awareness (not fully asleep or awake). Sleepwalking disorders can range from sitting up in bed to complex behaviors, such as driving a car. Sleepwalkers are unaware of their surroundings and can fall down or put themselves in danger. Despite the myths, it is not dangerous to awaken a sleepwalker. However, the person will not typically recall the sleepwalking event and may be confused or disoriented.

## Confusional Arousals

We all have experienced that strange and confused feeling when we first wake up. Confusional arousal is a sleep disorder that causes a person to act that way for a prolonged period. Episodes usually start when someone is abruptly woken up. The person does not wake up completely and so remains in a foggy state of mind. The person with confusional arousal may have difficulty understanding situations around them, react slowly to commands, or react aggressively as the first response to others.

## WHAT CAN YOU DO FOR PARASOMNIAS?

Many people with parasomnias see an improvement by improving their sleep habits. Some healthy sleep tips include the following:
- Ensure you are getting enough sleep.
- Keep a regular schedule of going to bed and waking up.
- Avoid alcohol or other sedatives at night that might make it hard for you to wake up completely.
- Avoid caffeine or smoking.
- Keep the bedroom quiet to avoid getting disturbed.

Make sure that persons suffering from parasomnias remain safe. Some tips for bedroom safety with a parasomnia include the following:
- Avoid large objects that can fall by the bedside.
- Make sure there are no objects on the floor that can be tripped over.
- Close and lock bedroom doors and windows to ensure a person cannot go outside.
- Consider an alarm or bell on the door.
- Close shades over windows in case they are hit to protect a person from glass.
- Remove potentially dangerous objects and weapons in the bedroom.
- Avoid significant elevation and bunk beds. Consider mattresses on the ground and ground-floor bedrooms.[1]

---

[1] "Parasomnia," U.S. Department of Veterans Affairs (VA), August 14, 2015. Available online. URL: www.paloalto.va.gov/services/pulmonary/parasomnia.asp. Accessed March 27, 2023.

# Chapter 26 | **Sleep-Related Movement Disorders**

**Chapter Contents**

Periodic limb movement disorder (PLMD) is a sleep disorder where a person repeatedly moves their arms and legs while sleeping. These movements can last minutes or hours and happen every 20–40 seconds.

Around 4–11 percent of the population is affected by PLMD, which can happen at any age but is more frequent in older individuals. The movements occur during light non-rapid eye movement (non-REM) sleep and can also be detected in other sleep disorders such as narcolepsy and obstructive sleep apnea (OSA). PLMD can interrupt sleep, causing tiredness during the day.

People with PLMD may not be aware of this disorder, as they may only experience symptoms such as waking up at night or feeling tired during the day. PLMD can be diagnosed by observing the person's sleep or conducting a sleep study. Many people with PLMD also have restless legs syndrome (RLS), but PLMD is a separate condition.

## CAUSES AND RISK FACTORS OF PERIODIC LIMB MOVEMENT DISORDER

The exact cause of PLMD is unknown, but low iron levels or nerve problems caused by other illnesses, such as diabetes, may play a role. Researchers have not uncovered the cause of primary PLMD although some believe it may be linked to abnormalities in regulating nerve impulses from the brain to the limbs. PLMD affects males and females equally and can affect people of any age. However, the incidence of PLMD increases with age and affects 34 percent of people over 60.

Underlying medical conditions, including the following, cause secondary PLMD:
- diabetes
- iron deficiency anemia
- spinal cord injury
- RLS
- sleep apnea

- narcolepsy
- REM sleep behavior disorder
- sleep-related eating disorder
- multiple system atrophy

Certain medications have also been found to increase the risk or worsen symptoms of PLMD, including antidepressants such as amitriptyline (Elavil) and lithium, dopamine-receptor antagonists such as Haldol, and withdrawal from sedatives such as Valium.

## DIAGNOSIS OF PERIODIC LIMB MOVEMENT DISORDER
Diagnosis of PLMD begins with a visit to a sleep specialist. Patients are typically asked to keep a sleep diary for several weeks, to evaluate their sleep using a rating system, such as the Epworth Sleepiness Scale, and to provide a complete medical history, including any medications taken. In most cases, patients will then undergo an overnight sleep study, during which a polysomnogram keeps track of brain activity, heartbeat, breathing, and limb movement. In addition to diagnosing PLMD and other sleep disorders, the sleep specialist can help identify other potential causes of sleep problems, such as medical conditions, medications, substance abuse, or mental health disorders.

Other medical tests can be used to detect underlying causes of PLMD, such as diabetes, anemia, or metabolic disorders. Doctors may take blood samples to check hormone levels, organ function, and blood chemistry. They may also look for infections or traces of drugs that can contribute to secondary PLMD. If no underlying cause can be found, the patient may be referred to a neurologist to rule out nervous system disorders and confirm the diagnosis of PLMD.

## TREATMENT FOR PERIODIC LIMB MOVEMENT DISORDER
Many people with PLMD do not experience symptoms or require treatment. When sleep disruption makes treatment necessary, however, several medications are available to help reduce the

movements or help the patient sleep through them. Some of the medications commonly prescribed to treat PLMD include:

- benzodiazepines, such as clonazepam (Klonopin), which suppress muscle contractions
- anticonvulsant agents such as gabapentin (Neurontin), which also reduce muscle contractions
- dopaminergic agents such as levodopa/carbidopa (Sinemet) and pergolide (Permax), which increase the levels of the neurotransmitter dopamine in the brain and are also used to treat Parkinson disease (PD) and RLS
- gamma-aminobutyric acid (GABA) agonists, such as baclofen (Lioresal), which inhibit the release of neurotransmitters in the brain that stimulate muscle contractions

While there is no cure for PLMD, medical treatments are available to help manage its symptoms. People with primary PLMD may experience the condition in the long term, with occasional periods of improved sleep. Secondary PLMD, caused by an underlying condition, can be fully treated by addressing the underlying issue. If an individual is experiencing trouble sleeping or suspects they have PLMD, it is essential to seek medical attention. A doctor may refer them to a specialist for further treatment, and attending follow-up appointments is crucial to managing any health issues.

## References

Cafasso, Jacquelyn. "What Is Periodic Limb Movement Disorder?" Healthline Media LLC., September 17, 2018. Available online. URL: www.healthline.com/health/sleep-disorder-periodic-limb-movement. Accessed April 11, 2023.

Foley, Logan. "Periodic Limb Movements Disorder," Sleep Foundation, March 2, 2023. Available online. URL: www. sleepfoundation.org/periodic-limb-movement-disorder. Accessed April 11, 2023.

"Periodic Limb Movements," American Academy of Sleep Medicine (AASM), September 2020. Available online. URL: https://sleepeducation.org/sleep-disorders/periodic-limb-movements/#what-are-perioodic-limb-movements. Accessed April 11, 2023.

"Periodic Limb Movement Disorder," WebMD, May 14, 2022. Available online. URL: www.webmd.com/sleep-disorders/periodic-limb-movement-disorder. Accessed April 11, 2023.

"Periodic Limb Movement Disorder (PLMD) in Adults," Cleveland Clinic, July 21, 2012. Available online. URL: https://my.clevelandclinic.org/health/diseases/14177-periodic-limb-movement-disorder-plmd-in-adults. Accessed April 11, 2023.

## Section 26.2 | Restless Legs Syndrome

## WHAT IS RESTLESS LEGS SYNDROME?

Restless legs syndrome (RLS)—also known as "Willis-Ekbom disease," primary RLS, and idiopathic RLS—is a neurological disorder that causes unpleasant or uncomfortable sensations in your legs and an irresistible urge to move them. Symptoms commonly occur in the late afternoon or evening hours and are often most intense at night when you are resting. RLS can severely disrupt your sleep, making it difficult to fall asleep or return to sleep after waking up. Moving the legs or walking typically relieves the discomfort, but the sensations often recur once the movement stops.

RLS is both a sleep disorder because the symptoms are triggered by resting and attempting to sleep and a movement disorder because people with RLS are forced to move their legs in order to relieve symptoms.

It is estimated that up to 7–10 percent of the United States population may have RLS, which can begin at any age. It occurs in both males and females although females are more likely to have it. Many individuals who are severely affected are middle-aged or older, and

278

the symptoms typically become more frequent and last longer with age. RLS is generally a lifelong condition for which there is no cure. However, treatments are available to ease symptoms.

## COMMON SIGNS AND SYMPTOMS OF RESTLESS LEGS SYNDROME

If you have RLS, you may feel an irresistible urge to move, which is accompanied by uncomfortable sensations in your lower limbs that are unlike normal sensations experienced by someone without the disorder. The sensations in your legs may feel like aching, throbbing, pulling, itching, crawling, or creeping. These sensations less commonly affect the arms and rarely the chest or head. Although the sensations can occur on just one side of your body, they most often affect both sides.

Common characteristics of RLS include the following:

- Sensations that begin after rest. They typically occur when you are inactive and sitting for extended periods (e.g., when taking a trip by plane or watching a movie).
- Relief of discomfort with movement. You may need to keep your legs (or other affected parts of the body) in motion to minimize or prevent the sensations. You might need to pace the floor or constantly move your legs while sitting.
- Worsening of symptoms at night with a distinct symptom-free period in the early morning. You might have difficulty falling asleep and staying asleep. You may also note a worsening of symptoms if your sleep is further reduced by events or activity.

RLS symptoms may vary from day to day, in severity and frequency, and from person to person. With moderately severe RLS, your symptoms might only occur once or twice a week but often result in a significant delay of sleep onset, with some disruption of daytime function. In severe cases of RLS, the symptoms occur more than twice a week.

RLS can cause you to experience the following:

- changes in mood
- exhaustion and daytime sleepiness

- problems concentrating
- impaired memory
- decreased productivity
- depression and anxiety

You might experience remissions—periods in which symptoms decrease or disappear for weeks or months—usually during the early stages of the disorder. In general, however, symptoms often reappear and become more severe over time.

## IS PERIODIC LIMB MOVEMENT OF SLEEP THE SAME OR DIFFERENT FROM RESTLESS LEGS SYNDROME?

More than 80 percent of people with RLS also experience periodic limb movement of sleep (PLMS). PLMS is characterized by involuntary leg (and sometimes arm) twitching or jerking movements during sleep that typically occur every 15–40 seconds, sometimes throughout the night. Although many individuals with RLS also develop PLMS, most people with PLMS do not experience RLS.

## WHO IS MORE LIKELY TO HAVE RESTLESS LEGS SYNDROME?

In most cases, the cause of RLS is unknown. However, RLS often runs in families, and specific gene variants have been associated with the condition. Low levels of iron in the brain may also be responsible for RLS.

RLS may also be related to a dysfunction in a part of your brain that controls movement. The basal ganglia uses the brain chemical dopamine to produce smooth, purposeful muscle activity and movement. Disruption of dopamine levels in the brain frequently results in involuntary movements. Individuals living with the movement disorder Parkinson disease (PD) have an increased risk of developing RLS.

RLS also appears to be related to or accompany the following factors or underlying conditions:
- end-stage renal disease and hemodialysis
- neuropathy (nerve damage)
- sleep deprivation and other sleep conditions, such as sleep apnea

- pregnancy or hormonal changes, especially in the last trimester. In most cases, symptoms usually disappear within four weeks after delivery
- use of alcohol, nicotine, and caffeine

Certain medications may aggravate your RLS symptoms, such as some antinausea drugs, antipsychotic drugs, antidepressants that increase serotonin, and cold and allergy medications that contain older antihistamines.

## HOW IS RESTLESS LEGS SYNDROME DIAGNOSED AND TREATED?
### Diagnosing Restless Legs Syndrome

There is no specific test for RLS, so the condition is diagnosed by a doctor's evaluation. The five basic criteria for clinically diagnosing RLS include the following:

- A strong and often overwhelming need or urge to move your legs is often associated with abnormal, unpleasant, or uncomfortable sensations.
- The urge to move your legs starts or gets worse during rest or inactivity.
- The urge to move your legs is at least temporarily and partially or totally relieved by movements.
- The urge to move your legs starts or is aggravated in the evening or night.
- The above four features are not due to any other medical or behavioral condition.

A neurological and physical exam, plus information about your medical and family history and a list of current medications, may be helpful. You should talk with your doctor about the frequency, duration, and intensity of your symptoms—if movement helps relieve them; how much time it takes to fall asleep; any pain related to symptoms; and any tendency toward daytime sleep patterns and sleepiness, disturbance of sleep, or daytime function.

Blood tests may rule out other conditions that may be causing your RLS symptoms, such as kidney failure, low iron levels, and other causes of sleep disruption, such as sleep apnea and pregnancy.

In fact, about 25 percent of pregnant females develop RLS, but the symptoms often disappear after giving birth.

Diagnosing RLS in children may be especially difficult as it may be hard for children to describe their symptoms. Pediatric RLS can sometimes be misdiagnosed as "growing pains" or attention deficit hyperactivity disorder.

## Treating Restless Legs Syndrome

There is no cure for RLS, but some symptoms can be treated. Moving your affected limb(s) may provide temporary relief. Sometimes, RLS symptoms can be controlled by treating an associated medical condition, such as peripheral neuropathy, diabetes, or iron deficiency anemia.

Medications for RLS include the following:

- **Antiseizure drugs**. Antiseizure drugs are the first-line prescription drugs for those with RLS. The U.S. Food and Drug Administration (FDA) approved gabapentin enacarbil for the treatment of moderate-to-severe RLS. Other antiseizure drugs, such as pregabalin, can decrease such sensory disturbances and nerve pain.
- **Dopaminergic agents**. These drugs, which increase dopamine in the brain, can reduce symptoms of RLS when taken at night. The medications ropinirole, pramipexole, and rotigotine are FDA-approved to treat moderate-to-severe RLS. Levodopa plus carbidopa may be effective when used intermittently but not daily because long-term use of dopaminergic drugs can eventually worsen symptoms and cause other complications.
- **Opioids**. Drugs such as methadone, codeine, hydrocodone, or oxycodone are sometimes prescribed to treat individuals with more severe symptoms of RLS who do not respond well to other medications.
- **Benzodiazepines**. Medications such as clonazepam and lorazepam are generally prescribed to treat anxiety, muscle spasms, and insomnia and can help individuals get more restful sleep.

- **Iron supplements**. Low iron in the brain is one of the most common causes of RLS. Taking iron supplements in the form of a pill or injection can increase the iron levels in the brain.

The following lifestyle changes and activities may provide some relief if you have mild-to-moderate RLS:
- Avoid or decrease the use of alcohol, nicotine, and caffeine.
- Change or maintain a regular sleep pattern.
- Try moderate, regular exercise.
- Massage the legs or take a warm bath.
- Apply a heating pad or ice pack.
- Use foot wraps specially designed for people with RLS or vibration pads to the back of the legs.
- Do aerobic and leg-stretching exercises of moderate intensity.

## WHAT ARE THE LATEST UPDATES ON RESTLESS LEGS SYNDROME?

The National Institute of Neurological Disorders and Stroke (NINDS) is the primary federal funding agency for research on RLS. The NINDS is a component of the National Institutes of Health (NIH), a leading supporter of biomedical research in the world.
- Researchers are investigating changes in the brain's signaling pathways that are likely to contribute to RLS. In particular, researchers suspect that impaired transmission of dopamine in the brain's basal ganglia may play a role. Researchers also hope to discover genetic relationships in RLS and to better understand what causes the disease.
- NINDS-funded researchers are studying the role of epigenetics in RLS development. Epigenetic changes can switch genes on or off, which can broadly impact both health and disease. Evidence suggests that iron deficiency during pregnancy, infancy, and childhood increases the risk of developing RLS later in life. Scientists hope that understanding epigenetic

changes associated with iron deficiency can offer new information on how to prevent RLS.

- The NINDS also supports research on why the use of dopamine agents to treat RLS, PD, and other movement disorders can lead to impulse control disorders, with the aim to develop new or improved treatments that avoid this adverse side effect.
- NINDS-funded researchers are using advanced magnetic resonance imaging (MRI) to measure brain chemical changes in the brain's arousal system in individuals with RLS to develop new research models and ways to correct the overactive arousal process.
- Scientists currently do not fully understand the mechanisms through which iron gets into the brain and how those mechanisms are regulated. NINDS-funded researchers are studying the role of endothelial cells— part of the protective lining called the "blood-brain barrier" that separates circulating blood from the fluid surrounding brain tissue—in the regulation of cerebral iron metabolism. Results may offer new insights into treating the cognitive and movement symptoms associated with RLS.
- Researchers are also testing nondrug therapies such as a compact, wearable, noninvasive nerve stimulation device designed to treat RLS during sleep.

## HOW CAN YOU OR YOUR LOVED ONE HELP IMPROVE CARE FOR PEOPLE WITH RESTLESS LEGS SYNDROME?

Consider participating in a clinical trial, so clinicians and scientists can learn more about RLS. Clinical research uses human volunteers to help researchers learn more about a disorder and perhaps find better ways to safely detect, treat, or prevent disease.

All types of volunteers are needed—those who are healthy or may have an illness or disease—of all different ages, sexes, races, and ethnicities to ensure that study results apply to as many people as possible and that treatments will be safe and effective for everyone who will use them.[1]

## Section 26.3 | **Sleepwalking or Somnambulism**

Somnambulism, commonly called "sleepwalking," is a type of parasomnia that is characterized by undesirable physical events that disrupt sleep before, during, or upon waking up. During sleepwalking, individuals get up and walk around while still in a state of sleep. This condition is more prevalent in children than adults. According to the National Center for Biotechnology Information, approximately 1.5 percent of adults have experienced sleepwalking episodes beyond childhood.

Sleepwalking is more likely to occur in individuals with a family history of the condition, those who are sleep deprived, or those who experience repeated nighttime awakenings. Sleepwalking incidents can lead to injuries, and individuals who sleepwalk may experience poor sleep quality and daytime sleepiness. According to the National Institutes of Health, 6.9 percent of people have experienced at least one sleepwalking episode.

## CAUSES OF SLEEPWALKING

Sleepwalking occurs during the non-rapid eye movement (non-REM) sleep stage. Recurrent sleepwalking can indicate an underlying sleep disorder and may be caused by many factors, including:

- hereditary factors
- sleep deprivation
- stress
- fever

---

[1] "Restless Legs Syndrome," National Institute of Neurological Disorders and Stroke (NINDS), February 7, 2023. Available online. URL: www.ninds.nih.gov/health-information/disorders/restless-legs-syndrome. Accessed March 29, 2023.

- sleep schedule disruptions
- breathing disorders, such as obstructive sleep apnea (OSA)
- gastroesophageal reflux disease (GERD)

Other underlying medical conditions that can contribute to sleepwalking include:
- restless legs syndrome (RLS)
- Parkinson disease (PD)
- chronic migraine
- medications such as antidepressants, antipsychotics, and sleep-inducing drugs

## SYMPTOMS OF SLEEPWALKING

Sleepwalking frequently occurs within the first few hours of falling asleep and seldom happens during naps. Although sleepwalking episodes typically persist for several minutes, they may last longer and can happen on a regular or sporadic basis.

Individuals who sleepwalk exhibit symptoms of simple or complex behaviors, such as walking, running, moving furniture, preparing food, eating, engaging in sexual activity, or urinating in inappropriate locations. Occasionally, the behavior may be more complicated, such as attempting to operate a vehicle or showing violent tendencies. Throughout a sleepwalking episode, an individual may have open eyes with a vacant look, be minimally responsive, or have unclear speech. Sleepwalkers may also experience sleep terrors.

Sleepwalkers typically do not respond to attempts to get their attention and may appear dazed or distant. They may either return to bed and fall asleep or wake up confused while still outside of bed. A notable symptom of sleepwalking is that the individual usually has no recollection of the episode upon waking up. Therefore, they often learn of their sleepwalking from family or roommates. Sleepwalkers may be challenging to rouse during an episode and may be disorientated or confused upon awakening. They may have difficulty functioning during the day due to disrupted sleep.

## DIAGNOSIS OF SLEEPWALKING

Sleepwalking typically does not require examinations or testing. Still, if episodes occur frequently, health-care providers may perform tests to rule out other disorders that could be confused with sleepwalking, such as seizures. Moreover, individuals with a history of emotional problems may need a mental health evaluation to identify potential causes, such as anxiety or stress.

Health-care providers typically review the patient's medical history and symptoms to diagnose sleepwalking. The evaluation may involve a physical examination to identify sleep disorders, panic attacks, or other conditions that might be mistaken for sleepwalking. The doctor may also ask the patient and their sleep partner to complete a questionnaire about their sleep behaviors and discuss the patient's symptoms.

Health-care providers may sometimes suggest polysomnography, a sleep study conducted in a sleep laboratory overnight. This study entails placing sensors on the patient's body to monitor their brain waves, blood oxygen level, heart rate, breathing, and eye and leg movements while they sleep. Patients may also be videotaped to document their behavior during various sleep cycles to diagnose sleepwalking better.

## TREATMENT FOR SLEEPWALKING

Sleepwalking typically does not require active treatment since it occurs infrequently and poses minimal risks to the sleepwalker and those around them. Nonetheless, treatment may be necessary if sleepwalking leads to potential harm, disrupts the sleep of family members, or causes embarrassment.

Treatment for sleepwalking varies depending on the patient's age, frequency of occurrence, and severity of the episodes. The primary step is removing potential safety risks, such as tripping hazards, and locking away sharp objects or weapons. Additional treatment may involve addressing underlying medical conditions, modifying medications, or utilizing anticipatory awakenings, where the person is awoken approximately 15 minutes before their usual sleepwalking time and remains awake briefly before returning to sleep.

Improving sleep hygiene can also help reduce the risk of sleep-walking. Cognitive behavioral therapy (CBT) may assist in preventing stress-related episodes. In some cases, medication such as benzodiazepines or antidepressants may be necessary, but it is essential to consult a health-care provider before taking them. Seeking medical attention is highly recommended to determine the likely cause and create a personalized treatment plan if dangerous activities occur while sleepwalking or other symptoms are present.

## References

"Sleepwalking," Cleveland Clinic, January 22, 2020. Available online. URL: https://my.clevelandclinic.org/health/diseases/14292-sleepwalking. Accessed April 17, 2023.

"Sleepwalking," Mayo Foundation for Medical Education and Research (MFMER), July 21, 2017. Available online. URL: www.mayoclinic.org/diseases-conditions/sleepwalking/symptoms-causes/syc-20353506. Accessed April 17, 2023.

"Sleep Walking," University of Pennsylvania, May 4, 2021. Available online. URL: www.pennmedicine.org/for-patients-and-visitors/patient-information/conditions-treated-a-to-z/sleep-walking. Accessed April 17, 2023.

Stanborough, Rebecca Joy. "What Causes Sleepwalking?" Healthline Media, July 21, 2020. Available online. URL: www.healthline.com/health/why-do-people-sleepwalk. Accessed April 17, 2023.

Suni, Eric. "Sleepwalking: What Is Somnambulism?" Sleep Foundation, March 17, 2023. Available online. URL: www.sleepfoundation.org/parasomnias/sleepwalking. Accessed April 17, 2023.

# Part 4 | Other Health Problems That Often Affect Sleep

# Chapter 27 | Mental Health Disorders and Sleep Issues

## Chapter Contents

## Section 27.1 | Attention Deficit Hyperactivity Disorder and Sleep

### WHAT IS ATTENTION DEFICIT HYPERACTIVITY DISORDER?

Attention deficit hyperactivity disorder (ADHD) is a problem of not being able to focus, being overactive, not being able to control behavior, or a combination of these. For these problems to be diagnosed as ADHD, they must be out of the normal range for a person's age and development.

### CAUSES OF ATTENTION DEFICIT HYPERACTIVITY DISORDER

Attention deficit hyperactivity disorder usually begins in childhood but may continue into the adult years. It is the most commonly diagnosed behavioral disorder in children. ADHD is diagnosed much more often in boys than in girls.

It is not clear what causes ADHD. A combination of genes and environmental factors likely plays a role in the development of the condition. Imaging studies suggest that the brains of children with ADHD are different from those of children without ADHD.

### SYMPTOMS OF ATTENTION DEFICIT HYPERACTIVITY DISORDER

Symptoms of ADHD fall into the following three groups:
- not being able to focus (inattentiveness)
- being extremely active (hyperactivity)
- not being able to control behavior (impulsivity)

Some people with ADHD have mainly inattentive symptoms. Some have mainly hyperactive and impulsive symptoms. Others have a combination of different symptom types. Those with mostly inattentive symptoms are sometimes said to have attention deficit disorder (ADD). They tend to be less disruptive and are more likely not to be diagnosed with ADHD.

Inattentive symptoms include the following:
- failing to give close attention to details or making careless mistakes in schoolwork
- having difficulty keeping attention during tasks or play

- not seeming to listen when spoken to directly
- not following through on instructions and failing to finish schoolwork or chores and tasks
- having problems organizing tasks and activities
- avoiding or disliking tasks that require sustained mental effort (such as schoolwork)
- often losing toys, assignments, pencils, books, or tools needed for tasks or activities
- being easily distracted
- being often forgetful in daily activities

Hyperactivity symptoms include the following:
- fidgeting with hands or feet or squirming in the seat
- leaving the seat when remaining seated is expected
- running about or climbing in inappropriate situations
- having problems playing or working quietly
- acting as if "on the go" or "driven by a motor"
- talking excessively

Impulsivity symptoms include the following:
- blurting out answers before questions have been completed
- having difficulty awaiting their turn
- interrupting or intruding on others (butting in conversations or games)[1]

## HOW DOES SLEEP AFFECT ATTENTION DEFICIT HYPERACTIVITY DISORDER?

Sleep deprivation among adolescents is a common problem in the United States, and researchers have found substantial links between ADHD and sleep issues. Adolescents who are diagnosed with ADHD tend to experience problems such as trouble falling asleep, staying asleep, and disrupted sleep. The National Sleep

[1] MentalHealth.gov, "Attention Deficit Hyperactivity Disorder (ADHD)," U.S. Department of Health and Human Services (HHS), August 22, 2017. Available online. URL: www.mentalhealth.gov/what-to-look-for/behavioral-disorders/adhd. Accessed March 23, 2023.

Foundation (NSF) studies have found that 50 percent of children and teens with ADHD suffer from sleep-disordered breathing and have more daytime sleepiness when compared to just 22 percent of other children and teens. Sleep issues can aggravate ADHD symptoms, and a few studies have even suggested that regular sleep patterns can help eliminate hyperactivity among some young people.

Interestingly, lack of sleep affects children and teens quite differently than it affects adults. While adults who get very little sleep generally become lethargic, young people tend to get high-strung and inattentive and often display disruptive behavior. As a result, sleep disorders in children and teens can lead to more serious issues in school, at home, and in social situations.

Here are some tips to help teens with ADHD get better sleep:

- Caffeine is a major stimulant; therefore, avoiding caffeinated beverages and foods can help ensure proper sleep.
- Consistent habits, such as specific bedtimes, waking times, and a healthy diet, can be helpful.
- A dark, quiet, and cozy room helps promote undisturbed sleep.
- Avoid sleep medication, which can result in daytime grogginess and lead to dependency.
- Daily exercise can help teens sleep better.
- Take a warm bath before bedtime to encourage relaxation.

# References

"ADHD and Sleep," Sleep Foundation, March 17, 2023. Available online. URL: www.sleepfoundation.org/mental-health/adhd-and-sleep. Accessed March 23, 2023.

Bhandari, Smitha "ADHD and Sleep Disorders," WebMD, November 18, 2014. Available online. URL: www.webmd.com/add-adhd/childhood-adhd/adhd-sleep-disorders. Accessed March 23, 2023.

"Diagnosing ADHD in Adolescence," CHADD, n.d. Available online. URL: https://chadd.org/for-parents/

diagnosing-adhd-in-adolescence. Accessed March 23, 2023.

Karen Spruyt, David Gozal, "Sleep Disturbances in Children with Attention-Deficit/Hyperactivity Disorder," *Expert Review of Neurotherapeutics*, 11, no. 4 (2011): 565–577. https://doi.org/10.1586/ern.11.7.

## Section 27.2 | **Depression and Sleep**

## WHAT IS DEPRESSION?

Depression (also known as "major depression," "major depressive disorder," or "clinical depression") is a common but serious mood disorder. It causes severe symptoms that affect how a person feels, thinks, and handles daily activities, such as sleeping, eating, or working. To be diagnosed with depression, the symptoms must be present for at least two weeks.

There are different types of depression, some of which develop due to specific circumstances:

- **Major depression**. It includes symptoms of depressed mood or loss of interest, most of the time for at least two weeks, that interfere with daily activities.
- **Persistent depressive disorder**. It (also called "dysthymia" or "dysthymic disorder") consists of less severe symptoms of depression that last much longer, usually for at least two years.
- **Perinatal depression**. It is a depression that occurs during or after pregnancy. Depression that begins during pregnancy is prenatal depression, and depression that begins after the baby is born is postpartum depression.
- **Seasonal affective disorder**. It is a depression that comes and goes with the seasons, with symptoms typically starting in the late fall and early winter and going away during the spring and summer.

- **Depression with symptoms of psychosis**. It is a severe form of depression in which a person experiences psychosis symptoms, such as delusions (disturbing, false fixed beliefs) or hallucinations (hearing or seeing things others do not hear or see).

People with bipolar disorder (formerly called "manic depression" or "manic-depressive illness") also experience depressive episodes, during which they feel sad, indifferent, or hopeless, combined with a very low activity level. But a person with bipolar disorder also experiences manic (or less severe hypomanic) episodes, or unusually elevated moods, in which they might feel very happy, irritable, or "up," with a marked increase in the activity level.

Other types of depressive disorders found in the *Diagnostic and Statistical Manual of Mental Disorders, Fifth Edition* (*DSM-5*) include disruptive mood dysregulation disorder (diagnosed in children and adolescents) and premenstrual dysphoric disorder (that affects women around the time of their period). Figure 27.1 shows the episodes of mania and depression.

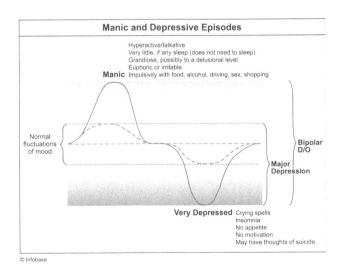

© Infobase

**Figure 27.1.** Manic and Depressive Episodes

*Infobase*

## WHO GETS DEPRESSION?

Depression can affect people of all ages, races, ethnicities, and genders. Women are diagnosed with depression more often than men, but men can also be depressed. Because men may be less likely to recognize, talk about, and seek help for their feelings or emotional problems, they are at a greater risk of depression symptoms being undiagnosed or undertreated. Studies also show higher rates of depression and an increased risk of the disorder among members of the lesbian, gay, bisexual, transgender, queer or questioning, intersex, asexual, and more (LGBTQIA+) community.

## WHAT ARE THE SIGNS AND SYMPTOMS OF DEPRESSION?

If you have been experiencing some of the following signs and symptoms most of the day, nearly every day, for at least two weeks, you may be suffering from depression:

- persistent sad, anxious, or "empty" mood
- feelings of hopelessness or pessimism
- feelings of irritability, frustration, or restlessness
- feelings of guilt, worthlessness, or helplessness
- loss of interest or pleasure in hobbies and activities
- decreased energy, fatigue, or feeling slowed down
- difficulty concentrating, remembering, or making decisions
- difficulty sleeping, waking early in the morning, or oversleeping
- changes in appetite or unplanned weight changes
- physical aches or pains, headaches, cramps, or digestive problems that do not have a clear physical cause and do not go away with treatment
- thoughts of death or suicide or suicide attempts

Not everyone who is depressed experiences every one of these symptoms. Some people experience only a few symptoms, while others experience many symptoms. Symptoms associated with depression interfere with day-to-day functioning and cause significant distress for the person experiencing them.

Depression can also involve other changes in mood or behavior that include the following:
- increased anger or irritability
- feeling restless or on edge
- becoming withdrawn, negative, or detached
- increased engagement in high-risk activities
- greater impulsivity
- increased use of alcohol or drugs
- isolating from family and friends
- inability to meet the responsibilities of work and family or ignoring other important roles
- problems with sexual desire and performance

Depression can look different in men and women. Although men, women, and people of all genders can feel depressed, how they express those symptoms and the behaviors they use to cope with them may differ. For example, some men (as well as women) may show symptoms other than sadness, instead seeming angry or irritable. And, although increased use of alcohol or drugs can be a coping strategy for any person with depression, men may be more likely to use alcohol or drugs to cope.

In some cases, mental health symptoms appear as physical problems, for example, a racing heart, tightened chest, ongoing headaches, or digestive issues. Men are often more likely to see a health-care provider about these physical symptoms than their emotional ones.

Because depression tends to make people think more negatively about themselves and the world, some people may also have thoughts of suicide or self-harm.

Several persistent symptoms, in addition to low mood, are required for a diagnosis of depression, but people with only a few symptoms may also benefit from treatment. The severity and frequency of symptoms and how long they last will vary depending on the person, the illness, and the stage of the illness.

If you experience signs or symptoms of depression and they persist or do not go away, talk to a health-care provider. If you see signs or symptoms of depression in someone you know, encourage them to seek help from a mental health professional.

## WHAT ARE THE RISK FACTORS FOR DEPRESSION?

Depression is one of the most common mental disorders in the United States. Research suggests that genetic, biological, environmental, and psychological factors play a role in depression.

Depression can happen at any age, but it often begins in adulthood. Depression is now recognized as occurring in children and adolescents although children may express more irritability than sadness. Many chronic mood and anxiety disorders in adults begin as high levels of anxiety in childhood.

Depression, especially in midlife or older age, can co-occur with other serious medical illnesses, such as diabetes, cancer, heart disease, and Parkinson disease. These conditions are often worse when depression is present, and research suggests that people with depression and other medical illnesses tend to have more severe symptoms of both illnesses. The Centers for Disease Control and Prevention (CDC) has also recognized that having certain mental disorders, including depression and schizophrenia, can make people more likely to get severely ill from COVID-19.

Sometimes, a physical health problem, such as thyroid disease, or medications taken for a physical illness cause side effects that contribute to depression. A health-care provider experienced in treating these complicated illnesses can help work out the best treatment strategy.

Other risk factors for depression include the following:
- personal or family history of depression
- major negative life changes, trauma, or stress

## HOW IS DEPRESSION TREATED?

Depression, even in the most severe cases, can be treated. The earlier treatment begins, the more effective it is. Depression is usually treated with medication, psychotherapy, or a combination of the two.

Some people may experience treatment-resistant depression, which occurs when a person does not get better after trying at least two antidepressant medications. If treatments such as medication and psychotherapy do not reduce depressive symptoms or the need for rapid relief from symptoms is urgent, brain stimulation therapy may be an option to explore.

No two people are affected the same way by depression, and there is no "one-size-fits-all" treatment. Finding the treatment that works best for you may take trial and error.

## Medications

Antidepressants are medications commonly used to treat depression. They work by changing how the brain produces or uses certain chemicals involved in mood or stress. You may need to try several different antidepressants before finding the one that improves your symptoms and has manageable side effects. A medication that has helped you or a close family member in the past will often be considered first.

Antidepressants take time—usually four to eight weeks—to work, and problems with sleep, appetite, and concentration often improve before mood lifts. It is important to give a medication a chance to work before deciding whether it is the right one for you.

New medications, such as intranasal esketamine, can have rapidly acting antidepressant effects, especially for people with treatment-resistant depression. Esketamine is a medication approved by the U.S. Food and Drug Administration (FDA) for treatment-resistant depression. Delivered as a nasal spray in a doctor's office, clinic, or hospital, it acts rapidly, typically within a couple of hours, to relieve depression symptoms. People who use esketamine will usually continue taking an oral antidepressant to maintain the improvement in their symptoms.

Another option for treatment-resistant depression is to take an antidepressant alongside a different type of medication that may make the antidepressant more effective, such as an antipsychotic or anticonvulsant medication. Further research is needed to identify the best role of these newer medications in routine practice.

If you begin taking an antidepressant, do not stop taking it without talking to a health-care provider. Sometimes, people taking antidepressants feel better and stop taking the medications on their own, and their depression symptoms return. When you and your health-care provider have decided it is time to stop a medication, usually after a course of 9–12 months, the provider will help you slowly and safely decrease your dose. Abruptly stopping a medication can cause withdrawal symptoms.

In some cases, children, teenagers, and young adults under 25 years may experience an increase in suicidal thoughts or behavior when taking antidepressants, especially in the first few weeks after starting or when the dose is changed. The FDA advises that patients of all ages taking antidepressants be watched closely, especially during the first few weeks of treatment.

If you are considering taking an antidepressant and are pregnant, planning to become pregnant, or breastfeeding, talk to a health-care provider about any health risks to you or your unborn or infant and how to weigh those risks against the benefits of available treatment options.

## Psychotherapies

Several types of psychotherapy (also called "talk therapy" or "counseling") can help people with depression by teaching them new ways of thinking and behaving and how to change habits that contribute to depression. Evidence-based approaches to treating depression include cognitive behavioral therapy (CBT) and interpersonal therapy (IPT).

The growth of telehealth for mental health services, which offers an alternative to in-person therapy, has made it easier and more convenient for people to access care in some cases. For people who may have been hesitant to look for mental health care in the past, telemental health services might be an easier first step than traditional mental health services.

## Brain Stimulation Therapies

If medication or psychotherapy does not reduce symptoms of depression, brain stimulation therapy may be an option to explore. There are now several types of brain stimulation therapy, some of which have been authorized by the FDA to treat depression. Other brain stimulation therapies are experimental and still being investigated for treating mental disorders such as depression.

Although brain stimulation therapies are less frequently used than medication and psychotherapy, they can play an important role in treating mental disorders in people who do not respond to other treatments. These therapies are used for most mental disorders only after medication and psychotherapy have been tried and usually continue to be used alongside these treatments.

Brain stimulation therapies act by activating or inhibiting the brain with electricity. The electricity is given directly through electrodes implanted in the brain or indirectly through electrodes placed on the scalp. The electricity can also be induced by applying magnetic fields to the head.

The brain stimulation therapies with the largest bodies of evidence include the following:

- electroconvulsive therapy (ECT)
- repetitive transcranial magnetic stimulation (rTMS)
- vagus nerve stimulation (VNS)
- magnetic seizure therapy (MST)
- deep brain stimulation (DBS)

ECT and rTMS are the most widely used brain stimulation therapies, with ECT having the longest history of use. The other therapies are newer and, in some cases, still considered experimental. Other brain stimulation therapies may also hold promise for treating specific mental disorders.

ECT, rTMS, and VNS have authorization from the FDA to treat severe, treatment-resistant depression. They can be effective for people who have not been able to feel better with other treatments or for whom medications cannot be used safely and in severe cases where a rapid response is needed, such as when a person is catatonic, suicidal, or malnourished.

Although ECT involves using electricity to induce seizures, in rTMS, a magnet is used to activate the brain. Unlike ECT, in which stimulation is more generalized, in rTMS, the stimulation is targeted to a specific brain site. Both procedures are noninvasive and do not require surgery to perform. In contrast, VNS is usually a surgical procedure that involves implanting a device under the skin to activate the vagus nerve.

Additional types of brain stimulation therapy are being investigated for treating depression and other mental disorders. Talk to a health-care provider and make sure you understand the potential benefits and risks before undergoing brain stimulation therapy.

## Alternative Treatments

The FDA has not approved any natural products for depression. Although research is ongoing, some people use natural products, including vitamin D and the herbal dietary supplement St. John's wort, for depression. However, these products can come with risks. For instance, dietary supplements and natural products can limit the effectiveness of some medications or interact in dangerous or even life-threatening ways with them.

Do not use vitamin D, St. John's wort, or other dietary supplements or natural products without talking to a health-care provider. Rigorous studies must be conducted to test whether these and other natural products are safe and effective.

Daily morning light therapy is a common treatment choice for people with seasonal affective disorder. Light therapy devices are much brighter than ordinary indoor lighting and considered safe, except for people with certain eye diseases or taking medications that increase sensitivity to sunlight. As with all interventions for depression, evaluation, treatment, and follow-up by a health-care provider are strongly recommended. Research into the potential role of light therapy in treating nonseasonal depression is ongoing.[2]

## DEPRESSION AMONG U.S. WOMEN

Depression is one of the most common psychiatric disorders. In the United States, depressive disorders were the second leading cause of years lived with disability in 2010. Women are more likely to have depression than men. During 2013–2016, 10.4 percent of

[2] "Depression," National Institute of Mental Health (NIMH), April 2023. Available online. URL: www.nimh.nih.gov/health/topics/depression. Accessed May 1, 2023.

U.S. women aged 20 or older had depression in a given two-week period and were almost twice as likely as men (5.5%) to have had depression. Although this sex difference persists throughout the female lifespan, it seems to vary according to the reproductive stage (puberty, the week or so before menstruation, after pregnancy, and perimenopause). Female hormonal fluctuation may be a trigger for depression. Depression is associated with decreased physical, cognitive, and social function; it is often chronic and impairs the quality of life. Depression is predicted to be the leading cause of disease burden by 2030, and it is already the leading cause of disease burden in young adult women worldwide. Therefore, treatment and prevention of depression have become an important topic in the field of public health.

Sleep is an important determinant of a person's overall health and well-being. Sleep, as a critical health-related factor, plays a role in the development of many diseases and even all-cause mortality. Sleep disturbance is one of the most common health complaints among young adults. Although seven to nine hours of sleep per night on weeknights is recommended for young and midlife adults, 40 percent of U.S. adults have reported fewer than seven hours of sleep per night. Of young adults aged 19–29, 67 percent reported not getting enough sleep to function properly. Many psychosocial, biological, and environmental factors contribute to insufficient sleep and sleep disturbance among young adults. The high prevalence of sleep-related disturbances may be partially due to increased academic, social, and work demands. Female sex is also a risk factor for sleep problems. Several studies showed that young adult women are twice as likely as young men to have poor sleep. Thus, young women appear to be a particularly vulnerable population to both sleep problems and depression.

Previous studies suggested an association between depression and sleep disturbances in older people and an association between sleep disturbances and poor quality of life among women. Less research has been conducted among young adults who are at particular risk of sleep problems and alterations in circadian timing as a result of developmental and social influences. This age group is at an important stage of life when early interventions or treatment

305

of sleep problems may have clinical implications. Little research has explored the relationship between sleep and depression among young women, even though the correlates of depression may differ between young women and older women. Understanding the relationships between sleep and depression and correlates among young women may increase the potential to intervene and improve mental health outcomes before they become clinically concerning. The objective of this study was to assess the relationship between trouble sleeping and depression among U.S. women aged 20–30 and to determine whether trouble sleeping increased the odds of depression in this population. Researchers hypothesized that ever having trouble sleeping would be associated with depression among women in this age group.

## WHAT IS ALREADY KNOWN ON THIS TOPIC?

Sleep problems are associated with depression; however, little is known about this association among young women in the United States.

## WHAT IS ADDED BY THIS REPORT?

Women aged 20–30 who reported having trouble sleeping were 4.1 times significantly more likely to have experienced depression in the previous two weeks after accounting for several covariates.

## WHAT ARE THE IMPLICATIONS FOR PUBLIC HEALTH PRACTICE?

Regular screening and treatment for sleep disturbances are needed among U.S. women aged 20–30 to reduce the prevalence of depression among this population.[3]

---

[3] "Trouble Sleeping and Depression among US Women Aged 20 to 30 Years," Centers for Disease Control and Prevention (CDC), April 2, 2020. Available online. URL: www.cdc.gov/pcd/issues/2020/19_0262.htm. Accessed May 1, 2023.

## Section 27.3 | Generalized Anxiety Disorder and Sleep

## WHAT IS GENERALIZED ANXIETY DISORDER?

Occasional anxiety is a normal part of life. Many people may worry about things such as health, money, or family problems. But people with generalized anxiety disorder (GAD) feel extremely worried or nervous more frequently about these and other things—even when there is little or no reason to worry about them. GAD usually involves a persistent feeling of anxiety or dread that interferes with how you live your life. It is not the same as occasionally worrying about things or experiencing anxiety due to stressful life events. People living with GAD experience frequent anxiety for months, if not years. GAD develops slowly. It often starts around the age of 30 although it can occur in childhood. The disorder is more common in women than in men.

## WHAT ARE THE SIGNS AND SYMPTOMS OF GENERALIZED ANXIETY DISORDER?

People with GAD may:

- worry excessively about everyday things
- have trouble controlling their worries or feelings of nervousness
- know that they worry much more than they should
- feel restless and have trouble relaxing
- have a hard time concentrating
- startle easily
- have trouble falling asleep or staying asleep
- tire easily or feel tired all the time
- have headaches, muscle aches, stomachaches, or unexplained pains
- have a hard time swallowing
- tremble or twitch
- feel irritable or "on edge"
- sweat a lot, feel light-headed, or feel out of breath
- have to go to the bathroom frequently

Children and teens with GAD often worry excessively about:
- their performance in activities such as school or sports
- catastrophes, such as earthquakes or war
- the health of others, such as family members

Adults with GAD are often highly nervous about everyday circumstances, such as:
- job security or performance
- health
- finances
- health and well-being of their children or other family members
- being late
- completing household chores and other responsibilities

Both children and adults with GAD may experience physical symptoms such as pain, fatigue, or shortness of breath that make it hard to function and that interfere with daily life.

Symptoms may fluctuate over time and are often worse during times of stress, for example, with a physical illness, during school exams, or during a family or relationship conflict.

## WHAT CAUSES GENERALIZED ANXIETY DISORDER?

The risk of GAD can run in families. Several parts of the brain and biological processes play a key role in fear and anxiety. By learning more about how the brain and body function in people with anxiety disorders, researchers may be able to develop better treatments. Researchers have also found that external causes, such as experiencing a traumatic event or being in a stressful environment, may put you at a higher risk of developing GAD.

## HOW IS GENERALIZED ANXIETY DISORDER TREATED?

If you think you are experiencing symptoms of GAD, talk to a health-care provider. After discussing your history, a health-care provider may conduct a physical exam to ensure that an unrelated physical problem is not causing your symptoms. A health-care provider may refer you to a mental health professional, such as a psychiatrist, psychologist, or clinical social worker. The first step to effective treatment is to get a diagnosis, usually from a mental health professional.

GAD is generally treated with psychotherapy (sometimes called "talk therapy"), medication, or both. Speak with a health-care provider about the best treatment for you.

## Psychotherapy

Cognitive behavioral therapy (CBT), a research-supported type of psychotherapy, is commonly used to treat GAD. CBT teaches you different ways of thinking, behaving, and reacting to situations that help you feel less anxious and worried. CBT has been well studied and is the gold standard for psychotherapy.

Another treatment option for GAD is acceptance and commitment therapy (ACT). ACT takes a different approach than CBT to negative thoughts and uses strategies such as mindfulness and goal setting to reduce your discomfort and anxiety. Compared to CBT, ACT is a newer form of psychotherapy treatment, so fewer data are available on its effectiveness. However, different therapies work for different types of people, so it can be helpful to discuss what form of therapy may be right for you with a mental health professional.

## Medication

Health-care providers may prescribe medication to treat GAD. Different types of medication can be effective, including the following:

- antidepressants, such as selective serotonin reuptake inhibitors (SSRIs) and serotonin-norepinephrine reuptake inhibitors (SNRIs)
- antianxiety medications, such as benzodiazepines

SSRI and SNRI antidepressants are commonly used to treat depression, but they can also help treat the symptoms of GAD. They may take several weeks to start working. These medications may also cause side effects, such as headaches, nausea, or difficulty sleeping. These side effects are usually not severe for most people, especially if the dose starts off low and is increased slowly over time. Talk to your health-care provider about any side effects that you may experience.

Benzodiazepines, which are antianxiety sedative medications, can also be used to manage severe forms of GAD. These medications can be very effective in rapidly decreasing anxiety, but some people build up a tolerance to them and need higher doses to get the same effect. Some people even become dependent on them. Therefore, a health-care provider may prescribe them only for brief periods of time if you need them.

Buspirone is another antianxiety medication that can be helpful in treating GAD. Unlike benzodiazepines, buspirone is not a sedative and has less potential to be addictive. Buspirone needs to be taken for three to four weeks for it to be fully effective.

Both psychotherapy and medication can take some time to work. Many people try more than one medication before finding the best one for them. A health-care provider can work with you to find the best medication, dose, and duration of treatment for you.

## Support Groups

Some people with anxiety disorders might benefit from joining a self-help or support group and sharing their problems and achievements with others. Support groups are available both in person and online. However, any advice you receive from a support group member should be used cautiously and does not replace treatment recommendations from a health-care provider.

## Healthy Habits

Practicing a healthy lifestyle can also help combat anxiety although this alone cannot replace treatment. Researchers have found that implementing certain healthy choices in daily life—such as reducing caffeine intake and getting enough sleep—can reduce anxiety symptoms when paired with standard care—such as psychotherapy and medication.

Stress management techniques, such as exercise, mindfulness, and meditation, can also reduce anxiety symptoms and enhance the effects of psychotherapy.

## HOW CAN YOU SUPPORT YOURSELF AND OTHERS WITH GENERALIZED ANXIETY DISORDER?
### Educate Yourself
A good way to help yourself or a loved one who may be struggling with GAD is to seek information. Research the warning signs, learn about treatment options, and keep up-to-date with current research.

### Communicate
If you are experiencing GAD symptoms, have an honest conversation about how you are feeling with someone you trust. If you think that a friend or family member may be struggling with GAD, set aside time to talk with them to express your concern and reassure them of your support.

### Know When to Seek Help
If your anxiety, or the anxiety of a loved one, starts to cause problems in everyday life—such as at school, at work, or with friends and family—it is time to seek professional help.[4]

## COGNITIVE BEHAVIORAL THERAPY FOR INSOMNIA
People with GAD commonly experience sleep problems. CBT can be an effective tool in helping to improve sleep. A therapist will first do a thorough assessment of insomnia to get a better understanding of what might be causing it. A common practice for CBT for insomnia (CBT-I) is to instill good sleep hygiene practices, which might

---

[4] "Generalized Anxiety Disorder: When Worry Gets Out of Control," National Institute of Mental Health (NIMH), 2022. Available online. URL: www.nimh.nih.gov/health/publications/generalized-anxiety-disorder-gad. Accessed April 4, 2023.

include going to bed and waking up around the same time every day, taking time to wind down before bed, not drinking caffeine from the mid-afternoon on, not using alcohol before bedtime (can disrupt sleep rhythms), not using electronics in bed, and not doing work in bed. Another important facet of CBT-I is making sure the bed is not associated with stress and anxiety, which means having the person with insomnia get out of bed and do something relaxing and calming if they have not fallen asleep after approximately 15 minutes. They can return to bed after they feel sleepy again.

A therapist will also use cognitive techniques, such as decatastrophizing, to help a person address anxious thoughts associated with sleep. Often people who have insomnia have fearful thoughts about sleep (e.g., "I'll never get a good night's sleep again," or "What if I don't sleep tonight?"), which is counterproductive to sleep. It is important that these thoughts are addressed because they increase anxiety, making it harder to fall asleep. A therapist might assign "worry time" during the day or early evening. During this time, the person will allow themselves to worry and/or plan as much as they need to do in order to get their worries out of their system before bed. Finally, a person might be instructed to do relaxation or mindfulness activities to help them wind down before going to sleep.

## Medication: What You Should Know

- The most widely recommended medications for GAD are antidepressant medications. Other medications that may be used include buspirone and benzodiazepines.
- These medications are thought to work by modulating gamma-aminobutyric acid (GABA), serotonin, norepinephrine, or dopamine, which are neurotransmitters believed to regulate anxiety and mood.
- All medications may cause side effects, but many people have no side effects or minor side effects with their antianxiety medications. The side effects people typically experience are tolerable and subside in a few days. Check with your doctor if any of the common side effects listed persist or become bothersome. In rare cases, these medications can cause severe side effects. Contact your

doctor immediately if you experience one or more severe symptoms.

- When taking medications for GAD, if you forget to take a dose, this is a safe rule of thumb: If you missed your regular time by four hours or less, you should take that dose when you remember it. If it is more than four hours after the dose should have been taken, just skip the forgotten dose and resume your medication at the next regularly scheduled time. Never double up on doses of your medication to "catch up" on those you have forgotten.

## Antidepressant Medications

- Antidepressant medications, while initially developed for depression, have been found to be successful in treating anxiety disorders and are commonly used to treat GAD. While many available antidepressants are listed below, the evidence for their effectiveness in treating GAD varies considerably. You should discuss medication choices with your doctor.
- Antidepressant medications impact levels of various neurotransmitters in the brain (serotonin, norepinephrine, and/or dopamine) though it is still uncertain if that is the mechanism by which they work to reduce symptoms of anxiety and depression.
- Antidepressants must be taken as prescribed for three to four weeks before you can expect to see the start of positive changes in your symptoms. And it may take several months to see maximum effects. So do not stop taking your medication because you think it is not working only after a week or two. Give it time and discuss it with your doctor.
- Once you have responded to treatment, it is important to continue treatment. It is recommended that treatment continue for 9–12 months once a good response has been achieved. Discontinuing treatment earlier may lead to a relapse of symptoms. If you have a more severe or chronic

case of GAD, your doctor might recommend longer-term treatment.

- To prevent anxiety from coming back or worsening, do not abruptly stop taking your medication, even if you are feeling better. Stopping your medication too soon or abruptly can cause a relapse. Medication should only be stopped (and usually tapered slowly) under your doctor's supervision. If you want to stop taking your medication, talk to your doctor about how to correctly stop it.[5]

## Section 27.4 | Posttraumatic Stress Disorder and Sleep

Many people have trouble sleeping sometimes. This is even more likely, though, if you have posttraumatic stress disorder (PTSD). Trouble sleeping and nightmares are two symptoms of PTSD.

## WHY DO PEOPLE WITH POSTTRAUMATIC STRESS DISORDER HAVE SLEEP PROBLEMS?

They may be "on alert." Many people with PTSD may feel as if they need to be on guard or "on the lookout" to protect themselves from danger. It is difficult to have a restful sleep when you feel the need to be always alert. You might have trouble falling asleep, or you might wake up easily in the night if you hear any noise.

They may worry or have negative thoughts. Your thoughts can make it difficult to fall asleep. People with PTSD often worry about general problems or worry that they are in danger. If you often have trouble getting to sleep, you may start to worry that you will not be able to fall asleep. These thoughts can keep you awake.

---

[5] Mental Illness Research, Education and Clinical Centers (MIRECC), "What Is Generalized Anxiety Disorder?" U.S. Department of Veterans Affairs (VA), 2019. Available online. URL: www.mirecc.va.gov/visn22/gad.pdf. Accessed May 16, 2023.

They may use drugs or alcohol. Some people with PTSD use drugs or alcohol to help them cope with their symptoms. In fact, using too much alcohol can get in the way of restful sleep. Alcohol changes the quality of your sleep and makes it less refreshing. This is true of many drugs as well.

They may have bad dreams or nightmares. Nightmares are common for people with PTSD. Nightmares can wake you up in the middle of the night, making your sleep less restful. If you have frequent nightmares, you may find it difficult to fall asleep because you are afraid you might have a nightmare.

They may have medical problems. There are medical problems that are commonly found in people with PTSD, such as chronic pain, stomach problems, and pelvic area problems in women. These physical problems can make going to sleep difficult.

## WHAT CAN YOU DO IF YOU HAVE PROBLEMS?

There are a number of things you can do to make it more likely that you will sleep well.

### Change Your Sleeping Area

Too much noise, light, or activity in your bedroom can make sleeping harder. Creating a quiet, comfortable sleeping area can help. Here are some things you can do to sleep better:

- Use your bedroom only for sleeping and sex.
- Move the TV and radio out of your bedroom.
- Keep your bedroom quiet, dark, and cool. Use curtains or blinds to block out light. Consider using soothing music or a white noise machine to block out noise.

### Keep a Bedtime Routine and Sleep Schedule

Having a bedtime routine and a set wake-up time will help your body get used to a sleeping schedule. You may want to ask others in your household to help you with your routine.

- Do not do stressful or energizing things within two hours of going to bed.

- Create a relaxing bedtime routine. You might want to take a warm shower or bath, listen to soothing music, or drink a cup of tea with no caffeine in it.
- Use a sleep mask and earplugs if light and noise bother you.
- Try to get up at the same time every morning, even if you feel tired. That will help set your sleep schedule over time, and you will be more likely to fall asleep easily when bedtime comes. On weekends, do not sleep more than an hour past your regular wake-up time.

## Try to Relax If You Cannot Sleep

- Imagine yourself in a peaceful, pleasant scene. Focus on the details and feelings of being in a place that is relaxing.
- Get up and do a quiet activity, such as reading, until you feel sleepy.

## Watch Your Activities during the Day

Your daytime habits and activities can affect how well you sleep. Here are some tips:

- Exercise during the day. Do not exercise within two hours of going to bed, though, because it may be harder to fall asleep.
- Get outside during daylight hours. Spending time in sunlight helps reset your body's sleep and wake cycles.
- Cut out or limit what you drink or eat that has caffeine in it, such as coffee, tea, cola, and chocolate.
- Do not drink alcohol before bedtime. Alcohol can cause you to wake up more often during the night.
- Do not smoke or use tobacco, especially in the evening. Nicotine can keep you awake.
- Do not take naps during the day, especially close to bedtime.
- Do not drink any liquids after 6 p.m. if you wake up often because you have to go to the bathroom.

- Do not take medicine that may keep you awake or make you feel hyper or energized right before bed. Your doctor can tell you if your medicine may do this and if you can take it earlier in the day.

## Talk to Your Doctor

If you cannot sleep because you are in pain or have an injury, you often feel anxious at night, or you often have bad dreams or night-mares, talk to your doctor.

There are a number of medications that are helpful for sleep problems associated with PTSD. Depending on your sleep symptoms and other factors, your doctor may prescribe some medication for you. There are also other skills you can learn to help improve your sleep.[6]

[6] National Center for Posttraumatic Stress Disorder (NCPTSD), "Sleep and PTSD," U.S. Department of Veterans Affairs (VA), October 17, 2019. Available online. URL: www.ptsd.va.gov/understand/related/sleep_ptsd.asp. Accessed April 21, 2023.

# Chapter 28 | **Neurological Problems Affecting Sleep**

**Chapter Contents**

## Section 28.1 | **The Link between Alzheimer Disease and Sleep**

Alzheimer disease (AD) is a brain disorder that slowly destroys memory and thinking skills and, eventually, the ability to carry out the simplest tasks. In most people with AD, symptoms first appear later in life. Estimates vary, but experts suggest that more than 6 million Americans, most of them aged 65 or older, may have dementia caused by AD.

AD is ranked as the seventh leading cause of death in the United States and is the most common cause of dementia among older adults.

Dementia is the loss of cognitive functioning—thinking, remembering, and reasoning—and behavioral abilities to such an extent that it interferes with a person's daily life and activities. Dementia ranges in severity from the mildest stage, when it is just beginning to affect a person's functioning, to the most severe stage, when the person must depend completely on others for help with basic activities of daily living.

The causes of dementia can vary, depending on the types of brain changes that may be taking place. Other dementias include Lewy body dementia, frontotemporal disorders, and vascular dementia. It is common for people to have mixed dementia—a combination of two or more types of dementia. For example, some people have both AD and vascular dementia.

AD is named after Dr. Alois Alzheimer, a German psychiatrist and neuropathologist and a colleague of Emil Kraepelin. In 1906, Dr. Alzheimer noticed changes in the brain tissue of a woman who had died of an unusual mental illness. Her symptoms included memory loss, language problems, and unpredictable behavior. After she died, he examined her brain and found many abnormal clumps (now called "amyloid plaques") and tangled bundles of fibers (now called "neurofibrillary tangles," or "tau tangles").

These plaques and tangles in the brain are still considered some of the main features of AD. Another feature is the loss of connections between neurons in the brain. Neurons transmit messages between different parts of the brain and from the brain to muscles and organs in the body.

## HOW DOES ALZHEIMER DISEASE AFFECT THE BRAIN?

Scientists continue to unravel the complex brain changes involved in AD. Changes in the brain may begin a decade or more before symptoms appear. During this very early stage of AD, toxic changes are taking place in the brain, including abnormal buildups of proteins that form amyloid plaques and tau tangles. Previously healthy neurons stop functioning, lose connections with other neurons, and die. Many other complex brain changes are thought to play a role in AD as well.

The damage initially appears to take place in the hippocampus and the entorhinal cortex, which are parts of the brain that are essential in forming memories. As more neurons die, additional parts of the brain are affected and begin to shrink. By the final stage of AD, the damage is widespread, and brain tissue has shrunk significantly.[1]

## DOES POOR SLEEP RAISE THE RISK OF ALZHEIMER DISEASE?

Studies confirm what many people already know: Sleep gets worse with age. Middle-aged and older adults often sleep less deeply, wake more frequently at night, or awake too early in the morning. Could these problems be related to the risk of cognitive decline or AD?

Scientists are beginning to probe the complex relationship between the brain changes involved in poor sleep and those in very early-stage AD. It is an intriguing area of research, given that both risk of disturbed sleep and risk of AD increase with age.

"Nearly 60 percent of older adults have some kind of chronic sleep disturbance," said Phyllis Zee, Ph.D., a sleep expert at Northwestern University's Feinberg School of Medicine, Chicago.

It has long been known that people with AD often have sleep problems—getting their days and nights mixed up, for example. Now scientists are probing the link between sleep and AD earlier in the disease process and in cognitively normal adults. They wonder if improving sleep with existing treatments might help

---

[1] National Institute on Aging (NIA), "Alzheimer's Disease Fact Sheet," National Institutes of Health (NIH), April 5, 2023. Available online. URL: www.nia.nih.gov/health/alzheimers-disease-fact-sheet. Accessed May 30, 2023.

memory and other cognitive functions—and perhaps delay or prevent AD.

## Which Comes First, Poor Sleep or Alzheimer Disease?

The chicken-and-egg question is whether AD-related brain changes lead to poor sleep or whether poor sleep somehow contributes to AD. Scientists believe the answer may be both.

Findings show that brain activity induced by poor sleep may influence AD-related brain changes, which begin years before memory loss and other disease symptoms appear.

Scientists funded by the National Institute on Aging (NIA) are studying the biological underpinnings of this relationship in animals and humans to better understand how these changes occur. Although evidence points to certain sleep problems as a risk factor for AD, Dr. Mack Mackiewicz, a program director in the Neurobiology of Aging and Neurodegeneration Branch in the Division of Neuroscience, says, "It is not known whether improving sleep will reduce the likelihood of developing AD." He adds, "There is no scientific evidence that sleep medications or other sleep treatments will reduce the risk for AD."

## Effects of Good and Bad Sleep

At any age, getting a good night's sleep serves a number of important functions for our bodies and brains. Although our bodies rest during sleep, our brains are active. The process is not totally understood, but researchers think that sleep might benefit the brain—and the whole body—by removing metabolic waste that accumulates in the brain during wakefulness. In addition, it has been shown that some memories are consolidated, moving from short-term to long-term storage during periods of deep sleep. Research shows that other sleep stages may also influence memory and memory consolidation.

Disturbed sleep—whether due to illness, pain, anxiety, depression, or a sleep disorder—can lead to trouble concentrating, remembering, and learning. A return to normal sleep patterns usually eases these problems. But, in older people, disturbed sleep may have more dire and long-lasting consequences.

"Scientists long believed that the initial buildup of the beta-amyloid protein in the brain, an early biological sign of AD, causes disturbed sleep," Dr. Mackiewicz said. Recently, though, evidence suggests the opposite may also occur—disturbed sleep in cognitively normal older adults contributes to the risk of cognitive decline and AD.

For example, in a study of older men free of dementia, poor sleep, including greater nighttime wakefulness, was associated with cognitive decline over a period of more than three years. Sleep was assessed through participants' reports and a device worn on the wrist that tracks movements during sleep.

Sleep disorders such as sleep apnea may pose an even greater risk of cognitive impairment. In a five-year study of older women, those with sleep-disordered breathing (SDB)—repeated arousals from sleep due to breathing disruptions, as happens in sleep apnea—had a nearly twofold increase in risk for mild cognitive impairment (a precursor to AD in some people) or dementia.

In addition, certain types of poor sleep seem to be associated with a risk of cognitive impairment, according to Kristine Yaffe, M.D., an American cognitive decline and dementia researcher at the University of California, San Francisco. These include hypoxia (low oxygen levels that can be caused by sleep disorders) and difficulty falling or staying asleep.

## What Is the Connection between Sleep and Alzheimer Disease?

Evidence of a link between sleep and the risk of AD has led to investigations to explain the brain activity that underlies this connection in humans. Some studies suggest that poor sleep contributes to abnormal levels of beta-amyloid protein in the brain, which in turn leads to the amyloid plaques found in the AD brain. These plaques might then affect sleep-related brain regions, further disrupting sleep.

Studies in laboratory animals show a direct link between sleep and AD. One study in mice, led by researchers at Washington University, St. Louis, showed that beta-amyloid levels naturally rose during wakefulness and fell during sleep. Mice deprived of sleep for 21 days showed significantly greater beta-amyloid plaques than those that slept normally. Increasing sleep had the opposite effect—it reduced the amyloid load.

A subsequent study, also by Washington University researchers, showed that when AD mice were treated with antibodies, beta-amyloid deposits decreased, and sleep returned to normal. Mice that received a placebo saline solution continued to sleep poorly. The results suggest that sleep disruption could be a sign of AD beginning in the brain, but not necessarily its cause.

Studies in humans have also addressed the relationship between sleep and biomarkers of AD. One study found that in cognitively normal older adults, poor sleep quality (more time awake at night and more daytime naps) was associated with lower beta-amyloid levels in cerebrospinal fluid, a preclinical sign of AD. Another study by researchers at the NIA and Johns Hopkins University, Baltimore, found that healthy older adults who reported short sleep duration and poor sleep quality had more beta-amyloid in the brain than those without such sleep problems.

## Emerging Insights: Stay Tuned

How exactly do poor sleep and AD influence each other? Research so far suggests a few possible mechanisms:

- Orexin, a molecule that regulates wakefulness and other functions, has been found to affect beta-amyloid levels in mice.
- Chronic hypoxia, insufficient oxygen in blood or tissue that is a feature of sleep apnea, increased the level of harmful beta-amyloid in the brain tissue of mice.
- Reduced slow-wave sleep leads to increased neuronal activity.

Other factors may also be involved. For example, it has been shown in laboratory animals that the glymphatic system, the brain's waste removal system, removes beta-amyloid during sleep. A mouse study suggests that sleeping in different positions impacts waste removal from the brain. Sleeping on the side cleared beta-amyloid more efficiently than sleeping on the back or belly, researchers found. They pointed to the glymphatic system as a possible pathway for intervention.

Further biological and epidemiological studies and clinical trials should cast more light on the mechanisms behind the sleep–AD connection and whether treating poor sleep might help delay or prevent cognitive decline in older adults.

"Sleep is something we can fix, and people with sleep problems should consult a doctor so that they can function at their best," Dr. Mackiewicz said. As for AD, for now, he said, improving sleep is "not the same as preventing AD. Researchers are committed to achieving a better understanding of this complex dynamic in hopes of making a difference in the lives of older adults."

Studies to examine the value of a good night's sleep in delaying or preventing AD are underway.[2]

## Section 28.2 | Sleep and Stroke

## WHAT IS A STROKE?

A stroke is sometimes called a "brain attack." A stroke happens when blood flow to part of the brain is blocked or when a blood vessel breaks, which can damage or kill cells in the brain. Stroke is a leading cause of death and long-term disability in adults. It can also cause brain damage. A stroke can cause long-term problems such as:

- memory problems or trouble thinking and speaking
- vision problems
- trouble walking or keeping your balance
- paralysis (not being able to move some parts of the body) and muscle weakness

[2] National Institute on Aging (NIA), "Does Poor Sleep Raise Risk for Alzheimer's Disease?" National Institutes of Health (NIH), February 29, 2016. Available online. URL: www.nia.nih.gov/news/does-poor-sleep-raise-risk-alzheimers-disease. Accessed March 30, 2023.

- trouble controlling or expressing emotions
- trouble with chewing and swallowing
- trouble controlling when you go to the bathroom

## WHAT ARE THE SIGNS OF A STROKE?

A stroke usually happens suddenly. But it can also happen over hours or even days. Signs of a stroke include the following:

- sudden dizziness, loss of balance, or trouble walking
- sudden confusion, trouble speaking, or trouble understanding what people are saying
- sudden trouble seeing in one or both eyes
- sudden numbness or weakness of the face, arm, or leg—especially on one side of the body
- sudden, severe headache with no known cause

Having a stroke is a medical emergency. Call 911 right away if you or someone else shows signs of a stroke. The acronym FAST can help you remember the most common signs of a stroke and what to do if you think you or someone else is having a stroke:

- F (face drooping)
- A (arm weakness)
- S (speech trouble)
- T (time to call 911)

Your chances of surviving and recovering from a stroke are better if you get emergency treatment right away.

## WHAT IS A MINI-STROKE?

A mini-stroke causes the same symptoms as a stroke, but the symptoms do not last as long. A mini-stroke is also called a "TIA," which stands for transient ischemic attack.

A TIA happens when blood flow to the brain is blocked for a short period of time—usually minutes to hours. If you have had a TIA, you are at a higher risk of having a larger stroke. Never ignore signs of a TIA. Call 911 right away if you or someone else shows signs of a mini-stroke.

## KNOW YOUR NUMBERS

Take the following steps today to reduce your risk of stroke:

- **Get your blood pressure checked**. High blood pressure is the most important risk factor for stroke, so it is important to get your blood pressure checked by a doctor or nurse regularly starting at the age of 18. It is also a good idea to check your own blood pressure at home if you have ever had high blood pressure. If your blood pressure is high, talk with your doctor or nurse about how to lower it.
- **Get your cholesterol checked**. Having high cholesterol can increase your risk of stroke. It is important to get your cholesterol checked at least every four to six years. Some people will need to get it checked more or less often. If your cholesterol is high, talk with your doctor about steps you can take to lower it.

## HEALTHY HABITS
### Quit Smoking

Quitting smoking is one of the best things you can do to prevent stroke. After you quit smoking, your risk of stroke and heart disease starts to go down.

### Get Active

Getting active can help lower your risk of stroke. Aim for:

- at least 150 minutes of moderate aerobic activity every week—try walking fast or biking
- muscle-strengthening activities two days a week—try lifting weights or doing push-ups

If that is more activity than you can do right now, do what you can. Even five minutes of physical activity has real health benefits. You can use this tool to build a personalized weekly activity plan.

## Get Enough Sleep

Sleep is important for staying healthy. Sleep apnea is a sleep disorder that causes people's breathing to pause during sleep and increases the risk of stroke.

## FOOD AND ALCOHOL
### Eat Healthy

Eating healthy can help keep your blood pressure and cholesterol under control. Try to fill half your plate with fruits and vegetables at meals. And be sure to cut down on foods high in sodium (salt) and saturated fat.

## Drink Alcohol Only in Moderation

Drinking too much alcohol can increase your risk of high blood pressure, which is a major cause of stroke. If you choose to drink alcohol, drink only in moderation. That means:
- one drink or less in a day for women
- two drinks or less in a day for men

## Take Steps to Prevent Type 2 Diabetes

Diabetes can increase your risk of stroke. Eating healthy and staying active can lower your risk of diabetes. If you have diabetes, talk with your doctor or nurse about ways to keep your blood sugar (glucose) in the normal range.

## TALK WITH YOUR DOCTOR
### Ask Your Doctor about Taking Aspirin Every Day

Taking aspirin regularly is not recommended for everyone. If you are aged 40–59 years, talk with your doctor to find out if taking aspirin is the right choice for you.

## Know Your Family's Health History

Your family's health history can give your doctor or nurse important information about your risk of stroke.[3]

## WHAT DO YOU NEED TO KNOW?

Sleep problems are common after a stroke. The good news is there are ways to improve your loved one's sleep. Both old and young adults need about seven to nine hours of sleep. Poor sleep is not a normal part of getting older. But, after a stroke, your loved one may have more sleep problems. Sleep is important for good health. Everyone should expect to get a good night's sleep.

## WHAT MIGHT BE CAUSING YOUR LOVED ONE'S SLEEP PROBLEMS?

More than half of stroke survivors have one of the following sleep problems.

### Sleep Apnea

This is a serious condition. Sleep apnea increases the risk of having a second stroke. It is caused by abnormal breathing patterns. Loud snoring, choking, and gasping sounds during sleep may mean that your loved one has sleep apnea. Tell your health-care team about these symptoms. There are good treatments.

### Change in Sleep–Wake Cycles

After a stroke, some survivors do not get sleepy at night. It may be difficult to wake the stroke survivor in the morning. This happens when the sleep–wake schedule is no longer affected by sunlight and the darkness of night. Talk with your health-care team. Bright light therapy may help.[4]

---

[3] Office of Disease Prevention and Health Promotion (ODPHP), "Reduce Your Risk of Stroke," U.S. Department of Health and Human Services (HHS), December 22, 2022. Available online. URL: https://health.gov/myhealthfinder/health-conditions/heart-health/reduce-your-risk-stroke#the-basics-tab. Accessed April 3, 2023.

[4] "Sleeping Problems—RESCUE Stroke Caregiving," U.S. Department of Veterans Affairs (VA), October 17, 2022. Available online. URL: www.stroke.cindrr.research.va.gov/en/fact_sheet_library/sleeping_problems.asp. Accessed May 9, 2023.

## Section 28.3 | **Multiple Sclerosis and Sleep Disorders**

Multiple sclerosis (MS) is a nervous system disease that affects your brain and spinal cord. It damages the myelin sheath, the material that surrounds and protects your nerve cells. This damage slows down or blocks messages between your brain and your body, leading to the symptoms of MS. They can include:

- visual disturbances
- muscle weakness
- trouble with coordination and balance
- sensations such as numbness, prickling, or "pins and needles"
- thinking and memory problems

No one knows what causes MS. It may be an autoimmune disease, which happens when your immune system attacks healthy cells in your body by mistake. MS affects women more than men. It often begins between the ages of 20 and 40. Usually, the disease is mild, but some people lose the ability to write, speak, or walk.

There is no single test for MS. Doctors use medical history, physical exam, neurological exam, magnetic resonance imaging (MRI), and other tests to diagnose it. There is no cure for MS, but medicines may slow it down and help control symptoms. Physical and occupational therapy may also help.[5]

## HOW DOES SLEEP IMPACT PEOPLE WITH MULTIPLE SCLEROSIS?

Sleep plays an important role in your physical health and well-being. Sleep supports healthy brain functioning, is involved in the healing and repair of your heart and blood vessels, regulates mood, reduces stress, and even helps your immune system defend your body against foreign or harmful substances. The average adult needs seven to nine hours of sleep each night to function well. Yet many people do not get adequate amounts of sleep.

---

[5] MedlinePlus, "Multiple Sclerosis," National Institutes of Health (NIH), June 1, 2021. Available online. URL: https://medlineplus.gov/multiplesclerosis.html. Accessed April 21, 2023.

People with MS often say they sleep poorly at night and are fatigued in the daytime. In the general population, the three most common sleep problems reported are insomnia, sleep apnea, and restless legs syndrome (RLS). Research suggests that people with MS have these problems even more often.

## Insomnia

Insomnia is characterized by problems getting to sleep, staying asleep, or waking up too early. Insomnia can have multiple causes and is a significant problem at some point for almost half of the people with MS. Insomnia can be caused by nighttime MS symptoms that disrupt sleep, such as pain, muscle spasms, and urinary frequency.

Medications, including some antidepressants (selective serotonin reuptake inhibitors (SSRIs)), stimulants used to treat daytime fatigue, and corticosteroids used to treat MS exacerbations, can also contribute to insomnia. Depression, which is common with MS, is also associated with insomnia. Although occasional self-medication of insomnia with over-the-counter (OTC) sleep medications containing antihistamines can help if you use them often, they will probably stop working and also make you sleepy or foggy during the day. Many approaches can be effective for treating insomnia, including adjusting your current medication regimen, addressing MS symptoms that are contributing to poor sleep, using nonmedication cognitive behavioral therapy (CBT) approaches, and, in resistant cases, using prescribed sleep-enhancing medications.

## Sleep Apnea

Sleep apnea affects at least one in five Americans and probably an even greater proportion of people with MS. Sleep apnea is characterized by repeatedly stopping breathing during sleep. The frequent pauses in breathing can cause fragmented sleep, as well as low blood oxygen levels. Untreated sleep apnea is associated with poor daytime functioning, mood and memory problems, and, if severe, cardiovascular disorders (CVD), such as heart disease and stroke. Sleep apnea may also lead to worsened fatigue, poor energy, and daytime tiredness common in people with MS. Treatment for sleep apnea can reduce these symptoms, which may have been attributed solely to MS.

## Restless Legs Syndrome

Restless legs syndrome is characterized by an uncomfortable urge to move your legs or, more rarely, other body areas. This urge is temporarily relieved by moving your legs. RLS symptoms are generally worst in the evening or at night. RLS is three times more common in people with MS than that in the general population. RLS may affect up to one-third of individuals with MS and is more common in those who are older, have had MS for longer, have primary progressive MS, and have a greater disability. The exact cause of RLS is not known, but RLS appears to be linked with iron metabolism in the brain. Checking for low iron levels with a blood test and replacing iron when low can improve symptoms. Decreasing the intake of caffeine, nicotine, and alcohol; massaging your legs; and taking warm baths before bedtime may decrease RLS symptoms. When these interventions fail, medications to treat RLS symptoms are available.

In summary, sleep problems, such as insomnia, sleep apnea, and RLS, are common in individuals with MS. These sleep problems may be troublesome on their own and may contribute to daytime fatigue and poorer quality of life and may be associated with greater disability. Fortunately, treatments are available for the most common sleep problems, so if you have poor quality, unrefreshing sleep, it is important that you discuss your symptoms with your health-care provider. Good sleep practices, such as keeping a regular bedtime and wake time, protecting your sleep time from other activities, setting up your bedroom only for sleep, and limiting caffeinated beverages, can also help. While symptoms may not completely resolve with treatment, substantial improvements in daytime functioning and an improved sense of well-being are possible.[6]

---

[6] "VA Multiple Sclerosis Centers of Excellence—Where There's a Will, There's a Way," U.S. Department of Veterans Affairs (VA), 2015. Available online. URL: www.va.gov/MS/Products/newsletters/Fall_2015_Newsletter. pdf. Accessed April 21, 2023.

## Section 28.4 | **Brain Protein Affects Aging and Sleep**

A study revealed how an aging-related protein in the brain affects sleep patterns. A better understanding of the connections between aging and sleep may lead to improved methods for treating or preventing certain diseases of aging.

Our sleep–wake cycle is governed by an internal circadian clock that is coordinated by a tiny brain region known as the "supra-chiasmatic nucleus" (SCN). The circadian clock adjusts to several cues in your surroundings, especially light and darkness. Animal studies have shown that disrupting the circadian cycle may trigger health problems, such as obesity and diabetes. In contrast, a stable circadian cycle that includes healthy, consistent sleep is associated with longer lifespans in mice.

Many people develop sleeping problems as they age. Studies have linked circadian activity with SIRT1, a protein known to be involved in the aging process. Researchers have been searching for ways to raise SIRT1 activity in the hope of warding off age-related diseases. Strategies include calorie restriction and the compound resveratrol found in grapes and wine.

To further explore the links between SIRT1 and the circadian clock, a research team led by Dr. Leonard Guarente, Ph.D., a Novartis professor of biology at the Massachusetts Institute of Technology, altered SIRT1 levels in the brain tissue of mice. Their study, funded in part by the National Institute on Aging (NIA) of the National Institutes of Health (NIH), appeared in the June 20, 2013, issue of *Cell*.

The team created genetically engineered mice that produce different amounts of SIRT1 in the brain. They studied groups of mice with normal levels of SIRT1, no SIRT1, and two groups with increased SIRT1—either 2 times or 10 times the normal amount. The researchers conducted "jet lag" experiments with the mice by shifting their light/dark cycles and observing their ability to adjust their sleep patterns.

Similar to previous findings, older mice with unaltered SIRT1 levels took much longer to adapt to shifting cycles than younger ones. Young mice lacking SIRT1 took twice as long to adapt as those with normal SIRT1 levels. Increasing SIRT1 levels, in contrast, had a protective effect. Old mice with 10 times the level of SIRT1 were able to adapt their sleep patterns much more quickly than normal SIRT1 mice of the same age.

A genetic analysis found that SIRT1 levels in the SCN affect the expression of genes involved in circadian control. All the circadian genes tested were expressed at significantly lower levels in mice lacking SIRT1. In contrast, the genes were expressed at higher levels in mice with more SIRT1. SIRT1 activated the two major circadian regulators, BMAL1 and CLOCK.

SIRT1 levels in the SCN declined with age in the mice—as did BMAL1 and other circadian regulatory proteins. These results suggest that SIRT1 plays a central role in the decline of circadian function as we age.

"What's now emerging is the idea that maintaining the circadian cycle is quite important in health maintenance," says Dr. Guarente, "and if it gets broken, there's a penalty to be paid in health and perhaps in aging." Further research will be needed to see whether dietary or other interventions that increase SIRT1 activity can help slow the onset and progression of sleep problems related to aging.[7]

---

[7] News and Events, "Brain Protein Affects Aging and Sleep," National Institutes of Health (NIH), July 15, 2013. Available online. URL: www.nih.gov/news-events/nih-research-matters/brain-protein-affects-aging-sleep. Accessed April 25, 2023.

# Chapter 29 | **Pain Disorders That Impact Sleep**

## Section 29.1 | **Pain and Sleep: An Overview**

Pain is the leading cause of insomnia. People who experience chronic pain—which include about 15 percent of the overall U.S. population and half of all elderly people—often have trouble falling asleep and staying asleep. In fact, about 65 percent of people with chronic pain report having disrupted sleep or nonrestorative sleep, resulting in an average deficit of 42 minutes between the amount of sleep they need and the amount they actually get. Shorter sleep duration and poorer sleep quality, in turn, exacerbate chronic pain and interfere with activities, work, mood, relationships, and other aspects of daily life.

## HOW DOES PAIN IMPACT SLEEP?

People who experience chronic pain often have trouble falling asleep. Most people prepare for sleep by eliminating distractions and trying to relax. This process may include preparing the covers and pillows, turning off the lights, quieting noises in the bedroom, and making themselves comfortable. When an individual experiences persistent pain, they may attempt to engage in other activities to distract themselves from the discomfort or reduce its intensity by concentrating on a different matter instead. As long as they are able to focus on working, socializing, preparing meals, performing household tasks, reading, watching television, or engaging in recreational activities, their perception of pain tends to decrease. When someone tries to fall asleep by removing distractions, their brain may end up fixating on the pain they are experiencing. As a result, the longer it takes for them to fall asleep, the more stressed they may feel and the worse their pain may become.

People dealing with pain also tend to have trouble sleeping through the night. Research has shown, for instance, that people with chronic back pain experience a number of microarousals—or changes from a deeper to a lighter stage of sleep—per hour each night. So, when someone with chronic pain keeps waking up frequently during the night, their normal sleep pattern gets disturbed. This disturbance makes their sleep quality poor, which means they do not get the rest they need to feel energized in the morning. As a result, they often experience drowsiness, diminished energy, depressed mood, and increased pain throughout the day.

In some cases, people with pain also have other medical problems that disrupt sleep, such as restless legs syndrome (RLS) or nocturnal leg cramps. People with RLS experience an uncomfortable tingling or tickling sensation in their legs at night. This sensation creates an uncontrollable urge to move the legs, which can result in involuntary kicking or jerking motions during sleep. The symptoms of RLS can contribute to problems falling asleep or staying asleep. They are sometimes relieved through massage, hot baths before bedtime, daily exercise, or eliminating caffeine or nicotine. They can also be treated with prescription medications.

Nocturnal leg cramps occur when a person's leg muscles suddenly tighten up and cause a lot of pain. This tightening of leg muscles usually happens when the person is sleeping or just about to fall asleep. They may affect the feet, calves, or thighs and last between a few seconds and several minutes. Dehydration is the most common cause of muscle cramps, so staying well-hydrated during the day can help prevent them from occurring. Overuse of the leg muscles is another factor that sometimes contributes to nocturnal cramping. Stretching before bedtime often helps with this problem. Deficiencies in calcium, magnesium, or potassium may also cause muscle cramps, so supplementing the intake of these minerals in the diet may also prove helpful.

## IMPROVING PAIN AND SLEEP

When pain impacts sleep, it is important to treat both problems together with a multidisciplinary approach. Since chronic pain and insomnia reinforce each other in a vicious cycle, treatments aimed at improving pain may also help improve sleep, while treatments aimed at improving sleep may also help improve pain. Many behavioral and psychological approaches are available to treat both pain and sleep issues.

Practices and habits that can lead to better quality sleep are known as "sleep hygiene." In many cases, people who experience chronic pain develop bad habits and poor sleep hygiene over time. Some of the practices that have proven safe and effective in improving sleep include the following:

- Develop a regular routine to help the body get into a consistent, healthy sleep–wake cycle. Having a consistent sleep schedule can help the body get into a regular routine, making it easier to fall asleep and wake up feeling rested.
- It is a good idea to try to stick to a consistent sleep schedule if possible. Chronic pain sufferers sometimes try to compensate for having trouble falling asleep by sleeping late the next morning, but this practice disrupts the sleep–wake pattern.
- Avoid taking naps during the day, which can make insomnia worse in the long run by disrupting the sleep–wake cycle.
- Do not go to bed unless sleepy. Instead, spend some time engaging in relaxing activities such as listening to music, reading a book, or meditating.
- Get out of bed if sleep does not come within 30 minutes. Trying to fall asleep for hours on end only increases anxiety levels and turns the bedroom into a stressful place. Instead, get up and return to a relaxing activity until a feeling of drowsiness occurs.
- Develop bedtime rituals to aid in relaxation and train the body to fall asleep. Suggestions include taking a warm bath or shower, listening to music, reading a book, or having a light snack.
- Avoid caffeine, nicotine, and alcohol before bedtime. Research has shown that such substances can be disruptive to a good night's sleep.
- Exercise at least four to six hours before bedtime. Although regular exercise can help ease chronic pain and promote good sleep, vigorous exercise within a few hours of bedtime can disrupt sleep.
- Create a comfortable, pleasant, relaxing sleep environment. People with chronic pain tend to be highly sensitive to environmental factors, such as

light, noise, temperature, mattresses, and bedding. As a result, choosing comfortable bedding, making sure the temperature is neither too hot nor too cold, and eliminating sources of distracting noise or light can make a big difference in helping them get a good night's sleep.

- Try alternative techniques such as meditation, yoga, deep breathing, deep muscle relaxation, or hypnosis to aid in chronic pain management and relaxation. These techniques can help people reduce stress, decrease the perception of pain, and improve sleep.

If these approaches are not effective in improving sleep, chronic pain sufferers should consult a doctor. A variety of medications are available to help address sleep problems. Before taking any sleep medication, however, patients must be sure to tell the doctor about any other medications they may be taking for chronic pain or other medical conditions.

## References

Deardorff, William. "Chronic Pain and Insomnia: Breaking the Cycle," Veritas Health, December 12, 2016. Available online. URL: www.spine-health.com/wellness/sleep/chronic-pain-and-insomnia-breaking-cycle. Accessed April 10, 2023.

"Pain and Sleep," National Sleep Foundation, April 29, 2022. Available online. URL: https://sleepfoundation.org/sleep-disorders-problems/pain-and-sleep. Accessed April 10, 2023.

Silberman, Stephanie. "What's Really Causing Your Sleepless Nights?" The Huffington Post, September 20, 2011. Available online. URL: www.huffpost.com/entry/insomnia-causes_b_904570. Accessed April 10, 2023.

## Section 29.2 | Fibromyalgia and Sleep Problems

## WHAT IS FIBROMYALGIA?

Fibromyalgia is a condition that causes pain all over the body (also referred to as widespread pain), sleep problems, fatigue, and often emotional and mental distress. People with fibromyalgia may be more sensitive to pain than people without fibromyalgia. This is called "abnormal pain perception processing." Fibromyalgia affects about 4 million U.S. adults, about 2 percent of the adult population. The cause of fibromyalgia is not known, but it can be effectively treated and managed.

## WHAT ARE THE SIGNS AND SYMPTOMS OF FIBROMYALGIA?

The most common symptoms of fibromyalgia are:
- pain and stiffness all over the body
- fatigue and tiredness
- depression and anxiety
- sleep problems
- problems with thinking, memory, and concentration
- headaches, including migraines

Other symptoms may include the following:
- tingling or numbness in hands and feet
- pain in the face or jaw, including disorders of the jaw known as "temporomandibular joint syndrome" (also known as "TMJ")
- digestive problems, such as abdominal pain, bloating, constipation, and even irritable bowel syndrome (also known as "IBS")

## WHAT ARE THE RISK FACTORS FOR FIBROMYALGIA?

The known risk factors include the following:
- **Age**. Fibromyalgia can affect people of all ages, including children. However, most people are diagnosed during middle age, and you are more likely to have fibromyalgia as you get older.

- **Lupus or rheumatoid arthritis**. If you have lupus or rheumatoid arthritis (RA), you are more likely to develop fibromyalgia.

Some other factors have been weakly associated with the onset of fibromyalgia, but more research is needed to see if they are real. These possible risk factors include the following:
- stressful or traumatic events, such as car accidents, posttraumatic stress disorder (PTSD)
- illness (such as viral infections)
- family history
- obesity

## HOW IS FIBROMYALGIA DIAGNOSED?
Doctors usually diagnose fibromyalgia using the patient's history, physical examination, x-rays, and blood work.

## HOW IS FIBROMYALGIA TREATED?
Fibromyalgia can be effectively treated and managed with medication and self-management strategies.

Fibromyalgia should be treated by a doctor or team of healthcare professionals who specialize in the treatment of fibromyalgia and other types of arthritis called "rheumatologists." Doctors usually treat fibromyalgia with a combination of treatments, which may include the following:
- medications, including prescription drugs and over-the-counter pain relievers
- aerobic exercise and muscle-strengthening exercise
- patient education classes, usually in primary care or community settings
- stress management techniques such as meditation, yoga, and massage
- good sleep habits to improve the quality of sleep
- cognitive behavioral therapy (CBT) to treat the underlying depression (CBT is a type of talk therapy meant to change the way people act or think.)

In addition to medical treatment, people can manage their fibromyalgia with the self-management strategies described below, which are proven to reduce pain and disability, so they can pursue the activities important to them.

## WHAT ARE THE COMPLICATIONS OF FIBROMYALGIA?

Fibromyalgia can cause pain, disability, and a lower quality of life (QOL). U.S. adults with fibromyalgia may have the following complications:

- **More hospitalizations**. If you have fibromyalgia, you are twice as likely to be hospitalized as someone without fibromyalgia.
- **Lower QOL**. Women with fibromyalgia may experience a lower QOL.
- **Higher rates of major depression**. Adults with fibromyalgia are more than three times more likely to have major depression than adults without fibromyalgia. Screening and treatment for depression are extremely important.
- **Higher death rates from suicide and injuries**. Death rates from suicide and injuries are higher among fibromyalgia patients, but overall mortality among adults with fibromyalgia is similar to the general population.
- **Higher rates of other rheumatic conditions**. Fibromyalgia often co-occurs with other types of arthritis, such as osteoarthritis, RA, systemic lupus erythematosus, and ankylosing spondylitis.

## HOW CAN YOU IMPROVE YOUR QUALITY OF LIFE?

- **Get physically active**. Experts recommend that adults be moderately physically active for 150 minutes per week. Walk, swim, or bike 30 minutes a day for five days a week. These 30 minutes can be broken into three separate 10-minute sessions during the day. Regular physical activity can also reduce the risk of developing other chronic diseases, such as heart disease and diabetes. You can exercise on your own or participate in a physical activity program recommended by the Centers for Disease Control and Prevention (CDC).

- **Go to recommended physical activity programs**. Those concerned about how to safely exercise can participate in physical activity programs that are proven effective for reducing pain and disability related to arthritis and improving mood and the ability to move. Classes take place at local Ys, parks, and community centers. These classes can help you feel better.
- **Join a self-management education class**. This helps people with arthritis or other conditions—including fibromyalgia—be more confident in how to control their symptoms and how to live well and understand how the condition affects their lives.[1]

## LIVING WITH FIBROMYALGIA

Having fibromyalgia can significantly impact your QOL and your ability to take part in everyday activities. There are things you can do to help you live with fibromyalgia, including the following:

- exercising
- educating yourself and getting support
- combating fatigue

### Exercising

Exercise is a mainstay of therapy for fibromyalgia. Although pain and fatigue may make exercise difficult, it is important for you to be as physically active as possible. Research shows that regular exercise is one of the most useful ways to combat fibromyalgia, and even modest levels are helpful. Aerobic activity can also improve sleep and lessen anxiety and depression.

---

[1] "Fibromyalgia," Centers for Disease Control and Prevention (CDC), January 6, 2020. Available online. URL: www.cdc.gov/arthritis/basics/fibromyalgia.htm. Accessed April 13, 2023.

You should start exercising at a low level and gradually increase over time. Low-impact aerobic activities—such as walking, biking, swimming, and water exercises—are especially helpful. Activities that engage the mind and body, such as yoga and tai chi, are also helpful. Physical therapists or exercise physiologists can prescribe an exercise program and provide ongoing support. Be sure to check with your doctor before beginning an exercise routine.

## Educating Yourself and Getting Support

Learn as much as you can about fibromyalgia and join an online or in-person support group that includes others who are dealing with it. Having a support network can help you manage difficult times.

Visit a mental health professional if emotional problems arise. Research has shown that a type of therapy called "CBT," which teaches skills for better controlling pain, can be helpful.

## Combating Fatigue and Sleep Deprivation

Persistent fatigue is one of the most troubling symptoms of fibromyalgia. The following strategies may help you sleep better and feel more rested:

- Create a relaxing sleep environment and establish a sleep routine.
- Go to sleep and get up at the same time every day.
- Reserve your bed for sleeping. Watching TV, reading, or using a laptop or phone in bed can keep you awake.
- Keep your bedroom comfortable. Try to keep your bedroom dark, quiet, and cool.
- Avoid stimulants such as caffeine and nicotine and limit alcohol intake.
- Wind down before bed. Avoid working or exercising close to bedtime. Try some relaxing activities that get you ready for sleep, such as listening to soft music, meditating, or taking a warm bath.
- Pace yourself during the day. You may not be able to do all the things you once did or not in the same amount of time. Try not to use up all your energy each day

because doing too much can make your symptoms worse.[2]

## Section 29.3 | Headaches and Sleep

## WHAT IS A HEADACHE?

Headache is our most common form of pain and a major reason cited for days missed at work or school as well as visits to the doctor. Without proper treatment, headaches can be severe and interfere with daily activities.

Headaches can range in frequency and severity of pain. Some individuals may experience headaches once or twice a year, while others may experience them more than 15 days a month. Some headaches may recur or last for weeks at a time. Pain can range from mild to disabling and may be accompanied by symptoms such as nausea or increased sensitivity to noise or light.

## WHY DO HEADACHES HURT?

The trigeminal nerve has three branches that conduct sensations from the scalp, the blood vessels inside and outside of the skull, the lining around the brain (the meninges), and the face, mouth, neck, ears, eyes, and throat.

The brain tissue itself lacks pain-sensitive nerves and does not feel pain. Headaches occur when pain-sensitive nerve endings called "nociceptors" react to headache triggers (such as stress, certain foods or odors, or the use of medicines) and send messages through the trigeminal nerve to the thalamus, the brain's "relay station" for pain sensations from all over the body. The following explains what each of these body parts does on a regular basis:

- The trigeminal nerve—1 of 12 pairs of cranial nerves that start at the base of the brain—sends information

---

[2] "Fibromyalgia," National Institute of Arthritis and Musculoskeletal and Skin Diseases (NIAMS), June 2021. Available online. URL: www.niams.nih.gov/health-topics/fibromyalgia. Accessed April 13, 2023.

about touch, pain, temperature, and vibration in the head and neck back to the brain.

- The thalamus controls the body's sensitivity to light and noise and sends messages to parts of the brain that manage awareness of pain and emotional response to it.
- Other parts of the brain may also be part of the process, causing nausea, vomiting, diarrhea, trouble concentrating, and other neurological symptoms.

## WHO IS MORE LIKELY TO GET A HEADACHE?

Anyone can experience a headache. Certain types of headache run in families. Migraines occur in both children and adults but affect adult women three times more often than men.

### Children and Headache

Headaches are common in children. Headaches that begin early in life can develop into migraines as the child grows older. Migraines in children or adolescents can develop into tension-type headaches at any time. Unlike adults with migraine, young children often feel migraine pain on both sides of the head and have headaches that usually last less than two hours. Children may look pale and appear restless or irritable before and during an attack. Other children may become nauseous, lose their appetite, or feel pain elsewhere in the body during the headache.

Headaches in children can be caused by a number of triggers, including the following:

- emotional problems, such as the tension between family members
- stress from school activities
- weather changes
- irregular eating and sleep
- dehydration
- certain foods and drinks

Of special concern are headaches that occur after a head injury or those accompanied by rash, fever, or sleepiness.

It may be difficult to identify the type of headache because children often have problems describing where it hurts, how often the headaches occur, and how long they last. Asking a child with a headache to draw a picture of where the pain is and how it feels can make it easier for the doctor to determine the proper treatment.

Migraine is often misdiagnosed in children. Clues to watch for include sensitivity to light and noise, which may be suspected when a child refuses to watch television or use the computer or when the child stops playing to lie down in a dark room. Observe whether or not a child is able to eat during a headache. Very young children may seem cranky or irritable and complain of abdominal pain (abdominal migraine).

Headache treatment in children and teens usually includes rest, fluids, and over-the-counter (OTC) pain relief medicines. Always consult with a physician before giving headache medicines to a child. Most tension-type headaches in children can be treated with OTC medicines that are marked for children with usage guidelines based on the child's age and weight. Headaches in some children may also be treated effectively using relaxation/behavioral therapy. Children with cluster headaches may be treated with oxygen therapy early in the initial phase of the attacks.

## Headache and Sleep Disorders

Headaches are often a secondary symptom of a sleep disorder. For example, tension-type headache is regularly seen in persons with insomnia or sleep–wake cycle disorders. Nearly 75 percent of individuals who suffer from narcolepsy complain of either migraine or cluster headaches. Migraines and cluster headaches appear to be related to the number of and transition between rapid eye movement (REM) and other sleep periods an individual has during sleep. Hypnic headache awakens individuals mainly at night but may also interrupt daytime naps. Reduced oxygen levels in people with sleep apnea may trigger early morning headaches.

Getting the proper amount of sleep can ease headache pain. Generally, too little or too much sleep can worsen headaches, as can overuse of sleep medicines. Daytime naps often reduce deep sleep at night and can produce headaches in some adults. Some sleep disorders and secondary headaches are treated using anti-depressants. Check with a doctor before using OTC medicines to ease sleep-associated headaches.

## HOW IS A HEADACHE DIAGNOSED AND TREATED?

Not all headaches require a physician's attention. But headaches can signal a more serious disorder that requires prompt medical care. Immediately call or see a physician if you or someone you are with experience any of these symptoms:

- sudden, severe headache that may be accompanied by a stiff neck
- severe headache accompanied by fever, nausea, or vomiting that is not related to another illness
- "first" or "worst" headache, often accompanied by confusion, weakness, double vision, or loss of consciousness
- headache that worsens over days or weeks or has changed in pattern or behavior
- recurring headaches in children
- headache following a head injury
- headache and a loss of sensation or weakness in any part of the body, which could be a sign of a stroke
- headache associated with convulsions and/or shortness of breath
- two or more headaches a week
- persistent headache in someone who has been previously headache-free, particularly in someone over age 50
- new headaches in someone with a history of cancer or human immunodeficiency virus (HIV)/acquired immunodeficiency syndrome (AIDS)

### Diagnosing Headache

How and under what circumstances a person experiences a head-ache can be key to diagnosing its cause. Keeping a headache journal can help a physician better diagnose your type of headache and determine the best treatment. After each headache, note:

- the time of day when it occurred
- its intensity and duration
- any sensitivity to light, odors, or sound
- activity immediately prior to the headache
- use of prescription and nonprescription medicines
- amount of sleep the previous night
- any stressful or emotional conditions
- any influence from weather or daily activity
- foods and fluids consumed in the past 24 hours
- any known health conditions at that time

Women should record the days of their menstrual cycles. Include notes about other family members who have a history of headaches or other disorders. A pattern may emerge that can be helpful in reducing or preventing headaches.

Once your doctor reviews your medical and headache history and conducts physical and neurological exams, lab screening and diagnostic tests may be ordered to either rule out or identify conditions that might be the cause of your headaches.

Blood and urine tests can help diagnose brain or spinal cord infections, blood vessel damage, and toxins that affect the nervous system. Testing the fluid that surrounds the brain and spinal cord can detect infections and bleeding in the brain (called a "brain hemorrhage") and measure any buildup of pressure within the skull.

Diagnostic imaging, such as computed tomography (CT) and magnetic resonance imaging (MRI), can detect irregularities in blood vessels and bones, certain brain tumors and cysts, brain damage from head injury, brain hemorrhage, inflammation, infection, and other disorders. Neuroimaging also gives doctors a way to see what is happening in the brain during headache attacks. An electroencephalogram (EEG) measures brain wave activity and can help diagnose brain tumors, seizures, head injury, and inflammation that may lead to headaches.

## Headaches and Their Types of Treatment

Primary headaches occur independently and are not caused by another medical condition. A cascade of events that affect blood vessels and nerves inside and outside the head causes pain signals to be sent to the brain. Brain chemicals called "neurotransmitters" are involved in creating head pain, as are changes in nerve cell activity.

Primary headache disorders are divided into the following four main groups:

- migraine
- tension-type headache
- trigeminal autonomic cephalgias (including cluster headache)
- miscellaneous primary headache

## MIGRAINE

Migraine headaches are characterized by recurrent attacks of moderate-to-severe throbbing and pulsating pain on one side of the head. The pain is caused by the activation of nerve fibers that reside within the wall of brain blood vessels traveling within the meninges.

Untreated attacks last from 4 to 72 hours. Other common symptoms are as follows:

- increased sensitivity to light, noise, and odors
- nausea
- vomiting

Routine physical activity, movement, or even coughing or sneezing can worsen headache pain.

Migraines occur most frequently in the morning, especially upon waking. Some people have migraines at predictable times, such as before menstruation or on weekends following a stressful week of work. Many people feel exhausted or weak following a migraine but are usually symptom-free between attacks.

A number of different factors can increase your risk of having a migraine. These factors, which trigger the headache process, vary from person to person and include the following:

- sudden changes in weather or environment
- too much or not enough sleep
- strong odors or fumes
- emotion
- stress
- overexertion
- loud or sudden noises
- motion sickness
- low blood sugar
- skipped meals
- tobacco
- depression
- anxiety
- head trauma
- hangover
- some medications
- hormonal changes
- bright or flashing lights

Medication overuse or missed doses may also cause headaches. Certain foods or ingredients, including the following, can trigger headaches; keeping a diet journal can help you identify your triggers:

- aspartame
- caffeine (or caffeine withdrawal)
- wine and other types of alcohol
- chocolate
- aged cheeses
- monosodium glutamate (MSG)
- some fruits and nuts
- fermented or pickled goods
- yeast
- cured or processed meats

## Migraine Treatment

Migraine treatment is aimed at relieving symptoms and preventing additional attacks. Quick steps to ease symptoms may include the following:

- napping or resting with eyes closed in a quiet, darkened room
- placing a cool cloth or ice pack on the forehead
- drinking lots of fluid, particularly if the migraine is accompanied by vomiting
- small amounts of caffeine to relieve symptoms during a migraine's early stages

Drug therapy for migraine is divided into acute and preventive treatment. Acute or "abortive" medications are taken as soon as symptoms occur to relieve pain and restore function. Preventive treatment involves taking medicines daily to reduce the severity of future attacks or keep them from happening. The U.S. Food and Drug Administration (FDA) has approved the drugs enenmab (Aimovig) for the preventive treatment of headaches and galcanezumab-gnlm (Emgality) injections to treat episodic cluster headaches. The FDA has also approved lasmiditan (Reyvow) and ubrogepant (Ubrelvy) tablets for short-term treatment of migraine with or without aura. Headache drug use should be monitored by a physician since some drugs may cause side effects.

Acute treatment for migraine may include any of the following drugs:

- Triptan drugs increase levels of the neurotransmitter serotonin in the brain. Serotonin causes blood vessels to constrict and lowers the pain threshold. Triptans are the preferred treatment for migraine because they can alleviate mmoderate-to-severe igraine pain.
- Ergot derivative drugs bind to serotonin receptors on nerve cells and decrease the transmission of pain messages along nerve fibers. They are most effective during the early stages of migraine.

- Nonprescription analgesics or OTC drugs such as ibuprofen, aspirin, or acetaminophen can ease the pain of less severe migraine headaches.
- Combination analgesics involve a mix of drugs, such as acetaminophen plus caffeine and/or a narcotic for migraine that may be resistant to simple analgesics.
- Nonsteroidal anti-inflammatory drugs can reduce inflammation and alleviate pain.
- Nausea relief drugs can ease queasiness brought on by various types of headaches.
- Narcotics are prescribed briefly to relieve pain. These drugs should not be used to treat chronic headaches.

Taking headache relief drugs more than three times a week may lead to medication overuse headache, in which the initial headache is relieved temporarily but reappears as the drug wears off. Taking more of the drug to treat the new headache leads to progressively shorter periods of pain relief and results in a pattern of recurrent chronic headaches. Headache pain ranges from moderate to severe and may occur with nausea or irritability. It may take weeks for these headaches to end once the drug is stopped.

Everyone with a migraine needs effective treatment at the time of the headaches. Some people with frequent and severe migraine need preventive medications. In general, prevention should be considered if migraines occur one or more times weekly or if migraines are less frequent but disabling. Preventive medicines are also recommended for individuals who take symptomatic headache treatment more than three times a week. Physicians will also recommend that a migraine sufferer take one or more preventive medications for two to three months to assess drug effectiveness unless intolerable side effects occur.

Several preventive medicines for migraine were initially marketed for conditions other than migraine:

- Anticonvulsants may be helpful for people with other types of headaches in addition to migraine. Although originally developed for treating epilepsy, these drugs increase levels of certain neurotransmitters and dampen pain impulses.

- Beta-blockers are used to treat high blood pressure and are often effective for migraine.
- Calcium channel blockers are used to treat high blood pressure treatment and help stabilize blood vessel walls. These drugs appear to work by preventing the blood vessels from either narrowing or widening, which affects blood flow to the brain.
- Antidepressants work on different chemicals in the brain; their effectiveness in treating migraine is not directly related to their effect on mood. Antidepressants may be helpful for individuals with other types of headaches because they increase the production of serotonin and may also affect levels of other chemicals, such as norepinephrine and dopamine.

Natural treatments for migraine include riboflavin (vitamin B2), magnesium, coenzyme Q10, and butterbur (plant extract).

Nondrug therapy for migraine includes biofeedback and relaxation training, both of which help individuals cope with or control the development of pain and the body's response to stress.

Lifestyle changes that reduce or prevent migraine attacks in some individuals include exercising, avoiding food and beverages that trigger headaches, eating regularly scheduled meals with adequate hydration, stopping certain medications, and establishing a consistent sleep schedule. Obesity increases the risk of developing chronic daily headaches, so a weight loss program is recommended for obese individuals.

## TENSION-TYPE HEADACHE

Tension-type headache is the most common type of headache. Its name indicates the role of stress and mental or emotional conflict in triggering the pain and contracting muscles in the neck, face, scalp, and jaw. Tension-type headaches may also be caused by:

- jaw clenching
- intense work
- missed meals
- depression

- anxiety
- not enough sleep

Sleep apnea may also cause tension-type headaches, especially in the morning. The pain is usually mild-to-moderate and feels as if constant pressure is being applied to the front of the face or to the head or neck. It may also feel as if a belt is being tightened around the head. Most often, the pain is felt on both sides of the head. People who suffer tension-type headaches may also feel overly sensitive to light and sound, but there is no preheadache aura as with migraine. Typically, tension-type headaches usually disappear once the period of stress or related cause has ended.

Tension-type headaches affect women slightly more often than men. The headaches usually begin in adolescence and reach peak activity in the 30s. They have not been linked to hormones and do not have a strong hereditary connection. The following are the two forms of tension-type headaches:

- Episodic tension-type headaches occur between 10 and 15 days per month, with each attack lasting from 30 minutes to several days. Although the pain is not disabling, the severity of the pain typically increases with the frequency of attacks.
- Chronic tension-type attacks usually occur more than 15 days per month over a three-month period. The pain, which can be constant over a period of days or months, strikes both sides of the head and is more severe and disabling than episodic headache pain. Chronic tension headaches can cause sore scalps—even combing your hair can be painful. Most individuals will have had some form of episodic tension-type headache prior to the onset of chronic tension-type headaches.

Depression and anxiety can cause tension-type headaches. Headaches may appear in the early morning or evening when conflicts in the office or at home are anticipated. Other causes include physical postures that strain head and neck muscles (such as holding your chin down while reading or holding a phone between your shoulder and ear), degenerative arthritis of the neck, and temporomandibular joint dysfunction (a disorder of the joints between the temporal bone located above the ear and the mandible, or lower jawbone).

The first step in caring for a tension-type headache involves treating any specific disorder or disease that may be causing it. For example, arthritis of the neck is treated with anti-inflammatory medication, and temporomandibular joint dysfunction may be helped by corrective devices for the mouth and jaw. A sleep study may be needed to detect sleep apnea and should be considered when there is a history of snoring, daytime sleepiness, or obesity.

A physician may suggest using analgesics, nonsteroidal anti-inflammatory drugs, or antidepressants to treat a tension-type headache that is not associated with a disease. Triptan drugs, barbiturates (drugs that have a relaxing or sedative effect), and ergot derivatives may provide relief to people who suffer from both migraine and tension-type headaches.

Alternative therapies for chronic tension-type headaches include biofeedback, relaxation training, meditation, and cognitive-behavioral therapy (CBT) to reduce stress. A hot shower or moist heat applied to the back of the neck may ease symptoms of infrequent tension headaches. Physical therapy, massage, and gentle exercise of the neck may also be helpful.

## TRIGEMINAL AUTONOMIC CEPHALGIAS

Some primary headaches are characterized by severe pain in or around the eye on one side of the face and autonomic (or involuntary) features on the same side, such as red and teary eyes, drooping eyelid, and runny nose. These disorders, called "trigeminal autonomic cephalgias," differ in attack duration and frequency and have episodic and chronic forms. Episodic attacks occur on a daily or near-daily basis for weeks or months with pain-free remissions. Chronic attacks occur on a daily or near-daily basis for a year or more with only brief remissions.

## Cluster Headache

The most severe form of primary headache involves sudden, extremely painful headaches that occur in "clusters," usually at the same time of the day and night for several weeks. They strike one side of the head, often behind or around one eye, and may be preceded by a migraine-like aura and nausea. The pain usually peaks 5–10 minutes after onset and continues at that intensity for up to three hours. The nose and the eye on the affected side of the face may get red, swollen, and teary. Some people will experience restlessness and agitation, changes in heart rate and blood pressure, and sensitivity to light, sound, or smell. These headaches often wake people from sleep.

Cluster headaches generally begin between the ages of 20 and 50 but may start at any age, occur more often in men than in women, and are more common in smokers than in nonsmokers. The attacks are usually less frequent and shorter than migraines. It is common to have one to three cluster headaches a day with two cluster periods a year, separated by months of freedom from symptoms. The cluster periods often appear seasonally, usually in the spring and fall, and may be mistaken for allergies. A small group of people develops a chronic form of the disorder, which is characterized by bouts of headaches that can go on for years with only brief periods (one month or less) of remission. Cluster headaches occur more often at night than during the day, suggesting they could be caused by irregularities in the body's sleep–wake cycle. Alcohol (especially red wine) and smoking can provoke attacks. Studies show a connection between cluster headaches and prior head trauma. An increased familial risk of these headaches suggests that there may be a genetic cause.

Treatment options include noninvasive vagus nerve stimulation (which uses a hand-held device to provide electrical stimulation to the vagus nerve through the skin), galcanezumab-gnlm injections, triptan drugs, and oxygen therapy (in which pure oxygen is inhaled through a mask to reduce blood flow to the brain). Certain antipsychotic drugs, calcium-channel blockers, and anticonvulsants can reduce pain severity and frequency of attacks. In extreme cases, electrical stimulation of the occipital nerve to prevent nerve signaling or surgical procedures that destroy or cut certain facial nerves may provide relief.

## Paroxysmal Hemicrania

Paroxysmal hemicrania is a rare form of primary headache that usually begins in adulthood. Pain and related symptoms may be similar to those felt in cluster headaches but with shorter duration. Attacks typically occur 5–40 times per day, with each attack lasting 2–45 minutes. Severe throbbing, claw-like, or piercing pain is felt on one side of the face-in, around or behind the eye, and occasionally reaching to the back of the neck. Other symptoms may include red and watery eyes, a drooping or swollen eyelid on the affected side of the face, and nasal congestion. Individuals may also feel dull pain, soreness, or tenderness between attacks or increased sensitivity to light on the affected side of the face.

Paroxysmal hemicrania has two forms:
- **Chronic**. Individuals experience attacks on a daily basis for a year or more.
- **Episodic**. The headaches may stop for months or years before recurring.

Certain movements of the head or neck, external pressure to the neck, and alcohol use may trigger these headaches. Attacks occur more often in women than in men and have no familial pattern.

The nonsteroidal anti-inflammatory drug indomethacin can quickly halt the pain and related symptoms of paroxysmal hemicrania, but symptoms recur once the drug treatment is stopped. Nonprescription analgesics and calcium-channel blockers can ease discomfort, particularly if taken when symptoms first appear.

## Short-Lasting, Unilateral, Neuralgiform Headache with Conjunctival Injection and Tearing

Short-lasting, unilateral, neuralgiform headache with conjunctival injection and tearing (SUNCT) is a very rare type of headache with bursts of moderate-to-severe burning, piercing, or throbbing pain that is usually felt in the forehead, eye, or temple on one side of the head. The pain usually peaks within seconds of onset and may follow a pattern of increasing and decreasing intensity. Attacks typically occur during the day and last from five seconds to four minutes per episode. Individuals generally have five to six attacks per hour and are pain-free between attacks. This primary headache is slightly more common in men than in women, with onset usually after age 50. SUNCT may be episodic, occurring once or twice annually with headaches that remit and recur, or chronic, lasting more than one year.

Symptoms include the following:
- reddish or bloodshot eyes (conjunctival injection)
- watery eyes
- stuffy or runny nose
- sweaty forehead
- puffy eyelids
- increased pressure within the eye on the affected side of the head
- increased blood pressure

SUNCT is very difficult to treat. Anticonvulsants may relieve some of the symptoms, while anesthetics and corticosteroid drugs can treat some of the severe pain felt during these headaches. Surgery and glycerol injections to block nerve signaling along the trigeminal nerve have poor outcomes and provide only temporary relief in severe cases. Doctors are beginning to use deep brain stimulation (involving a surgically implanted battery-powered electrode that emits pulses of energy to surrounding brain tissue) to reduce the frequency of attacks in severely affected individuals.[3]

## SLEEP GENE LINKED TO MIGRAINES

Migraines—pounding headaches sometimes preceded by a visual "aura" and often coupled with vomiting, nausea, distorted vision, and hypersensitivity to sound and touch—can be highly debilitating if recurrent and prolonged. They affect millions of Americans

[3] "Headache," National Institute of Neurological Disorders and Stroke (NINDS), March 8, 2023. Available online. URL: www.ninds.nih.gov/health-information/disorders/headache. Accessed April 13, 2023.

and an estimated 10–20 percent of the global population. Yet what predisposes individuals to them is somewhat of a mystery. Though there are certainly environmental triggers, the tendency for migraines to run in families suggests that there's likely an inherited component. Recently, a team of NIH-funded researchers, one of whom regularly suffered from migraines herself, found a gene that plays a part.

The clue that helped them identify the rogue gene came from a family that suffers from both migraines and a rare sleep disorder called "familial advanced sleep phase syndrome." The syndrome disrupts their sleep cycle, causing family members to fall asleep early, about 7 p.m., and rise around 4 a.m.

The researchers hunted for the cause of the sleep cycle disorder and discovered a mutation in the *casein kinase I delta* (*CKIδ*) gene. The gene produces an enzyme that is important for brain signaling and regulating our circadian rhythms. The particular mutation in this family seemed to reduce the activity of the *CKIδ* enzyme and made the researchers wonder whether the mutation was also responsible for causing migraines. To test the hypothesis, they engineered mice that carried the same mutation.

Just like the humans, the *CKIδ* mutant mice had disrupted sleep–wake cycles—but they were also more likely to suffer migraines compared to normal mice when given nitroglycerin. You cannot exactly ask a mouse if it has a headache. But, because migraines cause a range of sensory issues, there are other physical signs the researchers could monitor in the mice. In this case, the *CKIδ* mutant mice became more sensitive to pain, temperature, and touch than normal mice. This mirrors the experience of many migraine sufferers.

The *CKIδ* mutant mice were also more vulnerable to a type of brain activity called "cortical spreading depression" (CSD)—a wave of electrical silence that follows electrical stimulation. Brain cells called "astrocytes" from *CKIδ* mutants functioned differently from those from healthy mice, suggesting one possible mechanism through which the mutation wreaks havoc in the brain.

*CKIδ* affects several different proteins in the cell. The next step will be to tease apart which of these plays a role in triggering migraines. Once we understand how migraines begin, we have a better chance of identifying a new generation of drugs that can block that painful path.[4]

[4] "Sleep Gene Linked to Migraines," National Institutes of Health (NIH), May 21, 2013. Available online. URL: https://directorsblog.nih.gov/2013/05/21/sleep-gene-linked-to-migraines. Accessed April 13, 2023.

# Chapter 30 | Chronic Fatigue Syndrome and Sleep

## Chapter Contents

## Section 30.1 | Chronic Fatigue Syndrome in Children

Myalgic encephalomyelitis/chronic fatigue syndrome (ME/CFS) is a disabling and complex illness. Scientists do not know what causes it, and there is no cure or approved treatment for the illness. ME/CFS is often thought of as a problem in adults, but children (both adolescents and younger children) can also get ME/CFS.

- Not as much is known about ME/CFS in children because there have been few studies in this age group.
- Scientists estimate that up to 2 in 1,000 children suffer from ME/CFS.
- ME/CFS is more common in adolescents than in younger children.

### SYMPTOMS OF MYALGIC ENCEPHALOMYELITIS/CHRONIC FATIGUE SYNDROME IN CHILDREN

Children and adolescents with ME/CFS mostly have the same symptoms as adults. The following are some differences:
- Children, especially adolescents, with ME/CFS have orthostatic intolerance (dizziness and light-headedness and other symptoms that are triggered when standing up and sometimes also sitting upright) more often than adults. It is often the most unbearable symptom and may make other symptoms of ME/CFS worse.
- Sleep problems in young children may show up as a lack of their usual energy. In adolescents with ME/CFS, sleep problems may be hard to detect, as sleep cycles change during puberty. Many adolescents begin to stay up late and often have trouble waking up early. The demands of classes, homework, after-school jobs, and social activities also affect sleep. Common sleep complaints in children and adolescents with ME/CFS include:
  - difficulty falling or staying asleep
  - daytime sleepiness
  - intense and vivid dreaming

- Unlike adults with ME/CFS, children and adolescents with ME/CFS do not usually have muscle and joint pain. Yet headaches and stomach pain may be more common in this age group. Younger children may not be able to describe the pain well.
- In children, particularly in adolescents, ME/CFS is more likely to start after an acute illness, such as the flu or mononucleosis. Sometimes, ME/CFS in children might begin gradually.

## DIAGNOSIS OF MYALGIC ENCEPHALOMYELITIS/CHRONIC FATIGUE SYNDROME IN CHILDREN

As in adults, symptoms of ME/CFS in children and adolescents may appear similar to many other illnesses, and there is no test to confirm ME/CFS. This makes ME/CFS difficult to diagnose. The illness can be unpredictable. Symptoms may come and go, or there may be changes in how bad they are over time.

A diagnosis of ME/CFS requires at least six months of illness. However, children and other patients should be seen by doctors and get support as soon as they become ill. In other words, a child with some or all of the symptoms of ME/CFS should not wait for months to see a doctor. This six-month period is used to complete laboratory tests and other activities, including follow-up appointments, to check for other illnesses that have symptoms similar to ME/CFS. The six-month period also allows time for improvement for children with illnesses that have symptoms such as ME/CFS but that do not usually last as long as ME/CFS. It is also important that management of symptoms begins before six months have passed and that support and accommodations for children in school are considered and implemented during this time.

To diagnose ME/CFS, the child's doctor may undertake the following:

- Ask about the child's and family's medical history, including a review of any medications and recent illnesses.
- Do a thorough physical and mental status examination.
- Order blood, urine, or other tests.

To get a better idea about the child's illness, the doctor may ask many questions. Depending on the age of the child, the questions might be asked of the patient, parent/guardian, or both (together or independently). Questions might include the following:

- What is the child able to do now? How does it compare to what the child was able to do before?
- How long has the child been ill?
- Does the child feel better after sleeping or resting?
- What makes the child feel worse? What helps the child feel better?
- What symptoms keep the child from doing what he/she needs or wants to do?
- Does the child ever feel dizzy or light-headed? Has the child been falling more often than before?
- Does the child seem to have trouble remembering or focusing on tasks?
- What happens when the child tries to do activities that used to be normal?

Parents/guardians and patients may want to keep a journal for their ill child. This could help patients and families remember important details during their health-care visits. Keeping track of the child's activities and what leads to the worsening of the child's symptoms can help identify the effects of the illness on daily activities.

Doctors might refer patients to see a specialist, such as a neurologist, rheumatologist, or sleep specialist, to check for other conditions that can cause similar symptoms. These specialists might find other conditions that could be treated. Patients can have other conditions and still have ME/CFS. However, getting treatment for other conditions might help patients with ME/CFS feel better.

A number of factors can make diagnosing ME/CFS more difficult. For example:

- There is no laboratory test to confirm ME/CFS.
- Fatigue and other symptoms of ME/CFS are common to many illnesses.

- The illness is unpredictable, and symptoms may come and go.
- The type, number, and severity of ME/CFS symptoms vary from person to person.

When diagnosing ME/CFS in children and adolescents, it is useful to remember the following:
- Children and adolescents cannot always accurately describe their symptoms or how they feel.
- Parents may describe their child's symptoms differently from how the child describes her/his symptoms.

Children with ME/CFS may miss school, which may be mistaken for school phobia. But, unlike those with school phobia, children with ME/CFS are still ill and inactive on weekends and holidays. They may not be able to do their hobbies and take part in social activities as they did before the illness. They may also have a problem completing school assignments within the usual time. This might be a result of problems with thinking, learning, and memory caused by the illness.

## TREATMENT FOR MYALGIC ENCEPHALOMYELITIS/CHRONIC FATIGUE SYNDROME IN CHILDREN

As for adults, there is no cure or approved treatment for ME/CFS in children. However, some symptoms can be treated or managed. Treating these symptoms might provide relief for some patients with ME/CFS but not others. Other strategies, such as learning new ways to manage activity, can also be helpful.

Patients, their families, and health-care providers need to work together to decide which symptom causes the most problems. They should discuss the possible benefits and harms of any treatment plans, including medicines and other therapies. A treatment plan for a child who might have ME/CFS should focus on the most disruptive symptoms first.

The following are the symptoms that health-care providers might try to address.

## Post-Exertional Malaise

Post-exertional malaise (PEM) is the worsening of symptoms after even minor physical, mental, or emotional exertion. The symptoms typically get worse 12–48 hours after the activity and can last for days, weeks, or even longer.

PEM can be addressed by activity management, also called "pacing." The goal of pacing is for children with ME/CFS to learn to balance rest and activity to avoid PEM flare-ups caused by exertion that they cannot tolerate. To do this, patients need to find their individual limits for mental and physical activities. Then they need to plan activities and rest to stay within these limits. Some patients and doctors refer to staying within these limits as staying within the "energy envelope." The limits may be different for each patient. Keeping activity and symptom diaries may help patients find their personal limits, especially early on in the illness.

Patients with ME/CFS need to avoid "push-and-crash" cycles by carefully managing activity. "Push-and-crash" cycles are when someone with ME/CFS is having a good day and tries to push to do more than they would normally attempt (do too much, crash, rest, start to feel a little better, do too much once again). This can then lead to a "crash" (worsening of ME/CFS symptoms).

Any activity or exercise plan for children with ME/CFS needs to be carefully designed with input from each patient. While vigorous aerobic exercise is beneficial for many chronic illnesses, patients with ME/CFS do not tolerate such exercise routines. Standard exercise recommendations for healthy people can be harmful to patients with ME/CFS. However, it is important that patients with ME/CFS undertake activities that they can tolerate.

For patients with ME/CFS, it is important to find a balance between inactivity and excessive activity, which can make symptoms worse. This means a new way of thinking about daily activities. For example, daily chores and school activities may need to be broken down into smaller steps. A symptom diary can be very helpful for managing ME/CFS. Keeping daily track of how patients feel and what patients do may help find ways to make activities easier.

Rehabilitation specialists or exercise physiologists who know ME/CFS may help patients with adjusting to life with ME/CFS. Patients who have learned to listen to their bodies might benefit from carefully increasing exercise to improve fitness and avoid deconditioning. However, exercise is not a cure for ME/CFS.

Parents/guardians and doctors of children with ME/CFS can work with teachers and school administrators to adjust the school load for children with ME/CFS. While it is true that exercise can benefit children with certain chronic illnesses, children with ME/CFS should avoid activity that makes their symptoms worse.

### Dizziness and Light-Headedness (Orthostatic Intolerance)

Some children and adolescents with ME/CFS might also have symptoms of orthostatic intolerance that are triggered when—or made worse by—standing or sitting upright. These symptoms can include the following:

- frequent dizziness and light-headedness
- changes in vision (blurred vision, seeing white or black spots)
- weakness
- feeling like your heart is beating too fast or too hard, fluttering, or skipping a beat

For patients with these symptoms, their doctor will check their heart rate and blood pressure and may recommend they see a specialist, such as a cardiologist or neurologist.

For children with ME/CFS who do not have heart or blood vessel disease, their doctor might suggest patients increase daily fluid and salt intake and use support stockings. If symptoms do not improve, prescription medication can be considered.

### Sleep Problems

Good sleep habits are important for all people, including those with ME/CFS. When children try these tips but are still unable to sleep, their doctor might recommend taking medicine to help with sleep.

Children might continue to feel unrefreshed even after the medications help them get a full night of sleep. If so, they should consider seeing a sleep specialist. Most people with sleep disorders, such as sleep apnea (symptoms include brief pausing in breathing during sleep) and narcolepsy (symptoms include excessive daytime sleepiness), respond to therapy. However, for children with ME/CFS, not all symptoms may go away.

## Problems Concentrating, Thinking, and Remembering

Children with ME/CFS may have problems paying attention, thinking, remembering, and responding. For instance, after becoming ill, it may be hard for children to take notes and listen to their teacher at the same time.

For children with ME/CFS who have concentration problems, some doctors have prescribed stimulant medications, such as those typically used to treat attention deficit hyperactivity disorder (ADHD). While stimulants might help improve concentration for some patients with ME/CFS, they might lead to the "push-and-crash" cycle and worsen symptoms.

## Depression, Stress, and Anxiety

Adjusting to any chronic illness can sometimes lead to symptoms of depression and anxiety. Anxiety in children with ME/CFS is not caused by the illness itself. It can happen because of the changes the child must make to live with the illness. When health-care providers are concerned about a patient's psychological condition, they may recommend seeing a mental health professional.

Counseling may help reduce stress and some symptoms of depression and anxiety, such as sleep problems and headaches. Some children might benefit from antidepressants and antianxiety medications. However, doctors should use caution in prescribing these medications. Some drugs used to treat depression have other effects that might worsen other ME/CFS symptoms and cause side effects.

Some children with ME/CFS might benefit from trying techniques such as deep breathing and muscle relaxation, massage, and movement therapies (such as stretching, yoga, and tai chi). These can reduce stress and anxiety and promote a sense of well-being.

Although treating depression and anxiety can ease mental and emotional distress in some patients and can be very beneficial, it is not a cure for ME/CFS.

## Pain

Children with ME/CFS often have headaches and stomach pains. Doctors may want to check for food allergies and vision problems.

Gentle massage and heat may relieve pain for some patients. Parents/guardians should always talk to their child's health-care provider before trying any medication. Doctors may recommend trying over-the-counter (OTC) pain relievers, such as acetaminophen or ibuprofen.

It is important that health-care providers talk with family members and children about the child's lifestyle and behaviors to find out how the illness impacts the child's daily life. For example, the child's lack of energy may be because of ME/CFS or caused by normal changes in sleep cycles that often happen in puberty. Trying to understand what is causing the symptoms is important because it affects the treatment plan for the child.[1]

## Section 30.2 | Chronic Fatigue Syndrome in Adults

### WHAT IS MYALGIC ENCEPHALOMYELITIS/CHRONIC FATIGUE SYNDROME?

Myalgic encephalomyelitis/chronic fatigue syndrome (ME/CFS) is a disabling and complex illness. People with ME/CFS are often not able to do their usual activities. At times, ME/CFS may confine them to bed. People with ME/CFS have overwhelming fatigue that is not improved by rest. ME/CFS may get worse after any activity, whether it is physical or mental. This symptom is known as

---

[1] "ME/CFS in Children," Centers for Disease Control and Prevention (CDC), June 2, 2022. Available online. URL: www.cdc.gov/me-cfs/me-cfs-children/index.html. Accessed May 2, 2023.

"post-exertional malaise" (PEM). Other symptoms can include problems with sleep, thinking and concentrating, pain, and dizziness. People with ME/CFS may not look ill, but their condition may interfere in other ways that include the following:

- People with ME/CFS are not able to function the same way they did before they became ill.
- ME/CFS changes people's ability to do daily tasks, such as taking a shower or preparing a meal.
- ME/CFS often makes it hard to keep a job, go to school, and take part in family and social life.
- ME/CFS can last for years and sometimes leads to serious disability.
- At least one in four ME/CFS patients is bedbound or house bound for long periods during their illness.

Anyone can get ME/CFS. While most common in people between 40 and 60 years old, the illness affects children, adolescents, and adults of all ages. Among adults, women are affected more often than men. White persons are diagnosed more than other races and ethnicities. But many people with ME/CFS have not been diagnosed, especially among people from racial and ethnic minority groups.

The following are the data as noted in the Institute of Medicine (IOM) report:

- An estimated number of 836,000 to 2.5 million Americans suffer from ME/CFS.
- About 90 percent of people with ME/CFS have not been diagnosed.
- ME/CFS costs the U.S. economy about $17–$24 billion annually in medical bills and lost incomes.

Some of the reasons that people with ME/CFS have not been diagnosed include limited access to health care and a lack of education about ME/CFS among health-care providers.

- Most medical schools in the United States do not have ME/CFS as part of their physician training.
- The illness is often misunderstood and might not be taken seriously by some health-care providers.

- More education for doctors and nurses is urgently needed, so they are prepared to provide timely diagnosis and appropriate care for patients.

Researchers have not yet found what causes ME/CFS, and there are no specific laboratory tests to diagnose ME/CFS directly. Therefore, doctors need to consider the diagnosis of ME/CFS based on an in-depth evaluation of a person's symptoms and medical history. It is also important that doctors diagnose and treat any other conditions that can cause similar symptoms. Even though there is no cure for ME/CFS, some symptoms can be treated or managed.

## CAUSES OF MYALGIC ENCEPHALOMYELITIS/CHRONIC FATIGUE SYNDROME

Scientists have not yet identified what causes ME/CFS. It is possible that ME/CFS has more than one cause, meaning that patients with ME/CFS could have illnesses resulting from different causes (see below). In addition, it is possible that two or more triggers might work together to cause the illness.

Some of the areas that are being studied as possible causes of ME/CFS are as follows.

### Infections

People with ME/CFS often have their illness begin in a way that reminds them of getting the flu. This has made researchers suspect an infection may trigger ME/CFS. In addition, about 1 in 10 people who become infected with Epstein-Barr virus, Ross River virus, or *Coxiella burnetti* will develop a set of symptoms that meet the criteria for ME/CFS. People with these infections who had severe symptoms are more likely than those with mild symptoms to later develop ME/CFS symptoms. But not all people with ME/CFS have had these infections.

Other infections that have been studied in connection with ME/CFS are human herpesvirus 6, enterovirus, rubella, *Candida albicans*, bornavirus, mycoplasma, and human immunodeficiency virus (HIV). However, these infections have not been found to cause ME/CFS.

## Immune System Changes

It is possible that ME/CFS is caused by a change in the person's immune system and the way it responds to infection or stress. ME/CFS shares some features of autoimmune illnesses (diseases in which the immune system attacks healthy tissues in own body, such as rheumatoid arthritis). For example, both ME/CFS and most autoimmune diseases are more common in women, and both are characterized by increased inflammation. However, other signs of autoimmune diseases, such as tissue damage, are not found in patients with ME/CFS.

Scientists think that the immune system might be contributing to ME/CFS in other ways, including the following:

- **Chronic production of cytokines**. Cytokines are proteins that are produced by the immune system and regulate the behavior of other cells. Higher levels of cytokines for a prolonged period can lead to changes in the body's ability to respond to stress and might lead to the development of health conditions, including ME/CFS.

- **Low-functioning natural killer (NK) cells**. NK cells are cells of the immune system that help the body fight infections. Many patients with ME/CFS have NK cells with a lower functional ability to fight infections. Studies have found that the poorer the function of NK cells in ME/CFS patients, the worse the severity of the illness. NK cell function tests are hard to do, and their results are not reliable outside of research studies. Because of this problem, NK cell function testing is not yet useful for health-care providers. Also, low NK cell function can occur in other illnesses and thus cannot be used to diagnose ME/CFS.

- **Differences in markers of T-cell activation**. T-cells are cells of the immune system that help activate and suppress immune responses to infections. If they become too active or not active enough, the immune response does not work as it should. However, not all patients with ME/CFS appear to have these differences in markers of T-cell activation.

## Stress Affecting Body Chemistry

Physical or emotional stress affects the hypothalamic-pituitary-adrenal axis (HPA axis). The HPA axis is a complex network that controls our body's reaction to stress and regulates a lot of body processes such as the immune response, digestion, energy usage, and mood. This occurs through connections between two glands of the nervous system (hypothalamus and pituitary) and adrenal glands (small organs that reside on top of the kidneys). The glands release various hormones, such as corticotrophin-releasing hormone (CRH), cortisol, and others. When these hormones get out of balance, many body systems and functions, such as the immune response, can be negatively affected. Cortisol, also called the "stress hormone," helps lower inflammation and calm down the immune system. Low levels of cortisol thus may lead to an increase in inflammation and chronic activation of the immune system.

Patients with ME/CFS commonly report physical or emotional stress before they become ill. Some patients with ME/CFS have lower levels of cortisol than healthy people, but their cortisol levels are still within the normal range. Therefore, doctors cannot use cortisol levels to diagnose or treat ME/CFS.

## Changes in Energy Production

Scientists found differences between people with ME/CFS and healthy people in the way cells in their bodies get their energy. However, more studies are needed to figure out how these findings may be contributing to the illness.

## SYMPTOMS OF MYALGIC ENCEPHALOMYELITIS/CHRONIC FATIGUE SYNDROME

Symptoms of ME/CFS may appear similar to many other illnesses, and there is no test to confirm ME/CFS. This makes ME/CFS difficult to diagnose. The illness can be unpredictable. Symptoms may come and go, or there may be changes in how bad they are over time.

A doctor should be able to distinguish ME/CFS from other illnesses by doing a thorough medical exam. This includes asking many questions about the patient's health history and current illness and asking about the symptoms to learn how often they occur, how bad they are, and how long they have lasted. It is also important for doctors to talk with patients about how the symptoms affect their lives.

## Primary Symptoms

Also called "core" symptoms, three primary symptoms are required for diagnosis:

- The first symptom is greatly lowered ability to do activities that were usual before the illness. This drop in activity level occurs along with fatigue and must last six months or longer. People with ME/CFS have fatigue that is very different from just being tired. The fatigue of ME/CFS:
  - can be severe
  - is not a result of unusually difficult activity
  - is not relieved by sleep or rest
  - was not a problem before becoming ill (not lifelong)
- Worsening of ME/CFS symptoms after physical or mental activity that would not have caused a problem before the illness is the second symptom. This is known as "PEM." People with ME/CFS often describe this experience as a "crash," "relapse," or "collapse." During PEM, any ME/CFS symptoms may get worse or first appear, including difficulty thinking, problems sleeping, sore throat, headaches, feeling dizzy, or severe tiredness. It may take days, weeks, or longer to recover from a crash. Sometimes, patients may be housebound or even completely bedbound during crashes. People with ME/CFS may not be able to predict what will cause a crash or how long it will last. The following are a few examples:
  - Attending a child's school event may leave someone housebound for a couple of days and not able to do needed tasks, such as laundry.
  - Shopping at the grocery store may cause a physical crash that requires a nap in the car before driving home or a call for a ride home.

- Taking a shower may leave someone with ME/CFS bedbound and unable to do anything for days.
- Keeping up with work may lead to spending evenings and weekends recovering from the effort.
- People with ME/CFS may not feel better or less tired, even after a full night of sleep. Some people with ME/CFS may have problems falling asleep or staying asleep.

In addition to these core symptoms, one of the following two symptoms is required for diagnosis:

- **Problems with thinking and memory**. Most people with ME/CFS have trouble thinking quickly, remembering things, and paying attention to details. Patients often say they have "brain fog" to describe this problem because they feel "stuck in a fog" and are not able to think clearly.
- **Worsening of symptoms while standing or sitting upright**. This is called "orthostatic intolerance." People with ME/CFS may be light-headed, dizzy, weak, or faint while standing or sitting up. They may have vision changes such as blurring or seeing spots.

## Other Common Symptoms

Many, but not all, people with ME/CFS have other symptoms.

Pain is very common in people with ME/CFS. The type of pain, where it occurs, and how bad it is vary a lot. The pain people with ME/CFS feel is not caused by an injury. The most common types of pain in ME/CFS are:

- muscle pain and aches
- joint pain without swelling or redness
- headaches, either new or worsening

Some people with ME/CFS may also have:

- tender lymph nodes in the neck or armpits
- a sore throat that happens often
- digestive issues, such as irritable bowel syndrome (IBS)
- chills and night sweats

- allergies and sensitivities to foods, odors, chemicals, light, or noise
- muscle weakness
- shortness of breath
- irregular heartbeat

## DIAGNOSIS OF MYALGIC ENCEPHALOMYELITIS/CHRONIC FATIGUE SYNDROME

To diagnose ME/CFS, a patient's doctor or health-care provider will do the following:

- Ask about the medical history of the patient and their family.
- Do a thorough physical and mental status examination.
- Order blood, urine, or other tests.

To get a better idea about the illness, the health-care provider will ask many questions. Questions might include the following:

- What are you able to do now? How does it compare to what you were able to do before?
- How long have you felt this way?
- Do you feel better after sleeping or resting?
- What makes you feel worse? What helps you feel better?
- What happens when you try to push to do activities that are now hard for you?
- Are you able to think as clearly as you did before becoming ill?
- What symptoms keep you from doing what you need or want to do?

Patients may want to keep an activity journal. This could help them remember important details during their health-care visit. Doctors might refer patients to see a specialist, such as a neurologist, rheumatologist, or sleep specialist, to check for other conditions that can cause similar symptoms. These specialists might find other conditions that could be treated. Patients can have other conditions and still have ME/CFS. However, getting treatment for these conditions might help patients with ME/CFS feel better.

## TREATMENT FOR MYALGIC ENCEPHALOMYELITIS/CHRONIC FATIGUE SYNDROME

There is no cure or approved treatment for ME/CFS. However, some symptoms can be treated or managed. Treating these symptoms might provide relief for some patients with ME/CFS but not others. Other strategies, such as learning new ways to manage activity, can also be helpful.

Patients, their families, and health-care providers need to work together to decide which symptom causes the most problems. This should be treated first. Patients, families, and health-care providers should discuss the possible benefits and harms of any treatment plans, including medicines and other therapies.

Health-care providers need to support their patients' families as they come to understand how to live with this illness. Providers and families should remember that this process might be hard on people with ME/CFS.

Symptoms that health-care providers might try to address are as follows.

### Post-Exertional Malaise

Post-exertional malaise is the worsening of symptoms after even minor physical, mental, or emotional exertion. For some patients, sensory overload (light and sound) can induce PEM. The symptoms typically get worse 12–48 hours after the activity or exposure and can last for days or even weeks.

PEM can be addressed by activity management, also called "pacing." The goal of pacing is to learn to balance rest and activity to avoid PEM flare-ups, which can be caused by exertion that patients with ME/CFS cannot tolerate. To do this, patients need to find their individual limits for mental and physical activities. Then they need to plan activities and rest to stay within these limits. Some patients and doctors refer to staying within these limits as staying within the "energy envelope." The limits may be different for each patient. Keeping activity and symptom diaries may help patients find their personal limits, especially early on in the illness.

Being mindful of personal limits could prove to be a helpful coping skill for people living with ME/CFS. This enables them the ability to find a balance between activities and rest, giving them a sense of managing the illness rather than the illness controlling them. People living with ME/CFS may find that everyday activities such as buying groceries, brushing their teeth, or interacting with others may be enough to cause a relapse or "crash." It may not be possible to entirely avoid these situations, but people living with ME/CFS need to be aware of monitoring their own activity limits. When having a good day, it is tempting to try and "push" (increasing activity beyond what would normally attempt) to make up for lost time. However, this can then lead to a "crash" (worsening of ME/CFS symptoms); the cycle can then repeat itself after people start recovering from the crash.

Rehabilitation specialists or exercise physiologists who understand ME/CFS may help patients with adjusting to life with ME/CFS. Finding ways to make activities easier may be helpful, such as sitting while doing the laundry or showering, taking frequent breaks, and dividing large tasks into smaller steps. Some patients find heart rate monitors useful in keeping track of how hard their body is working as a way to prevent PEM. Patients who have learned to listen to their bodies might be able to increase their activity level. However, ME/CFS is unpredictable. PEM symptoms may not start right after exercise, making it important for each treatment plan to be tailored for each case. Exercise is not a cure for ME/CFS.

Any activity or exercise plan for people with ME/CFS needs to be carefully designed with input from each patient. While vigorous aerobic exercise can be beneficial for many chronic illnesses, patients with ME/CFS do not tolerate such exercise routines. Standard exercise recommendations for healthy people can be harmful to patients with ME/CFS. However, it is important that patients with ME/CFS undertake activities that they can tolerate, as described above.

## Sleep

Patients with ME/CFS often feel less refreshed and restored after sleep than they did before they became ill. Common sleep complaints include difficulty falling or staying asleep, extreme sleepiness, intense and vivid dreaming, restless legs, and nighttime muscle spasms.

Good sleep habits are important for all people, including those with ME/CFS. When people try these tips but are still unable to sleep, their doctor might recommend taking medicine to help with sleep. First, people should try over-the-counter sleep products. If this does not help, doctors can offer a prescription sleep medicine, starting at the smallest dose and using it for the shortest possible time.

People might continue to feel unrefreshed even after the medications help them get a full night of sleep. If so, they should consider seeing a sleep specialist. Most people with sleep disorders, such as sleep apnea (symptoms include brief pausing in breathing during sleep) and narcolepsy (symptoms include excessive daytime sleepiness), respond to therapy. However, for people with ME/CFS, not all symptoms may go away.

## Pain

People with ME/CFS often have deep pain in their muscles and joints. They might also have headaches (typically pressure-like) and soreness of their skin when touched.

Patients should always talk to their health-care provider before trying any medication. Doctors may first recommend trying over-the-counter pain relievers, such as acetaminophen, aspirin, or ibuprofen. If these do not provide enough pain relief, patients may need to see a pain specialist. People with chronic pain, including those with ME/CFS, can benefit from counseling to learn new ways to deal with pain.

Other pain management methods include stretching and movement therapies, gentle massage, heat, toning exercises, and water therapy for healing. Acupuncture, when done by a licensed practitioner, might help with pain for some patients.

## Depression, Stress, and Anxiety

Adjusting to a chronic, debilitating illness sometimes leads to other problems, including depression, stress, and anxiety. Many patients with ME/CFS develop depression during their illness. When present, depression or anxiety should be treated. Although treating depression or anxiety can be helpful, it is not a cure for ME/CFS.

Some people with ME/CFS might benefit from antidepressants and antianxiety medications. However, doctors should use caution in prescribing these medications. Some drugs used to treat depression have other effects that might worsen other ME/CFS symptoms and cause side effects. When health-care providers are concerned about the patient's psychological condition, they may recommend seeing a mental health professional.

Some people with ME/CFS might benefit from trying techniques such as deep breathing and muscle relaxation, massage, and movement therapies (such as stretching, yoga, and tai chi). These can reduce stress and anxiety and promote a sense of well-being.

## Dizziness and Light-headedness (Orthostatic Intolerance)

Some people with ME/CFS might also have symptoms of orthostatic intolerance that are triggered when—or made worse by—standing or sitting upright. These symptoms can include the following:

- frequent dizziness and light-headedness
- changes in vision (blurred vision, seeing white or black spots)
- weakness
- feeling like your heart is beating too fast or too hard, fluttering, or skipping a beat

For patients with these symptoms, their doctor will check their heart rate and blood pressure and may recommend they see a specialist, such as a cardiologist or neurologist.

For people with ME/CFS who do not have heart or blood vessel disease, the doctor might suggest patients increase daily fluid and salt intake and use support stockings. If symptoms do not improve, prescription medication can be considered.

## Memory and Concentration Problems

Memory aids, such as organizers and calendars, can help with memory problems. For people with ME/CFS who have concentration problems, some doctors have prescribed stimulant medications, such as those typically used to treat attention deficit hyperactivity disorder (ADHD). While stimulants might help improve concentration for some patients with ME/CFS, they might lead to the "push-and-crash" cycle and worsen symptoms. "Push-and-crash" cycles are when someone with ME/CFS is having a good day and tries to push to do more than they would normally attempt (do too much, crash, rest, start to feel a little better, do too much once again).

## LIVING WITH MYALGIC ENCEPHALOMYELITIS/CHRONIC FATIGUE SYNDROME

Strategies that do not involve the use of medications and might be helpful to some patients are as follows:

- **Professional counseling**. Talking with a therapist to help find strategies to cope with the illness and its impact on daily life and relationships.
- **Balanced diet**. A balanced diet is important for everyone's good health and would benefit a person with or without any chronic illness.
- **Nutritional supplements**. Doctors might run tests to see if patients lack any important nutrients and might suggest supplements to try. Doctors and patients should talk about any risks and benefits of supplements and consider any possible interactions that may occur with prescription medications. Follow-up tests to see if nutrient levels improve can help with treatment planning.
- **Complementary therapies**. Therapies such as meditation, gentle massage, deep breathing, or relaxation therapy might be helpful.

Patients should talk with their doctors about all potential therapies because many treatments that are promoted as cures for ME/CFS are unproven, are often costly, and could be dangerous.[2]

[2] "What Is ME/CFS?" Centers for Disease Control and Prevention (CDC), March 21, 2023. Available online. URL: www.cdc.gov/me-cfs/abvout/index.html. Accessed April 20, 2023.

# Chapter 31 | Cancer Patients and Sleep Disorders

## SLEEP DISORDERS IN PEOPLE WITH CANCER

Sleep disorders are common in people with cancer. As many as half of the people with cancer have problems sleeping. The sleep disorders most likely to affect people with cancer are insomnia and an abnormal sleep–wake cycle. There are many reasons you may have trouble sleeping, including the following:

- physical changes caused by cancer or surgery
- side effects of drugs or other treatments
- being in the hospital
- stress about having cancer
- health problems not related to cancer

Tumors may cause sleep problems. If you have a tumor, it may cause the following problems that make it hard to sleep:

- pressure from the tumor on nearby areas of the body
- gastrointestinal (GI) problems (nausea, constipation, diarrhea, being unable to control your bowels)
- bladder problems (irritation, being unable to control urine flow)
- pain
- fever
- cough
- trouble breathing

- itching
- feeling very tired

Certain drugs or treatments may affect sleep. Common cancer treatments and drugs can affect normal sleep patterns. How well you sleep may be affected by the following:
- hormone therapy (HT)
- corticosteroids
- sedatives and tranquilizers
- antidepressants
- anticonvulsants

Long-term use of certain drugs may cause insomnia. Stopping or decreasing the use of certain drugs can also affect normal sleep. Other side effects of drugs and treatments that may affect the sleep–wake cycle include the following:
- pain
- anxiety
- night sweats or hot flashes
- GI problems such as nausea, constipation, diarrhea, and being unable to control the bowels
- bladder problems, such as irritation or being unable to control urine
- breathing problems

Being in the hospital may make it harder to sleep. Getting a normal night's sleep in the hospital is difficult. The following may affect your sleep in a hospital:
- **Hospital environment**. You may be bothered by an uncomfortable bed, pillow, or room temperature; noise; or sharing a room with a stranger.
- **Hospital routine.** Sleep may be interrupted when doctors and nurses come in to check on you or give you drugs, other treatments, or exams.

Getting sleep during a hospital stay may also be affected by anxiety and age.

Stress caused by learning the cancer diagnosis often causes sleeping problems. Stress, anxiety, and depression are common reactions to learning you have cancer, receiving treatments, and being in the hospital. These are common causes of insomnia.

Other health problems not related to cancer may cause a sleep disorder. People with cancer can have sleep disorders that are caused by other health problems. Conditions such as snoring, headaches, and daytime seizures increase the chance of having a sleep disorder.

## ASSESSMENT OF SLEEP DISORDERS

An assessment is done for people with sleep disorders. An assessment is done to find problems that may be causing the sleep disorder and how it affects your life. People with mild sleep disorders may be irritable and unable to concentrate. People with moderate sleep disorders can be depressed and anxious. These sleep disorders may make it hard for you to stay alert and involve in activities during the day. You may not be able to remember treatment instructions and may have trouble making decisions. Being well-rested can improve energy and help you cope with the side effects of cancer and treatment.

People with cancer should have assessments done from time to time because sleep disorders may become more or less severe over time. A sleep disorder assessment includes a physical exam, health history, and sleep history. Your doctor will do a physical exam and take a medical history that includes the following:

- side effects of your cancer and cancer treatments
- medicines, including vitamins and other over-the-counter (OTC) drugs
- emotional effects of cancer and treatments
- diet
- exercise
- caregiver routines

You and your family can tell your doctor about your sleep history and patterns of sleep. A polysomnogram may be used to help diagnose the sleep disorder. A polysomnogram is a group of recordings taken during sleep that show:

- brain wave changes
- eye movements
- breathing rate
- blood pressure
- heart rate and electrical activity of the heart and other muscles

This information helps the doctor find the cause of your sleeping problems.

## TREATMENT FOR SLEEP DISORDERS

Treating sleep disorders may include supportive care for side effects of cancer or cancer treatment. Sleep disorders often occur along with cancer-related fatigue and may be related. Sleep disorders that are caused by the side effects of cancer or cancer treatment may be helped by relieving the symptoms of those side effects. It is important to talk about your sleep problems with your family and the health-care team so that education and support can be given. Supportive care may improve your quality of life and ability to sleep.

Cognitive behavioral therapy (CBT) may reduce anxiety and help you relax. CBT helps reduce anxiety about getting enough sleep. You learn to change negative thoughts and beliefs about sleep into positive thoughts and images in order to fall asleep more easily. It helps replace the anxiety of "I need to sleep" with the idea of "just relax." It may include the following:

- stimulus control
- sleep restriction
- relaxation therapy

### Stimulus Control

When you have sleep problems for a long time, just getting ready for bed or getting into bed to sleep may cause you to start worrying that you will have another sleepless night. That worry then makes it very hard to fall asleep. Stimulus control can help you learn to connect getting ready for bed and being in bed only with being asleep. By using the bed and bedroom only when you are sleepy, the bed and sleep are linked in your mind. Stimulus control may include the following changes in your sleeping habits:

- Go to bed only when sleepy and get out of bed if you do not fall asleep after a short time. Return to bed only when you feel sleepy.
- Use the bed and bedroom only for sleeping, not for other activities.

## Sleep Restriction

Sleep restriction decreases the time you spend in bed sleeping. This makes you more likely to feel sleepy the next night. The time you can set aside for sleeping is increased when your sleep improves.

## Relaxation Therapy

Relaxation therapy is used to relieve muscle tension and stress, lower blood pressure, and control pain. It may involve tensing and relaxing muscles throughout the body. It is often used with guided imagery (focusing the mind on positive images) and meditation (focusing thoughts). Self-hypnosis at bedtime can also help you feel relaxed and sleepy. Relaxation therapy exercises can make it easier for stimulus control and sleep restriction to work for you.

Learning good sleep habits is important. Good sleep habits help you fall asleep more easily and stay asleep. Habits and routines that may help improve sleep include the following.

## A Comfortable Bed and Bedroom

Making your bed and bedroom more comfortable may help you sleep. Some ways to increase bedroom comfort include the following:

- Keep the room quiet.
- Dim or turn off lights.

- Keep the room at a comfortable temperature.
- Keep skin clean and dry.
- Dress in loose, soft clothing.
- Keep bedding and pillows clean, dry, and smooth without wrinkles.
- Use blankets to keep warm.
- Use pillows to get into a comfortable position.

## Regular Bowel and Bladder Habits

Regular bowel and bladder habits reduce the number of times you have to get up during the night. Waking during the night to go to the bathroom may be reduced by doing the following:
- Drink more fluids during the day.
- Eat more high-fiber foods during the day.
- Avoid drinking a lot before bedtime.
- Empty your bowel and bladder before going to bed.

## Diet and Exercise

The following diet and exercise habits may improve sleep:
- Stay active during the day.
- Get regular exercise but do not exercise within three hours of bedtime.
- Eat a high-protein snack (such as milk or turkey) two hours before bedtime.
- Avoid heavy, spicy, or sugary foods before bedtime.
- Avoid drinking alcohol or smoking before bedtime.
- Avoid foods and drinks that have caffeine, including dietary supplements, to control appetite.

Other habits that may improve sleep include the following:
- Avoid naps.
- Avoid watching TV or working in the bedroom.
- Relax before bedtime.
- Go to sleep and wake up at the same hours every day, no matter how little you slept.

## Hospital Routines

Getting a good night's sleep in a hospital or other care facility can be hard to do. The good sleep habits listed above may help you. As a hospital patient, you may also do the following:

- Ask caregivers to plan care so that they wake you up the least number of times during the night.
- Ask for a back rub or massage to relieve pain or help you relax.

If treatment without drugs does not help, sleep medicines may be used for a short time. Treatment without drugs does not always work. Sometimes, CBTs are not available, or they do not help. Also, some sleep disorders are caused by conditions that need to be treated with drugs, such as hot flashes, pain, anxiety, depression, or mood disorders. The drug used will depend on your type of sleep problem (such as trouble falling asleep or trouble staying asleep) and the other medicines you are taking. All of your other medicines and health conditions will affect which sleeping medicines are safe and will work well for you.

Some drugs that help you sleep should not be stopped suddenly. Suddenly stopping them may cause nervousness, seizures, and a change in the rapid eye movement (REM) phase of sleep that increases dreaming, including nightmares. This change in REM sleep may be dangerous for people with peptic ulcers or heart conditions.

## SLEEP DISORDERS IN SPECIAL CASES
### People Who Have Pain

If pain disturbs your sleep, treatment to relieve the pain will be used before sleep medicines are used. Pain drugs, other drugs being taken, and any other health conditions may affect which sleeping medicines are prescribed.

## Older Patients

It is normal for older people to have insomnia. Changes related to age can cause lighter sleep, waking up more often during the night, and sleeping less total time. If you are an older person with cancer who is having trouble sleeping, the doctor will look for the specific causes, such as:

- physical health problems
- mental health problems, such as anxiety or depression
- loss of social support
- alcohol use (drinking)
- side effects of medicines
- conditions that commonly affect sleep, such as restless legs syndrome (RLS), cramping or jerking of the legs during sleep, and sleep apnea syndrome

Treating sleeping problems without drugs is tried first. The following may help improve sleep in older people with cancer:

- having meals at regular times
- avoiding naps during the day
- being more active during the day

Medicine may be used if nondrug treatments do not work. The doctor will look at all your medicines and health conditions before choosing a sleeping medicine. For some people, doctors will suggest a sleep disorder clinic for treatment.

## People Who Have Jaw Surgery

People who have surgery on the jaw may develop sleep apnea, which is a sleep disorder that causes the person to stop breathing for 10 seconds or more during sleep. Plastic surgery to rebuild the jaw may help prevent sleep apnea.[1]

---

[1] "Sleep Disorders (PDQ®)–Patient Version," National Cancer Institute (NCI), March 20, 2023. Available online. URL: www.cancer.gov/about-cancer/treatment/side-effects/sleep-disorders-pdq. Accessed March 31, 2023.

# Chapter 32 | **Importance of Sleep with Diabetes**

There are many reasons to get a good night's sleep. If you have diabetes, there are even more. A good night's sleep can feel like a luxury. Balancing school, work, physical activity, and your family may cause you to go to bed later than you like. One in three U.S. adults is not getting enough sleep, and over time, this can increase the risk of type 2 diabetes, heart disease, obesity, and depression.

If you have diabetes, too little sleep negatively affects every area of your management, including how much you eat, what you choose to eat, how you respond to insulin, and your mental health. Proper rest is not just important for your diabetes management—it may also put you in a better mood and give you more energy!

## HOW MUCH DO YOU NEED?
Being well-rested is important for people of all ages to stay in good health. How many hours of sleep you need changes as you age. The American Academy of Sleep Medicine (AASM) and the Sleep Research Society (SRS) recommend that adults should get at least seven hours of sleep per night. Children and teens need more sleep.

## COMPLICATIONS FROM LACK OF SLEEP

If you get less than seven hours of sleep per night regularly, your diabetes will be harder to manage. Too little sleep can:

- increase insulin resistance
- make you hungrier the next day and reduce how full you feel after eating
- make you more likely to reach for junk foods—those that are high in carbs and sugar
- make it harder to lose weight
- raise blood pressure and seriously increase the risk of a heart attack
- make your immune system less able to fight infections
- increase your risk of depression and anxiety

## TIPS TO GET MORE SLEEP

It is common to stay up late and get up early during the week and then sleep in on the weekend. You may hope to catch up on the hours you missed, but your brain cannot use these added hours.

One of the best things you can do is to wake up and go to bed at around the same time every day, even on weekends, making sure you get enough quality sleep consistently. These tips can help:

- Keep your bedroom dark, quiet, relaxing, and cool. Experts recommend a temperature of 65 degrees for your best rest.
- Remove electronic devices such as TVs, computers, and smartphones from the bedroom.
- Get some physical activity during the day.
- Mentally unwind and relax before bedtime.
- Have a routine that gets you ready for bed, such as taking a shower, reading, or writing in a journal.
- Get in bed only when you are tired.

And here are a few things to avoid:

- **Afternoon and evening caffeine**. It can affect your body for up to eight hours.

- **Alcohol in the evening**. It can affect how you breathe when you sleep. It can also wake you up and affect your sleep quality.
- **Large meals late at night**. Eating late can cause indigestion and higher blood sugar levels overnight.
- **Naps after 3 p.m**. This can make you less tired when it is time for bed.
- **Nicotine**. It acts like caffeine.[1]

[1] "Sleep for a Good Cause," Centers for Disease Control and Prevention (CDC), July 28, 2022. Available online. URL: www.cdc.gov/diabetes/library/features/diabetes-sleep.html. Accessed May 8, 2023.

# Chapter 33 | **Sleep and Chronic Disease**

As chronic diseases have assumed an increasingly common role in premature death and illness, interest in the role of sleep health in the development and management of chronic diseases has grown. Notably, insufficient sleep has been linked to the development and management of a number of chronic diseases and conditions, including type 2 diabetes, cardiovascular disease, obesity, and depression.

## DIABETES

Research has found that insufficient sleep is linked to an increased risk for the development of type 2 diabetes. Specifically, sleep duration and quality have emerged as predictors of levels of hemoglobin A1c, an important marker of blood sugar control. Recent research suggests that optimizing sleep duration and quality may be important means of improving blood sugar control in persons with type 2 diabetes.

## CARDIOVASCULAR DISEASE

Persons with sleep apnea have been found to be at an increased risk for a number of cardiovascular diseases. Notably, hypertension, stroke, coronary heart disease, and irregular heartbeats (cardiac arrhythmias) have been found to be more common among those with disordered sleep than their peers without sleep abnormalities. Likewise, sleep apnea and hardening of the arteries (atherosclerosis) appear to share some common physiological characteristics, further suggesting that sleep apnea may be an important predictor of cardiovascular disease.

## OBESITY

Laboratory research has found that short sleep duration results in metabolic changes that may be linked to obesity. Epidemiologic studies conducted in the community have also revealed an association between short sleep duration and excess body weight. This association has been reported in all age groups—but it has been particularly pronounced in children. It is believed that sleep in childhood and adolescence is particularly important for brain development and that insufficient sleep in youngsters may adversely affect the function of a region of the brain known as the "hypothalamus," which regulates appetite and the expenditure of energy.

## DEPRESSION

The relationship between sleep and depression is complex. While sleep disturbance has long been held to be an important symptom of depression, recent research has indicated that depressive symptoms may decrease once sleep apnea has been effectively treated and sufficient sleep restored. The interrelatedness of sleep and depression suggests it is important that the sleep sufficiency of persons with depression be assessed and that symptoms of depression be monitored among persons with a sleep disorder.[1]

---

[1] "Sleep and Chronic Disease," Centers for Disease Control and Prevention (CDC), September 13, 2022. Available online. URL: www.cdc.gov/sleep/about_sleep/chronic_disease.html. Accessed March 31, 2023.

# Chapter 34 | **Nocturia: When the Need to Urinate Interrupts Sleep**

Nocturia, also known as "nocturnal polyuria" or "frequent nighttime urination," is a problem that affects an estimated 33 percent of adults. Normally, hormones signal the bladder to produce less urine at night, so most people can sleep for six to eight hours without needing to get up to use the bathroom. Waking up once per night to empty the bladder is considered normal as well. People with nocturia, on the other hand, produce excessive amounts of urine and are regularly awakened several times per night by the need to urinate.

Waking up multiple times each night to use the bathroom can lead to chronic sleep deprivation. Since the incidence of nocturia increases with age, the majority of people affected are over the age of 60. Nocturia often appears as a symptom of underlying medical conditions, such as an enlarged prostate, diabetes, heart failure, or bladder problems. Nocturia should not be confused with enuresis—also known as "bed-wetting"—a condition in which urine is passed unintentionally during sleep. Nocturia also differs from urinary incontinence (UI), in which patients experience a lack of voluntary control over urination in the daytime.

## CAUSES OF NOCTURIA

The main causes of nocturia are excessive urine production and reduced bladder capacity. Many different factors and conditions can contribute to nocturia, including the following:

- **Age**. Elderly people are more prone to nocturia because the bladder gradually loses elasticity over time. In addition, levels of the hormones that signal the bladder to reduce urine production at night tend to decline with age. Nocturia commonly affects older men who have an enlarged prostate, which can press on the urethra and prevent the bladder from emptying completely, but it affects older women as well.
- **Diabetes**. Poorly controlled diabetes leads to sugar in the urine, which stimulates the production of additional urine.
- **Congestive heart failure and other circulatory problems**. When the heart cannot adequately pump blood through the body, fluid tends to build up in the legs (edema). Lying down at night reduces the burden on the heart and improves circulation, causing the fluid to fill the bladder.
- **Pregnancy**. The growing fetus takes up space usually occupied by the bladder and restricts its capacity to hold fluids.
- **Lower urinary tract conditions**. Infections of the urinary tract or kidneys can cause nocturia by irritating the bladder and decreasing its capacity to hold urine. Conditions such as cystitis can result in an overactive bladder. Bladder obstructions can prevent the full elimination of urine, which may increase the frequency of urination at night.
- **Constipation**. Excessive waste in the bowels or intestines can put pressure on the bladder.
- **Medications**. Certain drugs, such as diuretics, increase the production of urine. Other examples include cardiac glycosides, demeclocycline, lithium, methoxyflurane, phenytoin, and propoxyphene. It

is important to consult a doctor before stopping any prescribed medication, however, even if it causes nocturia as a side effect.

- **Diet**. Consuming excessive fluids before bedtime can contribute to nocturia. Alcohol and caffeinated beverages, in particular, act as diuretics to increase urine production.
- **Sleep disorders**. Obstructive sleep apnea (OSA) and other sleep disorders can disrupt the normal reduction in urine output at night.
- **Neurological disorders**. Conditions that affect the transmission of signals and hormones from the brain to the bladder—such as multiple sclerosis (MS), Parkinson disease (PD), or spinal cord injury—can result in nocturia.

## SYMPTOMS AND DIAGNOSIS OF NOCTURIA

Many experts consider nocturia to be a symptom rather than a health condition. As a result, doctors usually place an emphasis on diagnosing the underlying medical causes of frequent and excessive nighttime urination that disrupts sleep. To evaluate a patient with nocturia, medical practitioners generally collect detailed information about the problem as well as the patient's overall health. The patient may be asked to keep a record of their bladder activity for several days, including the amount of fluid consumed, the frequency of urination during the day and at night, the amount of urine output, and any leaking of urine or wetting the bed. The patient will also be asked about any medications they take regularly, how much alcohol and caffeine they consume each day, and any discomfort they may experience during urination. The doctor may order a urinalysis to evaluate kidney function and check for a urinary tract infection (UTI).

## PREVENTION AND TREATMENT OF NOCTURIA

Since nocturia is usually a symptom, most methods of treatment address the underlying medical conditions that contribute to frequent nighttime urination. Several of these conditions—such as an enlarged prostate or overactive bladder—can be managed with the help of medications. A number of lifestyle modifications can also help reduce urine production at night and prevent people from needing to get up to use the bathroom. Some of the recommended methods of prevention of and treatment for nocturia include the following:

- Avoid consuming fluids in the evening (but be sure that the total fluid intake is adequate during the day).
- Eliminate or reduce the consumption of caffeinated beverages and alcohol.
- Take an afternoon nap to improve circulatory function and drain fluids from the extremities consistently throughout the day.
- Wear compression stockings or elevate the legs to reduce fluid accumulation.
- Perform Kegel exercises to strengthen the pelvic muscles and improve bladder control (these exercises are particularly helpful for pregnant women and for men with an enlarged prostate).
- Take diuretic medications in the late afternoon—six hours before bedtime—so that their therapeutic effects are completed before nighttime.
- Eliminate UTI with antibiotic medications.
- Treat an enlarged prostate with medications such as tamsulosin (Flomax), finasteride, or dutasteride.
- Control an unstable or overactive bladder with anticholinergic medications such as oxybutynin, tolterodine, or solifenacin.
- Reduce urine production at night with medications such as desmopressin (DDAVP).

## References

Marchione, Victor. "Nocturia: Frequent Urination at Night," Doctors Health Press, 2016. Available online. URL: www.doctorshealthpress.com/general-health-articles/nocturia-frequent-urination-at-night. Accessed April 21, 2023.

"Nocturia," Cleveland Clinic, 2016. Available online. URL: http://my.clevelandclinic.org/health/diseases_conditions/ hic_Bladder_Irritating_Foods/hic_nocturia. Accessed April 21, 2023.

"Nocturia (Night-time Urination)," NetDoctor, October 4, 2012. Available online. URL: www.netdoctor.co.uk/ conditions/liver-kidney-and-urinary-system/a3031/nocturia- night-time-urination. Accessed April 21, 2023.

# Chapter 35 | **Connections between Sleep and Substance Use Disorders**

Most common mental disorders, from depression and anxiety to posttraumatic stress disorder (PTSD), are associated with disturbed sleep, and substance use disorders (SUDs) are no exception. The relationship may be complex and bidirectional: Substance use causes sleep problems, but insomnia and insufficient sleep may also be a factor raising the risk of drug use and addiction. Recognizing the importance of this once-overlooked factor, addiction researchers are paying increased attention to sleep and sleep disturbances and even thinking about ways to target sleep disruption in SUD treatment and prevention.

We now know that most kinds of substance use acutely disrupt sleep regulatory systems in the brain, affecting the time it takes to fall asleep (latency), duration of sleep, and sleep quality. People who use drugs also experience insomnia during withdrawal, which fuels drug cravings and can be a major factor leading to relapse. Additionally, because of the central role of sleep in consolidating new memories, poor-quality sleep may make it harder to learn new coping and self-regulation skills necessary for recovery.

The neurobiological mechanisms linking many forms of drug use and sleep disturbances are increasingly well understood. Dopamine is a neurochemical crucial for understanding the relationship between SUDs and sleep, for example. Drugs' direct or indirect stimulation of dopamine reward pathways accounts for their addictive properties, but dopamine also modulates alertness and is implicated in the sleep–wake cycle. Dopaminergic drugs are used to treat disorders of alertness and arousal such as narcolepsy. Cocaine and amphetamine-like drugs (such as methamphetamine) are among the most potent dopamine-increasing drugs, and their repeated misuse can lead to severe sleep deprivation. Sleep deprivation, in turn, downregulates dopamine receptors, which makes people more impulsive and vulnerable to drug taking.

In addition to their effects on dopamine, drugs also affect sleep through their main pharmacological targets. For instance, marijuana interacts with the body's endocannabinoid system by binding to cannabinoid receptors; this system is involved in regulating the sleep–wake cycle (among many other roles). Trouble sleeping is a very common symptom of marijuana withdrawal, reported by over 40 percent of those trying to quit the drug, and sleep difficulty is reported as the most distressing symptom. (Nightmares and strange dreams are also reported.) One in ten individuals who relapsed to cannabis use cited sleep difficulty as the reason.

Opioid drugs such as heroin interact with the body's endogenous opioid system by binding to mu-opioid receptors; this system also plays a role in regulating sleep. Morpheus, the Greek god of sleep and dreams, gave his name to morphia or morphine, the medicinal derivative of opium. Natural and synthetic opioid drugs can produce profound sleepiness, but they can also disrupt sleep by increasing transitions between different stages of sleep (known as "disruptions" in sleep architecture), and people undergoing withdrawal can experience terrible insomnia. Opioids in brainstem regions also control respiration, and when they are taken at high doses, they can dangerously inhibit breathing during sleep.

Addiction and sleep problems are intertwined in other, unexpected and complex ways. In a particularly fascinating finding published in *Science Translational Medicine* in 2018, a team of University of California, Los Angeles (UCLA) researchers studying the role of the wakefulness-regulating neuropeptide orexin in narcolepsy were examining human postmortem brain samples and found a brain with significantly more orexin-producing cells; this individual, they then learned, had been addicted to heroin. This serendipitous discovery led the team to analyze a larger sample of brain hypothalamic tissue from individuals with heroin addiction; these individuals had 54 percent more orexin-producing cells in their brains than nonheroin users. Administering morphine produced similar effects in rodents.

Further research on the overlaps between the brain circuits and signaling systems responsible for reward and those regulating sleep may help researchers understand individual differences in susceptibility to addiction and sleep disorders. The team believes that the future of addiction treatment lies in approaches that are more personalized and multidimensional, and this includes using combinations of medications and other interventions that target specific symptoms of the disorder. It could prove very useful to target an individual's sleep problems as one of the dimensions of treatment. For example, the National Institute on Drug Abuse (NIDA) is currently funding research to test the efficacy of suvorexant, an insomnia medication approved by the U.S. Food and Drug Administration (FDA) that acts as an antagonist at orexin receptors, in people with opioid use disorder.

The causal relationship between impaired sleep and drug misuse/addiction can also go in the other direction. People who suffer from insomnia may be at an increased risk for substance use because sufferers may self-medicate their sleep problems using alcohol or other drugs such as benzodiazepines that they may perceive as relaxing. Or they may use stimulant drugs to compensate for daytime fatigue caused by lost sleep. Impaired sleep may also increase the risk of drug use through other avenues, for instance, by impairing cognition. Consequently, sleep disorders and other barriers to getting sufficient sleep are important factors to target in prevention.

Early school start times, for instance, have been the focus of considerable debate in recent years, as teenagers may be particularly vulnerable to many health and behavioral effects of short sleep duration. Nora D. Volkow, M.D., director of the NIDA at the National Institutes of Health (NIH), wrote previously on this blog about research findings that fewer hours of sleep correlate with an increased risk of substance use and other behavior problems in teens. In this age group, tobacco, alcohol, and marijuana use are all associated with poorer sleep health, including lower sleep duration, again with possible bidirectionality of causation.

Longitudinal research is needed to better clarify the complex causal links between sleep, brain development, and mental health outcomes, including substance use. The Adolescent Brain and Cognitive Development (ABCD) study is examining these relationships in a large cohort of children who were recruited at the age of 9–10. This longitudinal study, now in its third year, is already beginning to produce valuable findings. A team of Chinese researchers using ABCD data recently published in *Molecular Psychiatry* their finding that kids with depressive problems had shorter sleep duration one year later, as well as a lower volume of brain areas associated with cognitive functions such as memory. We will learn much more as the ABCD study progresses.

Despite all we are learning, more research is needed on the relationship(s) between drug use, addiction, and sleep, in adults as well as young people. The NIDA is funding several projects to study various SUDs and sleep, as well as the neurobiology of reward and its relation to circadian rhythms. It is an area with great potential to prevent substance use as well as to treat one of the most debilitating side effects associated with SUDs.[1]

[1] "Connections between Sleep and Substance Use Disorders," National Institutes of Health (NIH), March 9, 2020. Available online. URL: https://nida.nih.gov/about-nida/noras-blog/2020/03/connections-between-sleep-substance-use-disorders. Accessed April 24, 2023.

# Part 5 | **Preventing, Diagnosing, and Treating Sleep Disorders**

# Chapter 36 | Sleep Hygiene: Tips for Better Sleep

## WHAT SHOULD YOU DO IF YOU CANNOT SLEEP?

It is important to practice good sleep habits, but if your sleep problems continue or if they interfere with how you feel or function during the day, you should talk to your doctor. Before visiting your doctor, keep a diary of your sleep habits for about 10 days to discuss at the visit.

Include the following in your sleep diary when you:

- go to bed
- go to sleep
- wake up
- get out of bed
- take naps
- exercise
- drink alcohol
- drink caffeinated beverages

Also, remember to mention if you are taking any medications (over-the-counter (OTC) or prescription) or supplements. They may make it harder for you to sleep.

## TIPS FOR BETTER SLEEP

Good sleep habits (sometimes referred to as "sleep hygiene") can help you get a good night's sleep.

Some habits that can improve your sleep health are as follows:

- Be consistent. Go to bed at the same time each night and get up at the same time each morning, including on the weekends.
- Make sure your bedroom is quiet, dark, relaxing, and at a comfortable temperature.
- Remove electronic devices, such as TVs, computers, and smartphones, from the bedroom.
- Avoid large meals, caffeine, and alcohol before bedtime.
- Get some exercise. Being physically active during the day can help you fall asleep more easily at night.[1]

[1] "What Do I Do If I Can't Sleep?" Centers for Disease Control and Prevention (CDC), September 13, 2022. Available online. URL: www.cdc.gov/sleep/about_sleep/sleep_hygiene.html. Accessed April 24, 2023.

# Chapter 37 | **Identifying Common Sleep Disruptors**

**Chapter Contents**

## Section 37.1 | **Common Causes of Disturbed Sleep**

Many factors can prevent a good night's sleep. These factors range from well-known stimulants, such as coffee, to certain pain relievers, decongestants, and other culprits. Many people depend on the caffeine in coffee, cola, or tea to wake them up in the morning or to keep them awake. Caffeine is thought to block the cell receptors that adenosine (a substance in the brain) uses to trigger its sleep-inducing signals. In this way, caffeine fools the body into thinking it is not tired. It can take as long as six to eight hours for the effects of caffeine to wear off completely. Thus, drinking a cup of coffee in the late afternoon may prevent you from falling asleep at night.

Nicotine is another stimulant that can keep you awake. Nicotine also leads to lighter than normal sleep, and heavy smokers tend to wake up too early because of nicotine withdrawal. Although alcohol is a sedative that makes it easier to fall asleep, it prevents deep sleep and rapid eye movement (REM) sleep, allowing only the lighter stages of sleep. People who drink alcohol also tend to wake up in the middle of the night when the effects of an alcoholic "nightcap" wear off.

Certain commonly used prescription and over-the-counter (OTC) medicines contain ingredients that can keep you awake. These ingredients include decongestants and steroids. Many medicines taken to relieve headaches contain caffeine. Heart and blood pressure medications known as "beta-blockers" can make it difficult to fall asleep and cause more awakenings during the night. People who have chronic asthma or bronchitis also have more problems falling asleep and staying asleep than healthy people, either because of their breathing difficulties or because of the medicines they take. Other chronic painful or uncomfortable conditions—such as arthritis, congestive heart failure, and sickle cell anemia—can disrupt sleep too.

A number of psychological disorders—including schizophrenia, bipolar disorder, and anxiety disorders—are well known for disrupting sleep. Depression often leads to insomnia, and insomnia can cause depression. Some of these psychological disorders are likely to disrupt REM sleep. Psychological stress also takes its toll on sleep, making it more difficult to fall asleep or stay asleep. People who feel stressed also tend to spend less time in deep sleep and REM sleep. Many people report having difficulties sleeping if, for example, they have lost a loved one, are going through a divorce, or are under stress at work.

Menstrual cycle hormones can affect how well women sleep. Progesterone is known to induce sleep and circulates in greater concentrations in the second half of the menstrual cycle. For this reason, women may sleep better during this phase of their menstrual cycle. On the other hand, many women report trouble sleeping the night before their menstrual flow starts. This sleep disruption may be related to the abrupt drop in progesterone levels that occurs just before menstruation. Women in their late forties and early fifties, however, report more difficulties sleeping (insomnia) than younger women. These difficulties may be linked to menopause when women have lower concentrations of progesterone. Hot flashes in women of this age may also cause sleep disruption and difficulties.

Certain lifestyle factors may also deprive a person of needed sleep. Large meals or vigorous exercise just before bedtime can make it harder to fall asleep. While vigorous exercise in the evening may delay sleep onset for various reasons, exercise in the daytime is associated with improved nighttime sleep.

If you are not getting enough sleep or are not falling asleep early enough, you may be overscheduling activities that can prevent you from getting the quiet relaxation time you need to prepare for sleep. Most people report that it is easier to fall asleep if they have time to wind down into a less active state before sleeping. Relaxing in a hot bath or having a hot, caffeine-free beverage before bedtime may help. In addition, your body temperature drops after a hot bath in a way that mimics, in part, what happens as you fall asleep. Probably for both these reasons, many people report that they fall asleep more easily after a hot bath.

Your sleeping environment can also affect your sleep. Clear your bedroom of any potential sleep distractions, such as noises, bright lights, a TV, a cell phone, or a computer. Having a comfortable mattress and pillow can help promote a good night's sleep. You also sleep better if the temperature in your bedroom is kept on the cool side.[1]

## Section 37.2 | Alcohol and Its Effects on Sleep

## ALCOHOL AND THE BODY
### Alcohol Entering the Body

After alcohol enters the stomach, it is absorbed quickly into the bloodstream through the stomach wall. The rest enters the bloodstream through the small intestine. How fast alcohol is absorbed into your bloodstream depends on several things. Higher concentrations of alcohol, such as shots, are absorbed faster than lower concentrations, such as light beer. Absorption is faster for a person who weighs less. If you ate while you consumed the alcohol, the absorption of alcohol will be slower than if you drink on an empty stomach.

### Alcohol Leaving the Body

Alcohol leaves your body in several ways. First, 90 percent of it is removed from the blood by the liver. Alcohol is then broken down into several chemicals, including carbon dioxide and water. The carbon dioxide and water come out in your urine. The final 10 percent is not removed by the liver and is expelled through sweat and breath. The reason why it is difficult to sober someone up is because the liver can only process about one drink per hour (this is slow, considering the body absorbs alcohol through the stomach lining in about 10 minutes). There is not much that can influence how fast your liver processes alcohol. That is why cold showers, hot coffee, or vomiting does not help.

---

[1] "Your Guide to Healthy Sleep," National Heart, Lung, and Blood Institute (NHLBI), August 2011. Available online. URL: www.nhlbi.nih.gov/files/docs/public/sleep/healthy_sleep.pdf. Accessed April 23, 2023.

## Tolerance

Over time, a person who drinks regularly has to drink more and more to feel the same effect as they did when they first began drinking. People develop a higher tolerance because they have adapted, both physically and psychologically, to having alcohol in their system. Low tolerance is similar to a built-in warning system to warn us when alcohol levels get too high in our body. A high tolerance may seem as if it is a good thing because it allows heavy drinkers to function when they have high levels of alcohol in their bodies, but it is not a good thing. People with a high alcohol tolerance short circuit this internal warning system. They do not experience negative reactions to the alcohol, and they continue drinking. Tolerant individuals are able to keep high levels of toxins in their bodies for long periods of time, which increases the stress on sensitive internal organs and the chances of developing long-term health problems. The good news about having a high tolerance is that you can decrease it (and the associated health risks) fairly easily. A high tolerance can be reversed gradually through either moderating the quantity and frequency of your drinking or taking a break from the alcohol for a few weeks.

A standard drink is defined as follows:
- one 12-oz beer
- one wine cooler
- one 5-oz glass of wine
- one shot of liquor
- one cocktail

## ALCOHOL INTOXICATION AND PERFORMANCE
### Sleep

The bottom line is that alcohol is bad for your sleep. Poor sleep can limit your ability to think, act quickly, and perform well. Alcohol intoxication shortens the time necessary to fall asleep, but sleep is usually disturbed and fragmented after just a few hours. Restful, restorative sleep decreases during the second half of the night. So heavy drinking compromises your sleep throughout the night. Poor sleep decreases the body's ability to function optimally and your physical endurance. If you want peak performance (at work, sports, or other engagements), either plan to abstain from alcohol use altogether or drink in moderation.

## Up-and-Down Response to Alcohol in Your Body

The up-and-down response refers to two different effects that alcohol produces. The up response is feeling stimulated or excited. This is followed by the down response of feeling depressed and tired. The initial up response is associated with low but rising blood alcohol levels (BALs). The BAL is the ratio of alcohol to blood in your bloodstream. Table 37.1 shows the alcohol's effects on the body.

**Table 37.1.** Alcohol Levels and Effects on the Body

| Blood Alcohol Level (%) | Effects of Alcohol on the Body |
|---|---|
| 0.02 | Light-to-moderate drinkers begin to feel some effect. |
| 0.04 | Most people begin to feel relaxed. |
| 0.06 | Judgment is somewhat impaired; people are less able to make rational decisions about their capabilities (e.g., driving). |
| 0.08 | There will be a definite impairment of muscle coordination and driving skills and an increased risk of nausea and slurred speech. It is considered as legal intoxication. |
| 0.10 | There will be clear deterioration of reaction time and control. |
| 0.15 | Balance and movement are impaired. There is a risk of blackouts and accidents. |
| 0.30 | Many people lose consciousness. There is a risk of death. |
| 0.45 | Breathing stops; death occurs. |

The down response is associated more with falling BALs. The up-and-down response is important because it allows you to test if "more" alcohol actually means "better." It also helps you understand how tolerance affects you physiologically when it comes to drinking alcohol. Over time, as BALs begin to fall, people experience the down effects of alcohol. This is the time when people begin to drink more in an attempt to get back their initial stimulated or excited state. However, the more alcohol that is consumed, the greater both the arousal and the depressant effects will be. At some point, the stimulating effects of a rising BAL will not amount to euphoria. The point at which an increase in BAL will not result in elevated mood or energy is known as the "point of diminishing returns." For most people, that point is a BAL of 0.05 percent.

## MODERATING YOUR DRINKING

Decide what you want from drinking alcohol and think about the pros and cons (short- and long-term) of moderating your use versus maintaining your usual drinking behavior. Also, consider what you absolutely want to avoid when you drink.

### Set Drinking Limits

- What is your upper limit on the number of drinks you consume per week?
- At what point do you decide you have had enough (consider a BAL limit)?
- What is the maximum number of days for drinking you will choose to give yourself?
- Use standard guidelines to determine what constitutes one drink as in 1.25 oz of 80-proof liquor, 4 oz of wine, 10 oz of beer with 5 percent alcohol (microbrews and "ice" beer), or 12 oz of beer with 4 percent alcohol (standard beer).

### Count Your Drinks and Monitor Your Drinking Behavior

Most people are surprised by what they learn when they actually count how much they drink. Simply observe your behavior—this is similar to standing outside yourself and watching how you are acting when you are drinking. Some people put bottle caps in their pockets while drinking to monitor how many beers they have had. You can also make tick marks with a pen on a napkin to monitor the number of drinks.

## Alter How and What You Drink
- Switch to drinks that contain less alcohol (e.g., light beers).
- Slow down your pace of drinking.
- Space drinks further apart.
- Alternate drinking nonalcoholic beverages with alcoholic drinks.

## Manage Your Drinking in the Moment
- Stay awake and on top of how you drink and what you are drinking when you are at a party.
- Choose what is right for you and ask a close friend to help you monitor your alcohol consumption.

## Safe Drinking Guideline
- for women, no more than three drinks/day or nine drinks/week
- for men, no more than four drinks/day or fourteen drinks/week[2]

## SLEEP AND ALCOHOL USE

Alcohol use also varied by usual hours of sleep although to a lesser extent than observed for cigarette smoking. Overall, about one in five adults (20%) had five or more drinks in one day in the past year. The prevalence of this behavior was slightly higher among adults who slept six hours or less (22%) than among adults who slept seven to eight hours (19%) or nine hours or more (19%). The association between having five or more drinks in one day and hours of sleep was most notable for men and for younger adults. Men who slept less than six hours were more likely to have had five or more drinks in one day (31%) than men who slept seven to eight hours

[2] Mental Illness Research, Education and Clinical Centers (MIRECC), "Alcohol Effects and Safer Drinking Habits," U.S. Department of Veterans Affairs (VA), June 2013. Available online. URL: www.mirecc.va.gov/cih-visn2/Documents/Patient_Education_Handouts/Alcohol_Effect_and_Safe_Drinking_Habits_Version_3.pdf. Accessed April 23, 2023.

(27%). Similarly, adults aged 18–44 years who slept less than six hours were more likely to have had five or more drinks in one day (33%) than adults in the same age group who slept seven to eight hours (26%) or nine hours or more (26%). Sleep was unrelated to having five or more drinks in one day among adults aged 45 years and over for whom the prevalence of consumption of this amount of alcohol was considerably lower.[3]

## Section 37.3 | Caffeine, Nicotine, and Food and Their Impact on Sleep

Caffeine has been called the most popular drug in the world. Millions of people consume it on a daily basis in the form of coffee, tea, soft drinks, energy drinks, chocolate, or certain medications. Many people depend on it to help them feel alert and energized throughout the day at work or at school. Some people become addicted to it and experience withdrawal symptoms such as headaches, fatigue, anxiety, and irritability if they do not get their daily dose. Yet most people do not think of caffeine as a drug or realize that it can interfere with sleep.

Caffeine is typically absorbed into the bloodstream within 15 minutes after it is consumed although it takes about an hour to reach peak levels. It acts as a stimulant to increase the heart rate and blood pressure and promote the production of adrenaline. As a result, caffeine temporarily increases alertness and reduces fatigue by suppressing sleep-inducing chemicals. These effects can last for four to six hours although it takes a full 24 hours for the body to eliminate caffeine completely.

By stimulating the body to remain awake, caffeine can also weaken the body's ability to sleep. Consuming too much caffeine may cause insomnia. Most people can safely consume up to 250 mg

[3] "Sleep Duration as a Correlate of Smoking, Alcohol Use, Leisure-Time Physical Inactivity, and Obesity among Adults: United States, 2004–2006," Centers for Disease Control and Prevention (CDC), May 2008. Available online. URL: www.cdc.gov/nchs/data/hestat/sleep04-06/sleep04-06.pdf. Accessed April 23, 2023.

per day, which is equivalent to two to three cups of coffee, without affecting their sleep. Consumption of 500 mg or more per day is considered excessive and can impair sleep.

Caffeine affects sleep in three ways: by making it harder to fall asleep, by reducing the quality of sleep, and by causing nocturia (frequent nighttime urination). These effects are particularly severe if the caffeine is consumed within four to six hours of bedtime. People with caffeine in their bloodstream are likely to feel jittery, anxious, or wired when they try to go to sleep. If they do manage to fall asleep, the stimulant effects of caffeine will make it difficult for their body to enter a deep, restorative phase of sleep. Finally, they are likely to wake up multiple times during the night to use the bathroom due to the diuretic effects of caffeine.

Although some people have a higher tolerance for caffeine than others, anyone who experiences difficulty sleeping may benefit from limiting caffeine consumption to less than 200 mg per day or eliminating it entirely. In addition, any caffeine consumption should take place early in the day—and at least six hours before bedtime. Ironically, cutting down on caffeine intake can cause withdrawal symptoms that can temporarily interfere with sleep. Although these symptoms subside over time as the body adjusts, people who are addicted to caffeine may want to reduce their consumption gradually rather than suddenly. Most people who eliminate caffeine find that they experience improvements in sleep afterward.

## NICOTINE AND SLEEP

Some people find smoking cigarettes relaxing and believe that smoking at bedtime or upon awakening in the middle of the night helps them sleep. But nicotine, the main addictive chemical in tobacco products, is actually a stimulant that can interfere with sleep. Smoking has countless other negative impacts on health, significantly increasing the risk of heart disease, lung disease, stroke, and cancer. In fact, smoking is the leading preventable cause of death in the United States. However, few people seem to recognize the impact of nicotine on sleep.

Like caffeine, nicotine is absorbed into the bloodstream quickly and acts as a stimulant, increasing the heart rate and breathing rate and releasing stress hormones in the body. The stimulant effects of nicotine persist for several hours, affecting brain waves, body temperature, and other systems. These effects make it more difficult to fall asleep and stay asleep. As a result, smokers tend to sleep lightly and spend less time in deep, restorative sleep than nonsmokers.

In addition to sleep disruptions from the stimulant effects of nicotine, which tend to occur in the early part of the night, smokers may also experience withdrawal symptoms closer to morning that interfere with sleep. These symptoms may include headaches, nausea, diarrhea or constipation, irritability, anxiety, fatigue, and depression. Although quitting smoking is the best way to avoid the negative effects of nicotine on sleep, the effects can be reduced by avoiding nicotine for at least two hours before bedtime.

## FOOD AND ALCOHOL AND SLEEP

Unlike caffeine and nicotine, alcohol is classified as a central nervous system depressant or sedative. Although consuming alcohol may help people relax and fall asleep more quickly, it actually disrupts sleep later in the night, leading to daytime drowsiness and poor concentration. People who drink alcohol before bedtime spend less time in deep, restorative rapid eye movement (REM) sleep. They are also likely to experience frequent awakenings, nocturia (frequent nighttime urination), headaches, night sweats, and nightmares. Experts recommend limiting alcohol consumption in general and avoiding drinking for at least four hours before bedtime.

Food also has the capacity to enhance or disrupt sleep. Eating a healthy, balanced diet has been shown to improve overall well-being, providing people with increased energy during the day and enabling them to sleep better at night. But eating large meals or spicy foods close to bedtime can have a negative impact on sleep. Experts recommend allowing two to three hours between the last large meal of the day and bedtime. Since going to bed hungry can also impair sleep, they also suggest eating a small, light snack or drinking a glass of milk as needed to assuage late-night hunger.

## References

"Caffeine, Food, Alcohol, Smoking, and Sleep," Sleep Health Foundation, May 21, 2013. Available online. URL: www.sleephealthfoundation.org.au/pdfs/CaffeineAlcohol-0713.pdf. Accessed May 4, 2023.

Stewart, Kristin. "The Chemistry of Caffeine, Nicotine, and Sleep," Everyday Health, January 7, 2013. Available online. URL: www.everydayhealth.com/sleep/101/improve-sleep.aspx. Accessed May 4, 2023.

## Section 37.4 | Opioid Misuse and Poor Sleep

The story of the U.S. opioid crisis is often told through numbers. And, for many that makes sense, because the numbers are staggering, more than 2 million Americans suffer from opioid use disorder (OUD), a serious but treatable chronic illness that claims the lives of more than 130 people every day. Many with OUD carry another burden; however, they are among the more than 50 million adults affected by chronic, often debilitating, pain and their addiction, often the fallout of their quest for relief.

## WHY FOCUS ON OPIOID USE AND SLEEP?

"Sleep deficiency, such as insufficient sleep duration, irregular sleep schedules, and poor sleep quality are prevalent comorbidities in individuals with OUD," Aaron D. Laposky, Ph.D., Program Director, Sleep and Neurobiology, said. "We need to determine if sleep deficiency contributes to the overuse of opioids, to addiction and to how individuals respond to medication treatments to overcome addiction." That way, he added, new therapeutic targets for the prevention and treatment of opioid addiction can be identified and investigated. Figure 37.1 shows the opiates binding to opiate receptors.

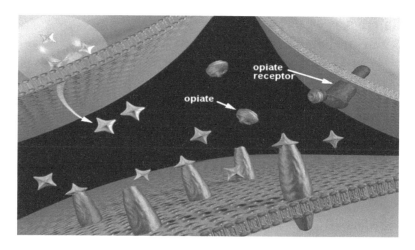

**Figure 37.1.** Opiates Binding to Opiate Receptors

*National Heart, Lung, and Blood Institute (NHLBI)*
*Note: Opiates binding to opiate receptors in the nucleus accumbens: increased dopamine.*

## ARE PEOPLE WHO MISUSE OPIOIDS MORE SUSCEPTIBLE TO SLEEP DISORDERS? CONVERSELY, ARE PEOPLE WITH SLEEP DISORDERS MORE PRONE TO OPIOID MISUSE?

The relationship between sleep and OUD is likely a two-way street, Dr. Laposky said. People with OUD often complain of sleep disturbance and insomnia, particularly during withdrawal and periods of abstinence following medication treatment, he said.

"While opioid exposure disrupts sleep, disturbance to sleep may trigger opioid overuse and dependence. New research supported by the HEAL Initiative will pinpoint how opioid use alters the regulation of sleep and how sleep deficiency may affect the propensity to misuse and become addicted to opioids," Dr. Laposky said.

## ARE RACIAL AND ETHNIC MINORITIES PARTICULARLY AFFECTED BY OPIOID-RELATED SLEEP DISORDERS?

American Indians/Alaska Natives and Whites have higher rates of nonmedical opioid use and overdose deaths, than African Americans and Latinos. These disparities make it difficult to fight the national epidemic.

"Studies suggest that sleep deficiency and untreated sleep disorders may be more common among minorities and women," Dr. Laposky said. "However, the direct contribution of racial and ethnic differences in sleep to opioid overuse, addiction and medication treatment outcomes are not yet well understood and require further study."

## ARE THERE COMMON PATHWAYS OR BIOLOGICAL MECHANISMS THAT COULD PROVIDE ANSWERS ABOUT THIS RELATIONSHIP?

Sleep deprivation, irregular sleep schedules, and poor-quality sleep weaken the network of circadian gene regulation in brain cells and affect how well the brain can adapt to stress. Impaired emotional regulation, increased risk-taking behavior, and greater sensitivity to pain increase susceptibility to substance use, Dr. Laposky said.

He explained the need to identify the mechanisms that directly connect sleep to the biological causes of OUD. Once that is done, he said, "we can explore these mechanisms as potential therapeutic targets in the prevention and treatment of opioid addiction."

Research has already started to make important connections, Dr. Laposky noted. Studies have demonstrated that sleep deprivation alters regions of the brain involved in reward (pleasure-seeking) mechanisms. There are indications that behavioral and molecular mechanisms that trigger OUDs may be directly influenced by the circadian clock. Lastly, opioid withdrawal and sleep are regulated by some of the same brain regions and neurochemical systems.[4]

---

[4] "NIH HEAL Initiative: Science Taking on Pain, Opioid Misuse—and Poor Sleep," National Heart, Lung, and Blood Institute (NHLBI), April 22, 2019. Available online. URL: www.nhlbi.nih.gov/news/2019/heal-initiative-science-taking-pain-opioid-misuse-and-poor-sleep. Accessed May 4, 2023.

# Chapter 38 | **Stress and Sleep**

Stress is a complex biological response that is designed to help people focus their attention, energy, and physical resources to deal with a problem or threat. Everyone faces sources of stress in their daily lives, such as traffic jams, work deadlines, relationship issues, or hectic schedules. In fact, surveys show that 70 percent of American adults experience stress, anxiety, or worry on a daily basis. Most people report that stress interferes with their lives, particularly by reducing the quantity and quality of their sleep.

People under stress often have trouble falling asleep because their minds race with thoughts rather than shut down. Sleep usually gives the brain a chance to rest by switching functions over from the active sympathetic nervous system to the calmer parasympathetic nervous system. Excessive worry prevents this switch from happening, so the brain remains on high alert. Stress also reduces the quantity of sleep by causing people to awaken frequently or toss and turn restlessly during the night. Among American adults, 43 percent report lying awake at night due to stress, with over half experiencing this problem more than once per week.

Stress also impacts the quality of sleep. Around 42 percent of American adults report feeling less satisfied with the quality of their sleep when they are under stress. In addition, people who experience ongoing stress have an increased risk of developing sleep disorders and insomnia. In fact, each additional source of stress in a person's life has been shown to increase their risk of insomnia by 19 percent. As a result, people with high levels of stress report sleeping only 6.2 hours per night on average, with only 33 percent feeling that they get enough sleep. People with lower levels of stress, on the other hand, sleep an average of 7.1 hours per night, and 79 percent feel that they get enough sleep.

Compounding the problem, research indicates that sleep deprivation leads to even higher levels of stress. Among people whose sleep is affected by stress or anxiety, 75 percent report that the lack of sleep increases their levels of stress and anxiety. People with high stress are also likely to feel the physical and emotional effects of getting too little sleep, such as fatigue, sluggishness, daytime drowsiness, trouble concentrating, irritability, lack of patience, and depression. When stress causes sleep problems and then sleep problems increase stress levels, people become locked in a vicious cycle that can be hard to break.

## MANAGING STRESS AND IMPROVING SLEEP

There are a number of stress management tools and techniques available to help people cope with anxiety and thus improve the quantity and quality of their sleep. Some helpful approaches for dealing with stress-related sleep issues include the following:

- **Identify sources of stress**. The first step in managing stress involves figuring out its main causes, which will vary by individual. Common sources of stress include one's job, health, and finances and experiencing trauma or going through a divorce.
- **Reduce exposure to stressors**. Once the main sources of stress have been identified, the next step is to find ways to handle them better. With job-related stress, for instance, it may be possible to delegate some responsibilities in order to reduce workload.
- **Adjust thought processes and expectations**. Often, the way of looking at a problem or situation can determine whether or not it is stressful. It is possible to change negative thought patterns and lower expectations in order to reduce stress. It is particularly important to avoid generalizing concerns and blowing small things out of proportion. Many self-help books and websites offer tips and exercises for managing negative thoughts. For instance, one approach might be to write down

worries and concerns and then throw away the paper in order to symbolically clear the mind.

- **Build a social support system.** Spending time relaxing with family and friends is a valuable way to reduce stress. Talking with supportive loved ones can also make problems seem more manageable or lead to positive new approaches and solutions.
- **Exercise**. Getting regular exercise is a proven way to relieve stress and improve mood. It can also lead to improvements in sleep. However, vigorous exercise should be undertaken at least two hours before bedtime to allow body temperature to return to normal.
- **Eat a healthy diet**. A healthy diet with plenty of fruits, vegetables, whole grains, and lean proteins promotes overall health, increases energy, and helps reduce stress. On the other hand, consuming refined sugars, caffeine, and alcohol can negatively impact sleep and leave people feeling sluggish.
- **Try relaxation techniques**. Deep breathing exercises can activate the parasympathetic nervous system and help calm nerves. Yoga, meditation, progressive muscle relaxation, and other techniques can also help quiet the mind and promote sleep.
- **Practice good sleep hygiene**. Since sleep problems increase stress levels, getting a good night's sleep is vital to effective stress management. Sleep hygiene methods that can improve the quality of sleep include making sleep a priority, blocking out eight full hours for sleep, establishing a regular sleep schedule and a relaxing bedtime routine, avoiding naps during the day, and creating a comfortable and inviting sleep environment.

If these steps are ineffective in reducing stress and improving sleep, it may be helpful to consult with a doctor. Therapists can help patients identify sources of stress and find productive ways of dealing with them. Sleep specialists can assess patients for sleep disorders and recommend approaches or medications to address the problem. Since stress and sleep often go hand in hand, both kinds of professional help may be needed to enable people to manage stress successfully and sleep soundly through the night.

## References

Holmes, Lindsay. "Five Ways Stress Wrecks Your Sleep (And What to Do about It)," Huffington Post, December 6, 2017. Available online. URL: http://www.huffingtonpost. com/entry/stress-and-sleep_n_5824506.html. Accessed May 4, 2023.

"Stress and Anxiety Interfere with Sleep," Anxiety and Depression Association of America, March 5, 2016. Available online. URL: www.adaa.org/understanding-anxiety/related-illnesses/other-related-conditions/stress/stress-and-anxiety-interfere. Accessed May 4, 2023.

"Tips to Reduce Stress and Sleep Better," WebMD, August 5, 2022. Available online. URL: www.webmd.com/sleep-disorders/tips-reduce-stress. Accessed May 4, 2023.

# Chapter 39 | Shift Work and Sleep

## Chapter Contents

In the current competitive economy, an increasing number of U.S. businesses operate to meet customer demand for 24/7 services. These around-the-clock operations are required in order to maintain a place in the global market where transactions with clients, suppliers, and colleagues can span multiple time zones. Consequently, for many women and men, the workday no longer fits the traditional 9-to-5 model. They may clock in at midnight and out at eight in the morning, or they may follow a rotating shift work schedule consisting of periodic day shifts, evening shifts, and night shifts.

Since our body clocks typically are set for a routine of daytime activity and nighttime sleep, working irregular shifts or night hours can be associated with disrupted or insufficient sleep. In turn, drowsiness, fatigue, and circadian rhythm disruption from too little sleep or interrupted sleep are associated with risks for dysfunction of the immune system, diabetes, cardiovascular disease (CVD), and other chronic health problems. As nontraditional schedules become more common, it becomes increasingly important to understand who may be at risk of unintended job-related outcomes and why. From that knowledge, employers, workers, and practitioners can better craft practical, effective interventions.

Scientists know little about the prevalence of sleep disorders broadly in the U.S. workforce because, to date, most studies have been limited to selected occupational groups, geographic areas, and types of sleep disorders. In a study published online earlier in the peer-reviewed journal *Occupational & Environmental Medicine* (oem.bmj.com/content/74/2/93.full), scientists designed a larger investigation that would not be subject to those limitations. Data were used from the National Health and Nutrition Examination Survey (NHANES), conducted by the National Center for Health Statistics (NCHS), one of the partner centers of the U.S. Centers for Disease Control and Prevention (CDC).

The NHANES was the first-ever study to use a nationally representative sample of the U.S. working population to examine the role of shift work in sleep quality, sleep-related activities of daily living (ADL), and insomnia.

The nationally representative sample included 6,338 adults, 18 years of age and older. They were asked to complete a survey questionnaire covering sleep duration, sleep disorders, sleep quality, impairment of sleep-related ADL, and insomnia. To determine the shift schedule worked by each individual, they were asked which choice best described the hours they usually worked: regular daytime (any hours between 6 a.m. and 6 p.m.), regular evening shift (any hours between 4 p.m. and midnight), regular night shift (any hours between 7 p.m. and 8 a.m.), rotating shift, or another schedule. Based on a recommendation by the National Sleep Foundation that adults should sleep seven to nine hours per night, researchers created two categories of sleep duration for the study: either less than seven hours referred to as short sleep duration or seven or more hours.

From a study of this large, nationally representative sample, the NCHS concluded that sleep-related problems were common among workers, especially among night-shift workers who had the highest risks for sleep problems. Moreover, these risks among night-shift workers persisted even after researchers adjusted for potentially confounding factors, such as long working hours, socio-demographic characteristics, and health/lifestyle/work factors. Findings included the following:

- 37.6 percent of the respondents reported short sleep duration, representing 54.1 million U.S. workers. Short sleep duration was more prevalent among night-shift workers (61.8% of those who reported short duration) than among daytime workers (35.9%).

- Daytime workers had the lowest prevalence (31%) of "prolonged sleep-onset latency," which is when at bedtime 30 or more minutes are required to go from full wakefulness to sleep—compared with the night shift (46.2%), evening shift (43%), and rotating shift (42.1%).

- Poor sleep quality was reported by 30.7 percent of night-shift workers, and moderate sleep quality was reported by 34.1 percent of workers on another schedule. Night- and evening-shift workers more frequently had difficulty falling asleep (21.7% and 21.2%, respectively, versus 12.7% of daytime workers). Night-shift workers had a higher prevalence of feeling excessively or overly sleepy during the day (22.3% versus 16.2%).

- Insomnia, which is defined as having both poor sleep quality and impaired sleep-related ADL, was reported by 18.5 percent of night-shift workers compared to 8.4 percent of daytime workers.
- Workers 60 years old or older had a lower prevalence of short sleep duration, impaired sleep-related ADL, and insomnia than those 30–59 years old.
- Female workers had a lower prevalence of short sleep duration but a higher prevalence of the other three sleep outcomes (poor sleep quality, impaired sleep-related ADL, and insomnia) than male workers.
- Obese workers had a higher prevalence of short sleep duration and poor sleep quality than those who were normal weight/underweight.
- Current smokers had a higher prevalence of short sleep duration, poor sleep quality, and insomnia (but not impaired sleep-related ADL) than nonsmokers.
- Workers who worked 48 hours or more per week had a higher prevalence of short sleep duration, poor sleep quality, and insomnia than those who worked less than 48 hours per week.
- Workers who frequently used sleeping pills had a higher prevalence of poor sleep quality, impaired sleep-related ADL, and insomnia (but not short sleep duration) than those who did not.
- A higher prevalence of all four sleep outcomes (short sleep duration, poor sleep quality, insomnia, and impaired sleep-related ADL) was observed among workers who were widowed, divorced, or separated; workers who reported fair or poor health; workers with symptomatic depression; and workers who had a physician-diagnosed sleep disorder—than among workers who did not have those characteristics.

441

Although the study was not subject to limitations of earlier investigations with smaller sample sizes, it was subject to other limitations inherent in the kind of investigation the NCHS conducted. As the NCHS notes, the limitations of their study are mitigated to some degree by the consistency of their methods and findings with those of other well-designed studies in the literature.

Particularly in light of the likely continuing increase in nontraditional working schedules, work-based prevention strategies and policies should be adopted to improve the quantity and quality of sleep among workers. Unfortunately, there is no single ideal strategy to successfully address the sleep risks of every demanding shift work situation. Instead, interventions often need to be customized to the specific employer and worker. These include designing new shift schedules with frequent rest breaks, avoiding night shifts that exceed eight hours, improving one's sleep environment, taking a long nap before a night shift begins, accelerating the modulation of circadian rhythms using bright lights, improving physical fitness, engaging in stress reduction activities, and strengthening family and social support.[1]

## STEPS YOU CAN TAKE TO HELP IMPROVE YOUR SLEEP

- **Make your room dark**. The darker, the better. As a shift worker, you are waking and sleeping against the natural rhythms of lightness and darkness—the most powerful regulators of our internal clocks. Your body wants to be active when it is light and craves rest when it is dark. Try using special room-darkening shades, lined drapes, or a sleep mask to simulate nighttime. Sleep without a night light, block the light that comes from your doorway, and, if your alarm clock is illuminated, cover it up.
- **Block outside sounds**. Sleep can be easily interrupted by sudden, unexpected sounds—the screech of a passing siren, a plane flying overhead, construction work, or a barking dog, to name a few. Use earplugs use a fan, or turn

---

[1] "Shift Work and Sleep," Centers for Disease Control and Prevention (CDC), April 26, 2021. Available online. URL: https://blogs.cdc.gov/niosh-science-blog/2016/10/05/shift-work-and-sleep. Accessed April 26, 2023.

the FM radio or TV to in-between stations, so the "shhhh" blocks out other noises and lulls you to sleep. (Just be sure to turn off the brightness on your TV or cover the screen.) You might even want to consider a "white noise" machine, which plays a steady stream of lulling sounds such as ocean waves.

- **Adjust your thermostat before going to bed**. A room that is too hot or too cold can disturb your sleep. Some research shows that 60–65 °F or 16–18 °C is ideal.
- **Keep a regular schedule**. Go to bed and get up at the same time every day. The best way to ensure a good night's sleep is to stick to a regular schedule, even on your days off, during holidays, or when traveling.
- **Maintain or improve your overall health**. Eat well and establish a regular exercise routine. It can be as simple as a 20- to 30-minute walk, jog, or swim or riding a bicycle three times a week. Exercising too close to bedtime may actually keep you awake because your body has not had a chance to unwind. Allow at least three hours between working out and going to bed.
- **Avoid caffeine several hours before bedtime**. Its stimulating effects will peak two to four hours later and may linger for several hours more. The result is diminished deep sleep and increased awakenings.
- **Avoid alcohol before going to sleep**. It may initially make you fall asleep faster, but it can make it much harder to stay asleep. As the immediate effects of the alcohol wear off, it deprives your body of deep rest, and you end up sleeping in fragments and waking often.
- **Know the side effects of medications**. Some medications can increase sleepiness and make it dangerous to drive. Other medications can cause sleeping difficulties as a side effect.
- **Change the time you go to sleep**. After driving home from work, do not go right to bed. Take a few hours to unwind and relax.
- **Develop a relaxing sleep ritual**. Before going to sleep, try taking a warm bath, listening to soothing music, or

reading until you feel sleepy—but do not read anything exciting or stimulating.

- **Do not solve the day's problems during bedtime**. Try to clear your mind. Make a list of things you are concerned about or need to do the next day so you do not worry about them when you are trying to sleep.
- **Set house rules**. Speak with your family about your sleep schedule and why your sleep time is so important. Establish guidelines for everyone in your household to help maintain a peaceful sleeping environment—such as wearing headphones to listen to music or watch TV and avoiding vacuuming, dishwashing, and noisy games.
- **Keep a sleep schedule**. Let family and friends know your sleep schedule and ask them to call or visit at times that are convenient for you. Plan ahead for activities together.
- **Switch off the phone**. Be sure unimportant calls do not wake you up. Unplug the phone in your bedroom and, if necessary, get a beeper so your family can reach you in an emergency.
- **Hang a "do not disturb" sign on your door**. Make sure your family understands the conditions under which they should wake you. Make a deal with them. If they let you sleep, you will be less grumpy! And make sure delivery people and solicitors understand your sleeping rules by hanging a "do not disturb" sign on your front door, too.

By following as many tips as possible, you should start to experience improvements in the quality of your sleep. It will not happen right away, but if you stick with it for a week or two, you will begin to notice positive changes. Staying alert on the job will be much easier. Drowsy driving will no longer be a problem. And you will be able to enjoy more quality time with your family—and they will enjoy you![2]

---

[2] "Wake Up and Get Some Sleep," National Highway Traffic Safety Administration (NHTSA), April 28, 2010. Available online. URL: https://one.nhtsa.gov/people/injury/drowsy_driving1/human/drows_driving/wbroch/wbroch_lg/wbroch_lg.html. Accessed April 26, 2023.

## Section 39.2 | **Sleep and Work**

We know that sleep is important. The need for sleep is biologically similar to the need to eat and drink, and it is critical for maintaining life and health and for working safely. Sleeping seven to eight hours a night is linked with a wide range of better health and safety outcomes. The National Institute for Occupational Safety and Health (NIOSH) has been actively involved in research to protect workers, workers' families, employers, and the community from the hazards linked to long work hours and shift work.

Why are more Americans getting less sleep? Work demands are one factor. The timing of a shift can strain a worker's ability to get enough sleep. Working at night or during irregular hours goes against the human body's biology, which is hardwired to sleep during the night and be awake and active during the day. Still, society needs certain workers around the clock to provide vital services in public safety, health care, utilities, food services, manufacturing, transportation, and others. The resulting shift work—any shift outside the normal daylight hours of 7 a.m. to 6 p.m.—is linked to poorer sleep, circadian rhythm disturbances, and strains on family and social life. It is not possible to eliminate shift work altogether, so the challenge is to develop strategies to make critical services available while keeping workers healthy and everyone around them safe. In addition to shift work, some data suggest that a growing number of employees are being asked to work long hours on a regular basis. Every extra hour on the job is one less spent attending to the person's off-the-job responsibilities. When the day is too full to fit everything in, it is often sleep that gets the short shrift.

## WHAT ARE THE RISKS OF LONG WORK HOURS AND SHIFT WORK?
### Risks for Workers
- sleep deprivation
- lack of adequate time to recover from work
- decline in mental function and physical ability, including emotional fatigue and a decline in the function of the body's immune system

- higher rates of depression, occupational injury, and poor perceived health
- higher prevalence of insomnia among shift workers with low social support
- increased risk of illness and injury
- strain on personal relationships, such as marriage and family life
- increased risk of long-term health effects, such as heart disease, gastrointestinal disorders, mood disturbances, and cancer

## Risks for Employers
- reduced productivity
- increase in errors
- absenteeism and presenteeism (present at work but not fully functioning because of health problems or personal issues)
- increased health-care and worker compensation costs
- workforce attrition due to disability, death, or moving to jobs with less demanding schedules

## Risks to the Community
Potential increase in errors by workers leads to:
- medical errors
- vehicle crashes
- industrial disasters

Research indicates that the effect of long work hours and shift work may be more complex than a simple direct relationship between a certain high number of work hours or shift schedule and risks. The effects appear to be influenced by a variety of factors, including characteristics of the worker and the job, worker control, pay, nonwork responsibilities, and other characteristics of the work schedule.

Both workers and employers share in the responsibility of reducing risks connected to poor sleep. Therefore, it is important for both workers and managers to make sleep a priority in their personal life and in the assignment of work.

## WHAT CAN EMPLOYERS DO TO ADDRESS THIS ISSUE?

- **Regular rest**. Establish at least 10 consecutive hours per day of protected time off-duty in order for workers to obtain seven to eight hours of sleep.
- **Rest breaks**. Frequent brief rest breaks (e.g., every one to two hours) during demanding work are more effective against fatigue than a few longer breaks. Allow longer breaks for meals.
- **Shift lengths**. Five 8-hour shifts or four 10-hour shifts per week are usually tolerable. Depending on the workload, 12-hour days may be tolerable with more frequent interspersed rest days. Shorter shifts (e.g., eight hours), during the evening and night, are better tolerated than longer shifts.
- **Workload**. Examine work demands with respect to shift length. Twelve-hour shifts are more tolerable for "lighter" tasks (e.g., desk work).
- **Rest days**. Plan one or two full days of rest to follow five consecutive 8-hour shifts or four 10-hour shifts. Consider two rest days after three consecutive 12-hour shifts.
- **Training**. Provide training to make sure that workers are aware of the ups and downs of shift work and that they know what resources are available to them to help with any difficulties they are having with the work schedule.
- **Incident analysis**. Examine near misses and incidents to determine the role, if any, of fatigue as a root cause or contributing cause to the incident.

## WHAT CAN WORKERS DO TO ADDRESS THIS ISSUE?

- Make sure you give yourself enough time to sleep after working your shift.
- Avoid heavy foods and alcohol before sleeping and reduce intake of caffeine and other stimulants several hours

beforehand since these can make it difficult to get quality sleep.

- Exercise routinely, as keeping physically fit can help you manage stress, stay healthy, and improve your sleep.
- Choose to sleep someplace dark, comfortable, quiet, and cool so you can fall asleep quickly and stay asleep.
- Seek assistance from an appropriate health-care provider if you are having difficulties sleeping.

## WHAT DOES THE FUTURE HOLD?

The NIOSH is working on several projects to reduce the risks associated with long working hours and shift work. The research of the Centers for Disease Control and Prevention (CDC) includes the following:

- studying new methods to better measure work hours
- surveillance to better understand the extent of the problem
- studies to estimate risks to workers and employers
- training interventions[3]

## Section 39.3 | Shift Work and Health Problems in Police Officers

Ensuring the safety of our community is a 24-hours-a-day, 7-days-a-week, 365-days-a-year kind of job. Weekends and holidays are included. Working at night (outside the normal daylight hours of 7 a.m.–6 p.m.) is known as "shift work," and it has been linked to certain health issues.

Police officers and detectives frequently work first, second, and third shifts, and it is common that these shifts rotate. The Buffalo Cardio-Metabolic Occupational Police Stress (BCOPS) study has been used to look at the relationships between shift work and

---

[3] "Sleep and Work," Centers for Disease Control and Prevention (CDC), April 26, 2021. Available online. URL: https://blogs.cdc.gov/niosh-science-blog/2012/03/08/sleep-and-work. Accessed April 25, 2023.

several health conditions among police officers. The BCOPS study began in 2004 as a collaboration between the National Institute for Occupational Safety and Health (NIOSH) and the University at Buffalo with tremendous support from the Buffalo, New York Police Department.

This section highlights BCOPS research findings from multiple studies over the past decade to share what has been learned, what these findings mean to officers and detectives, and what managers and officers can do to reduce the harmful effects of shift work.

## SHIFT WORK

Shift work is required in many occupations, but it is especially common among those who work in protective services. Shift work includes working nights or rotating day, evening, or night shifts.

Shift work has been linked to several physical and mental health problems, including the following:

- heart disease
- cancer
- depression
- reduced immune functions
- injury
- sleep issues (sleeping less and not getting quality sleep)

Understanding how shift work is associated with health problems is key to determining how to eliminate or reduce the negative effects.

## HEALTH CONCERNS RELATED TO SHIFT WORK AMONG POLICE OFFICERS

Workers in other occupations who work nights or have rotating day, night, or evening shifts have reported several health concerns. Researchers assessed many of these same health concerns among police officers using BCOPS data.

Here are some key findings from the BCOPS study:

- Shift work may lead to poor sleep quality among officers. Getting a good night's sleep is particularly important for police officers, who work and drive long hours under high-risk and uncontrolled environments and often need to make on-the-spot decisions in complex situations. Researchers found poor sleep quality was 70 percent higher among officers working the night shift and 49 percent higher among those working the afternoon shift than among officers on the day shift.

- Shift work may increase job-related injuries and absences among officers. Researchers found officers who worked night shifts had two times the rate of long-term injury leave (90 or more days leave) than those who worked the afternoon and three times the rate of leave than those who worked day shifts.

- Shift work may increase stress and depression among officers. Researchers found that work-related stress was more prevalent among police officers working the afternoon or night shift than the day shift. Officers working these two shifts reported more stressful events than those who worked the day shift. Officers who worked the evening/night shift were about four times more likely to report depressive symptoms than those working the day shift. Officers reporting higher stress also tended to have higher levels of depressive symptoms.

- Shift work may affect officers' immune system. Researchers found officers working long-term night shifts had greater numbers of white blood cells than day-shift police officers, which indicates that shift work may have a negative effect on the immune system. Shift work is associated with biological changes that may indicate an increased risk of heart disease among officers. Among the BCOPS police officers, researchers examined changes in biological signals of cardiovascular disease (CVD) while also considering the body mass index. Researchers found that officers working night shifts had higher levels of signs of inflammation than day-shift police officers. Increased levels of inflammation may lead to an increased risk of CVD.

Researchers also found officers on night and afternoon shifts were more likely to be absent from work due to sickness; this was particularly evident among overweight officers. This is consistent with what other studies have found. Both obesity and shift work are risk factors for adverse health outcomes. Their combined effects may lead to a greater risk of absence due to sickness.

## WHAT MANAGERS CAN DO TO LESSEN THE EFFECTS OF SHIFT WORK

Reduce double shifts, where possible, to prevent fatigue. Fatigue is likely to impact performance, increasing the risk of accidents and injuries.

- Provide training and information on shift work so your workers are aware of the potential effects on their health and work performance. The NIOSH offers a 30-minute online training for emergency responders on reducing risks associated with long work hours.
- Make sure your workers have access to appropriate health-care and counseling services to support their health and well-being. The U.S. Department of Justice (DOJ) has law enforcement mental health and wellness program resources.
- Develop and promote the use of a workplace health promotion program. These programs can reduce chronic disease risk, lower health-care costs and absenteeism, and increase employee productivity.

## WHAT POLICE OFFICERS CAN DO TO LESSEN THE EFFECTS OF SHIFT WORK

- Exercise regularly and eat a healthy diet to reduce your stress levels and improve your quality of sleep.

- Protect your sleep—keep a regular sleep routine, avoid heavy foods and alcohol before sleep, and block out noise and lights when trying to sleep.
- Discuss concerns about the effects of shift work on your health with a health professional. Follow medical advice to ensure you are staying healthy.[4]

## Section 39.4 | Daylight Saving: Helping Workers to Prevent Sleep Deprivation

Spring forward, fall back.

We all know the saying to help us remember to adjust our clocks for daylight saving time changes. But what can we do to help workers adjust to the effects of the time change? A few studies have examined these issues, but many questions remain on this topic, including the best strategies to cope with time changes.

By moving the clocks ahead one hour in the spring, we lose one hour, which shifts work times and other scheduled events one hour earlier. This pushes most people to have a one-hour earlier bedtime and wake-up time. In the fall, time moves back one hour. We gain one hour that shifts work times and other scheduled events one hour later, thereby pushing most people to have a one-hour later bedtime and wake-up time.

It can take about one week for the body to adjust to the new times for sleeping, eating, and activity. Until they have adjusted, people can have trouble falling asleep, staying asleep, and waking up at the right time. This can lead to sleep deprivation and reduction in performance, increasing the risk of mistakes, including vehicle crashes. Workers can experience somewhat higher risks to both their health and safety after the time changes. A study by Inge Kirchberger, PhD Senior Researcher, Central Hospital of Augsburg

---

[4] "Shiftwork May Lead to Health Problems among Police Officers: What Can Be Done? Using Buffalo Cardio-Metabolic Occupational Police Stress (BCOPS) Study Data to Examine First Responder Health," Centers for Disease Control and Prevention (CDC), May 24, 2022. Available online. URL: https://blogs.cdc.gov/niosh-science-blog/2022/05/16/police-and-shiftwork. Accessed May 10, 2023.

and colleagues reported men and persons with heart disease might be at higher risk for a heart attack during the week after the time changes in the spring and fall.

The reason for these problems is thought to be disruption to circadian rhythms and sleep. Circadian rhythms are daily cycles of numerous hormones and other body functions that prepare us for the expected times for sleeping, eating, and activity. Circadian rhythms have difficulty adjusting to an abrupt one-hour time change.

Other hazards for workers related to the time change in the fall include a sudden change in the driving conditions in the late-afternoon rush hour—from driving home from work during daylight hours to driving home in darkness. People may not have changed their driving habits to nighttime driving and might be at somewhat higher risk for a vehicle crash. Additionally, the spring time change leads to more daylight in the evening, which may disturb some people's sleep.

To help reduce risks about one and a half weeks before the time changes in the fall and spring, employers can relay the following points to help their workers:

- Remind workers that several days after the time changes are associated with somewhat higher health and safety risks due to disturbances to circadian rhythms and sleep.
- It can take one week for the body to adjust sleep times and circadian rhythms to the time change, so consider reducing demanding physical and mental tasks as much as possible that week to allow oneself time to adjust.
- Remind workers to be especially vigilant while driving, at work, and at home to protect themselves, as others around them may be sleepier and at risk of making an error that can cause a vehicle crash or other accident.
- The research found that people with existing heart disease may be at risk for a heart attack after the time change.
- Workers can improve their adaptation to the time change by using these suggestions. Circadian rhythms and sleep are strongly influenced by several factors,

including the timing of exposure to light and darkness, times of eating and exercise, and time of work. One way to help the body adjust is to gradually change the times for sleep, eating, and activity.

- For the spring time change, starting about three days before, one can gradually move up the timing of going to bed and waking up, meals, exercise, and exposure to light earlier by 15–20 minutes each day until these are in line with the new time. About one hour before bedtime, keep the lights dim and avoid electronic lit screens on computers, tablets, and so on to help the body adjust its internal clock in regard to bedtime and waking up.

- For the fall time change, starting about three days before, one can gradually move the timing of going to bed and waking up, meals, exercise, and exposure to light later by 15–20 minutes each day until these are in line with the new time. About one hour after waking up in the morning, keep the lights dim and avoid the electronic screens on computers, tablets, and so on to help the body adjust its internal clock in regard to bedtime and waking up.

- Being sleep-deprived before the time change will increase the health and safety risks, so make it a priority to get enough sleep and be well-rested several days before the time change.

## DOES THE TIME CHANGE AFFECT EVERYONE EQUALLY?

In short, no. People who sleep seven or less hours per day tend to have more problems with the time changes. Additionally, a person's natural tendency to get up early and go to bed early or get up late and go to bed late may also influence their ability to adjust to the one-hour time changes in the spring and fall. Those prone to naturally follow an "early to bed and early to rise" pattern (morningness) will tend to have more difficulties adjusting to the fall time change because this goes against their natural tendencies. Conversely, those who naturally follow a "late to bed and late to rise" routine (eveningness) will tend to have more trouble with the spring time change.

Morningness/eveningness tends to change as people age. Teenagers and young adults tend to be "evening" types, and researchers theorize this may be due to brain and body development at those ages. Younger workers, therefore, may have more difficulty adjusting to the spring time change. Morningness increases as people age, so older adults tend to be "morning" types. As a result, older workers may have more trouble adjusting to the fall time change. Finally, people who are on the extreme end of the eveningness or the morningness trait may tend to have more trouble adjusting their sleep to the time changes.[5]

## Section 39.5 | Lighting Interventions in Shift Workers

Shift work has been linked to poor sleep, chronic metabolic disorders (e.g., cardiovascular disease, diabetes, and obesity), several forms of cancer, depression, and an elevated risk of the occurrence of accidents. These risks are especially acute for those who work rotating shifts that involve working through the night, as sometimes occur in hospitals. Studies show that health-care workers are at greater risk for shift-work-related health and safety problems than their colleagues who work conventional daytime hours. To make matters more complex, nurses typically follow 12-hour shift schedules and can perform crucial tasks (e.g., monitoring unstable patients, etc.) when alertness levels are low and the pressure for sleep is high. Researchers from Mt. Sinai and Rensselaer Polytechnic Institute examined the effects of an experimental lighting intervention on levels of melatonin, task performance, activity–rest patterns, and subjective sleep quality.

---

[5] "Daylight Saving: Suggestions to Help Workers Adapt to the Time Change," Centers for Disease Control and Prevention (CDC), March 9, 2016. Available online. URL: https://blogs.cdc.gov/niosh-science-blog/2016/03/09/daylight-savings. Accessed May 5, 2023.

## BACKGROUND

Research conducted over the past 40 years has found a strong link between health problems and disruption of the human circadian system, which regulates our bodily processes such as sleeping by producing circadian rhythms that basically signal the body to do the right things at the right times. Because the human circadian system runs on a cycle that, for most people, is slightly longer than the solar day, it must be continually synchronized to keep the right things happening at the right times.

The circadian system's main synchronizer is the 24-hour pattern of light and dark reaching our eye retina, which sends those signals via the optic nerve to a cluster of cells in the brain's hypothalamus region called the "master biological clock," which in turn regulates circadian rhythms. Although several properties of light are known to influence the timing of the circadian system, a key property for this study is a light source's spectral composition or its wavelength. Short-wavelength light is the most effective of all light sources for stimulating the circadian system, perhaps best visualized as the blue light of the morning sky that energizes us for the coming day. Long-wavelength light, on the other hand, has negligible effects on the circadian system and is perhaps best visualized as the red sky at twilight that is followed by sleep.

## THE STUDY

In this study, they evaluated the effectiveness of experimental lighting interventions in terms of their effects on the participants' levels of the hormone melatonin, which is produced in darkness and prepares the body for sleep. Blue light suppresses melatonin production at night, while red light does not. But when experienced at sufficiently high levels at any time of day, both types of light can elicit a beneficial, immediate alerting effect that is similar to drinking a cup of coffee. They also assessed the lighting's effect on task performance, activity–rest patterns, and subjective sleep quality.

Their study took place in four hospitals in Albany, New York; Schenectady, New York; South Bend, Indiana; and Syracuse, New York. One of the interventions explored a novel lighting intervention (red light), delivered to the participants' retinas via personal light glasses, that was designed to increase alertness and improve performance without disrupting the secretion of melatonin. Based on their previous research, they hypothesized that the red light would be useful for promoting workplace alertness without negatively affecting sleep and the circadian system. Seventy-eight participants (49 on the day shift and 29 on the night shift) completed at least four weeks (two weeks baseline and two weeks intervention) of the study's 20-week protocol (refer to Figure 39.1).

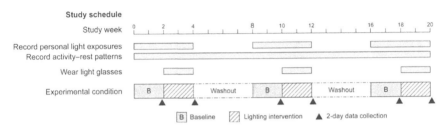

**Figure 39.1.** The Experimental Protocol

*Centers for Disease Control and Prevention (CDC)*

After the baseline data collection, participants were exposed to either 30 minutes of circadian-ineffective red light, circadian-effective blue light, or dim white light (the experimental control) during the beginning, middle, and end of their shifts for two consecutive weeks. On the last two shifts of the intervention period, the participants underwent computer-based auditory performance tests, submitted saliva samples for melatonin and cortisol assay prior to and immediately after the light exposures, and completed questionnaires relating to feelings of sleepiness during the testing, as well as sleep quality and sleep disturbance over the past week. Activity–rest patterns and personal light exposures were also continuously monitored via experimental devices routinely employed in this research.

Figure 39.2 shows the mean normalized melatonin levels by light color (baseline versus intervention).

The study's results were mostly positive and consistent with their hypotheses. Only the blue light suppressed participants' nighttime

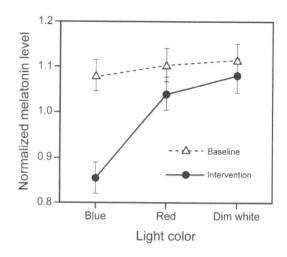

**Figure 39.2.** Normalized Melatonin Levels by Light Color

*Centers for Disease Control and Prevention (CDC)
Note: Mean normalized melatonin levels by light color (baseline versus intervention). As expected, exposure to the blue light suppressed the nurses' nighttime salivary melatonin levels compared to exposure to the red and dim white light, as well as to the recorded baseline level. The error bars represent the standard error of the mean.*

melatonin levels, as expected, but the performance testing results were mixed. While some positive effects of red light were shown at the end of the day shift and in the middle of the night shift, when workers are likely to be most tired, not all of the performance results were in the expected direction, and there were large amounts of missing data. This is understandable, given the challenges of gathering data from busy nurses while they were working. Sleep outcomes improved for night shift nurses exposed to the red and blue light compared to the dim control. Notably, the nurses who were exposed to the blue light experienced better-quality sleep, which is consistent with the hypothesis that blue light promotes synchronization between our circadian rhythms and the solar day's 24-hour pattern of light and dark.

This is the first field study to show that red light can be used to improve sleep and improve certain types of performance in real-life work situations without affecting nighttime melatonin levels. Future studies should focus on implementing the study's red-light intervention as less-intrusive, ambient workplace lighting to better ensure participant compliance.[6]

## Section 39.6 | Research on Work Schedules and Work-Related Sleep Loss

This section provides a brief overview of some of the work that the National Institute for Occupational Safety and Health (NIOSH) intramural scientists are carrying out to better understand these risks and ways to prevent them.

## NURSES/REPRODUCTION ISSUES/SHIFT WORK

The NIOSH studies are examining shift work and physical demands with respect to adverse pregnancy outcomes among nurses, specifically the association between work schedule and risk of spontaneous abortion, preterm birth, and menstrual function. This research was the first to look at shift work and pregnancy in U.S. nurses. The NIOSH researchers are collaborating with the Harvard Nurses' Health Study, which is the largest, ongoing prospective study of nurses. Results have shown that an increased risk of several reproductive outcomes, including spontaneous abortion, early preterm birth, and menstrual cycle irregularities, is related to shift work, particularly working the night shift. In addition, results show independent effects on reproductive outcomes from long working hours. The study hopes to establish a cohort of over 100,000 female

---

[6] "Lighting Interventions to Reduce Circadian Disruption in Rotating Shift Workers," Centers for Disease Control and Prevention (CDC), May 4, 2021. Available online. URL: https://blogs.cdc.gov/niosh-science-blog/2020/12/18/lighting-shift-work. Accessed May 10, 2023.

nurses of reproductive age. As this longitudinal study progresses, there will be increased opportunities to study the impact of occupational exposures on a wide variety of chronic disease outcomes, including cancers and heart disease.

## POLICE/SLEEP/SHIFT WORK/STRESS

A series of studies are being carried out to understand the connection between exposures to occupational stressors and health outcomes in police officers in Buffalo, New York. Early studies have already indicated that there are significant adverse health outcomes associated with sleep and shift work. One study found that the majority of officers reported feeling tired upon awakening (89.9%) and snoring (83.3%). The prevalence of snoring was 26 percent higher in night shift workers than that in other workers. A 2009 published study found that officers who worked nights and either had less than six hours of sleep or worked more overtime had a greater risk of injury and metabolic syndrome than officers working the day shift.

## TRUCKING/MANUFACTURING/WHITE-COLLAR WORKERS

Several studies examining large samples of workers have been published or are currently in progress. Information on driver fatigue and the quality, location, and length of sleep has been collected in a large national survey of long-haul truck drivers. Results from this survey are being used to determine the extent of sleep disorders (including sleep apnea) drivers experience and their relationship with health conditions and crashes. A series of studies examining long work hours have been published. In healthy daytime workers, emotional fatigue was associated with a decline in the function and quantity of natural killer cells, a white blood cell that is part of our first line of defense against cancer and viruses. A study found that long work hours combined with short sleep (less than six hours/day) or insufficient sleep was associated with depression, injury, and poor health that are largely associated with sleep problems rather than work hours itself. Among shift workers, those with low social support at work had two times higher prevalence of insomnia than those with high support even after considering the effects of workload.

## TRAINING

NIOSH scientists are developing and evaluating tailored training programs for managers and workers in manufacturing, mining, nursing, retail, and trucking to inform them of the importance of sleep and the risks linked to insufficient sleep, shift work, and long work hours and strategies to prevent these risks.

- The NIOSH has developed a comprehensive online training program for nurses. The program includes a short video and 12 modules. The training program is currently being pilot tested in senior nursing students and registered nurses enrolled in nursing graduate courses.
- For the trucking industry, the NIOSH has developed two public service announcements to broadcast over the radio and two brochures to raise awareness of the risks of long work hours and shift work, as well as what actions they can take to help manage their risks. A website for trucking is also under development.
- For the mining industry, the NIOSH is developing two presentations on shift work and sleep for mining trainers. A helmet sticker has also been developed to help further raise awareness of this issue.
- The NIOSH developed a series of six 30-minute webinars to educate workers and managers in manufacturing and retail about sleep.

## RISK ASSESSMENT

NIOSH scientists are exploring statistical and epidemiological issues to lay the groundwork for the quantitative risk assessment of work hours related to occupational illness and injury outcomes. This approach will use work hour data that is collected over a period of time. The project staff will examine how work hour patterns relate to a range of adverse outcomes, including, but not limited to, errors in the workplace. This work is in its early stages but is part of the effort to develop a quantitative risk assessment of work hours that can be used to refine policy and recommendations targeted at reducing illness and injury associated with long work hours, shift work, and other irregular work schedules.[7]

[7] "NIOSH Research on Work Schedules and Work-Related Sleep Loss," Centers for Disease Control and Prevention (CDC), April 26, 2021. Available online. URL: https://blogs.cdc.gov/niosh-science-blog/2012/03/09/sleep. Accessed May 10, 2023.

# Chapter 40 | **Discussing Sleep with Your Doctor**

Doctors might not identify sleep problems during routine office visits because patients are awake, so let your doctor know if you think you might have a sleep problem. For example, talk with your doctor if you often feel sleepy during the day, do not wake up feeling refreshed and alert, or are having trouble adapting to shift work.

## BE PREPARED

To get a better sense of your sleep problem, your doctor will ask you about your sleep habits. Before you see the doctor, think about how to describe your problems, including the following:
- how often you have trouble sleeping and how long you have had the problem
- when you go to bed and get up on workdays and days off
- how long it takes you to fall asleep, how often you wake up at night, and how long it takes you to fall back asleep
- whether you snore loudly and often or wake up gasping or feeling out of breath
- how refreshed you feel when you wake up and how tired you feel during the day
- how often you doze off or have trouble staying awake during routine tasks, especially driving

Your doctor may also ask questions about your personal routine and habits. For example, they may ask about your work and exercise routines. Your doctor may also ask whether you use caffeine, tobacco, alcohol, or any medicines (including over-the-counter (OTC) medicines).

## KEEP A SLEEP DIARY
To help your doctor, consider keeping a sleep diary for a few weeks:
- Write down when you go to sleep, wake up, and take naps. (e.g., you might note: Went to bed at 10 a.m.; woke up at 3 a.m. and could not fall back asleep; napped after work for two hours.)
- Write down how much you sleep each night, how alert and rested you feel in the morning, and how sleepy you feel at various times during the day.

## DIAGNOSTIC PROCEDURES THAT DOCTORS MAY CONSIDER
Doctors can diagnose some sleep disorders by asking questions about sleep schedules and habits and by getting information from sleep partners or parents. To diagnose other sleep disorders, doctors also use the results from sleep studies and other medical tests.

Sleep tests can help your doctor diagnose sleep-related breathing disorders such as sleep apnea, sleep-related seizure disorders, sleep-related movement disorders, and sleep disorders that cause extreme daytime tiredness such as narcolepsy. Doctors may also use sleep tests to help diagnose or rule out restless legs syndrome (RLS).

Your doctor will determine whether you need your sleep test at a sleep center or if you can do it at home with a portable device. Sleep tests at a sleep center usually last overnight. Removable sensors will be placed on your scalp, face, eyelids, chest, limbs, and finger. These sensors record your brain waves, heart rate, breathing effort and rate, oxygen levels, and muscle movements before, during, and after sleep. There is a small risk of irritation from the sensors, but this will go away after they are removed.

Your doctor may do a physical exam to rule out other medical problems that might interfere with sleep. You may need blood tests to check for thyroid problems or other conditions that can cause sleep problems.

## HOW IS SLEEP DEPRIVATION TREATED?

If your doctor diagnoses you with a sleep disorder, they may talk to you about healthy sleep habits. Your treatment options will depend on which type you have:

- For sleep apnea, the goals of treatment are to help keep your airways open during sleep. This may include a continuous positive airway pressure (CPAP) machine or other breathing devices, therapy, or surgery.
- For narcolepsy and insomnia, treatment options include medicines and behavior changes.[1]

---

[1] "Sleep Deprivation and Deficiency—Diagnosis," National Heart, Lung, and Blood Institute (NHLBI), March 24, 2022. Available online. URL: www.nhlbi.nih.gov/health/sleep-deprivation/diagnosis-treatment. Accessed May 5, 2023.

# Chapter 41 | **What You Need to Know about Sleep Studies**

Sleep studies, also called "polysomnography," are painless tests that measure how well you sleep and how your body responds to sleep problems. They are also used to help your doctor diagnose sleep disorders.

The most common type of sleep study records brain waves and monitors your heart rate, breathing, and the oxygen level in your blood during a full night of sleep.

Other ways to study your sleep include the following:

- Multiple sleep latency tests measure how quickly you fall asleep during a series of daytime naps and use sensors to record your brain activity and eye movements.
- Daytime maintenance of wakefulness test measures your ability to stay awake and alert.
- Activity monitors help doctors see how much you sleep and how well you sleep. They are worn at home for several days or sometimes weeks.

Your doctor will review your sleep test results and develop a treatment plan for any diagnosed sleep disorder. Untreated sleep disorders can raise your risk of heart failure, high blood pressure, stroke, diabetes, and depression. Sleep disorders have also been linked to an increased risk of injury and car accidents.[1]

---

[1] "Sleep Studies," National Heart, Lung, and Blood Institute (NHLBI), March 24, 2022. Available online. URL: www.nhlbi.nih.gov/health/sleep-studies. Accessed April 27, 2023.

## TYPES OF SLEEP STUDIES

Depending on your symptoms, your doctor will gather information and consider several possible tests when trying to diagnose a sleep disorder.

### Sleep History and Sleep Log

Your doctor will ask you how many hours you sleep each night, how often you awaken during the night and for how long, how long it takes for you to fall asleep, how well-rested you feel upon awakening, and how sleepy you feel during the day. Your doctor may ask you to keep a sleep diary for a few weeks. Your doctor may also ask you whether you have any symptoms of sleep apnea or restless legs syndrome, such as loud snoring, snorting or gasping, morning headaches, tingling or unpleasant sensations in the limbs that are relieved by moving them, and jerking of the limbs during sleep. Your sleeping partner may be asked whether you have some of these symptoms, as you may not be aware of them yourself.

### Polysomnogram

A sleep recording or polysomnogram (PSG) is usually done while you stay overnight at a sleep center or sleep laboratory. Electrodes and other monitors are placed on your scalp, face, chest, limbs, and finger. While you sleep, these devices measure your brain activity, eye movements, muscle activity, heart rate and rhythm, blood pressure, and how much air moves in and out of your lungs. This test also checks the amount of oxygen in your blood. A PSG test is painless. In certain circumstances, the PSG can be done at home. A home monitor can be used to record your heart rate, how air moves in and out of your lungs, the amount of oxygen in your blood, and your breathing effort.

### Multiple Sleep Latency Test

This daytime sleep study measures how sleepy you are and is particularly useful for diagnosing narcolepsy. The multiple sleep latency test (MSLT) is conducted in a sleep laboratory and is typically done after an overnight sleep recording (PSG). In this test, sleep-stage monitoring devices are placed on your scalp and face. You are asked to nap four or five times for 20 minutes every two hours during the day. Technicians note how quickly you fall asleep and how long it takes for you to reach various stages of sleep, especially rapid eye movement (REM) sleep, during your naps. Normal individuals either do not fall asleep during these short-designated nap times or take a long time to fall asleep. People who fall asleep in less than five minutes are likely to require treatment for a sleep disorder, as are those who quickly reach REM sleep during their naps. It is important to have a sleep specialist interpret the results of your PSG or MSLT.

## HOW TO FIND A SLEEP CENTER AND SLEEP SPECIALIST

If your doctor refers you to a sleep center or sleep specialist, make sure that center or specialist is qualified to diagnose and treat your sleep problem. To find sleep centers accredited by the American Academy of Sleep Medicine (AASM), go to www.aasmnet.org and click on "Find a Sleep Center" (under the patients and public menu) or call 708-492-0930. To find sleep specialists certified by the American Board of Sleep Medicine (ABSM), go to www.absm.org and click on "credential verification of diplomates of the ABSM."[2]

---

[2] "Your Guide to Healthy Sleep," National Heart, Lung, and Blood Institute (NHLBI), August 2011. Available online. URL: www.nhlbi.nih.gov/files/docs/public/sleep/healthy_sleep.pdf. Accessed April 27, 2023.

# Chapter 42 | **Treatment for Insomnia**

.

## Section 42.1 | How Is Insomnia Treated?

If your insomnia is caused by a short-term change in your sleep/wake schedule, such as with jet lag, your sleep schedule will probably return to normal on its own.

Chronic or long-term insomnia can be treated with steps you can try at home to sleep better, cognitive behavioral therapy (CBT), and prescription medicines.

If insomnia is a symptom or side effect of another health problem, your doctor may recommend treating the other health problem at the same time. When the other health problem is treated, secondary insomnia often goes away on its own. For example, if menopause symptoms, such as hot flashes, are keeping you awake, your doctor might try treating your hot flashes first. Research suggests that older women who use hormone replacement therapy (HRT), eat healthy foods based on a Mediterranean diet, and limit how much caffeine and alcohol they drink may have fewer sleep problems than women who do not do those things.

## HOW DOES COGNITIVE BEHAVIORAL THERAPY HELP TREAT INSOMNIA?

Research shows that CBT works as well as prescription medicine for many people who have chronic or long-term insomnia. CBT helps you change thoughts and actions that may get in the way of sleep.

This type of therapy is also used to treat conditions such as depression, anxiety disorders, and eating disorders. For success with CBT, you may need to see a therapist weekly for two months or more. CBT may involve the following:

- keeping a diary to track your sleep
- replacing negative thoughts about sleep with positive thinking, which includes linking being in bed to being asleep and not to the problems you have falling asleep
- talking with a therapist alone or in group sessions, which can help you identify and change any unhelpful thoughts and behaviors about sleep
- learning habits that can help you sleep better

## WHAT PRESCRIPTION MEDICINES TREAT INSOMNIA?

Prescription medicines can help treat short- or long-term insomnia. But your doctor or nurse may have you try CBT first rather than medicine to treat insomnia.

The types of prescription medicines used to treat insomnia include sedatives and certain kinds of antidepressants. Prescription sleep medicines can have serious side effects, including sleepiness during the daytime and an increased risk of falls for older adults. They can also affect women differently compared with men. In 2013, the U.S. Food and Drug Administration (FDA) required drug companies to lower the recommended dose for women of certain prescription sleep medicines with zolpidem because women's bodies do not break down the medicine as quickly as men's bodies do.

If you decide to use a prescription sleep medicine, do the following:

- Ask your doctor, nurse, or pharmacist about any warnings and potential side effects of the medicine.
- Take the medicine at the time of day your doctor tells you to.
- Do not drive or do other activities that require you to be alert and sober.
- Take only the amount of medicine prescribed by your doctor.
- Tell your doctor, nurse, or pharmacist about all other medicines you take, both over-the-counter (OTC) and prescription.
- Call your doctor or nurse right away if you have any problems while using the medicine.
- Do not drink alcohol.
- Do not take medicines that your doctor has not prescribed to you.
- Talk to your doctor or nurse if you want to stop using the sleep medicine and stop taking some sleep medicines gradually (a little at a time).

When taking sleep medicine, make sure to give yourself enough time to get a full night of sleep. A full night of sleep is usually at least seven hours. Ask your doctor or pharmacist to tell you about any side effects of taking sleep medicine, such as grogginess that may make it difficult to drive. Talk to your doctor or nurse if your insomnia symptoms continue longer than four weeks.

## CAN YOU TAKE AN OVER-THE-COUNTER MEDICINE FOR INSOMNIA?

Over-the-counter medicines, or sleep aids, may help some people with insomnia symptoms, but they are not meant for regular or long-term use. Many OTC sleep medicines contain antihistamines that are usually used to treat allergies.

If you decide to use an OTC sleep medicine, do the following:

- Ask your doctor, nurse, or pharmacist about any warnings and potential side effects of the medicine.
- Take the medicine at the time of day your doctor tells you to.
- Do not drive or do other activities that require you to be alert and sober.
- Take only the amount of medicine suggested by your doctor.
- Tell your doctor, nurse, or pharmacist about all other medicines you take, both OTC and prescription.
- Call your doctor or nurse right away if you have any problems while using the medicine.
- Do not drink alcohol.
- Do not use drugs that your doctor has not prescribed to you.

## CAN YOU TAKE A SUPPLEMENT OR NATURAL PRODUCT FOR INSOMNIA?

Some dietary supplements also claim to help people sleep. Manufacturers may label dietary supplements such as melatonin as "natural" products.

The U.S. Food and Drug Administration (FDA) does not regulate dietary supplements in the same way it regulates medicines. The FDA does not test supplements for safety or effectiveness (to see if the supplement is safe for humans and works in the way it is supposed to). The FDA can remove supplements from the market if they are found to be unsafe.

## DO COMPLEMENTARY OR ALTERNATIVE SLEEP AIDS WORK?

There is not enough scientific evidence to say whether most complementary and alternative sleep aids help treat insomnia.

- Certain relaxation techniques may be safe and effective in treating long-term insomnia. These techniques include using music, meditation, and yoga to relax the mind and body before sleeping.
- Some dietary supplements also claim to help people sleep. Manufacturers may label dietary supplements such as melatonin as a "natural" product. Most of these products have not been proven to help people with insomnia. Melatonin may be useful for treating short-term insomnia for shift workers or people who have jet lag, but you should probably not take it long-term.

The FDA does not regulate dietary supplements such as vitamins, minerals, and herbs in the same way it regulates medicines.

## WHY IS SLEEP IMPORTANT?

Sleep is essential for good health. During sleep, our bodies and brains repair themselves. Some research suggests our brains use the time during sleep to clear away toxins that build up during the day. Sleep is also important to our ability to learn and form memories. Not getting enough sleep puts people at risk for health problems, including high blood pressure, obesity, and depression.

## WHAT CAN YOU DO TO SLEEP BETTER?

It can be difficult to change everyday habits, but if you can stick with some of these changes, you might be able to improve your sleep. You may need to try these tips for several days in a row to improve sleep.

Try the following tips at home to improve sleep:

- Try to go to sleep at the same time each night or when you get sleepy.

## Treatment for Insomnia

- Try to get up at the same time each morning, regardless of how well you slept.
- Do not nap longer than 30 minutes or anytime between 3 p.m. and bedtime.
- Go outside every day for at least 15–20 minutes. The natural light will help you get into a natural pattern of sleeping.
- Before bedtime, try to avoid bright, artificial light from computer screens, mobile phones, or televisions. Do not allow electronic devices in the bedroom.
- Follow a regular, relaxing routine at the same time each night when you get ready for bed.
- Go to bed only after winding down and when you are ready to sleep. Do not read in bed, listen to music, or do other activities that engage your mind and can keep you awake.
- Keep your bedroom dark, quiet, and cool for sleeping. Use a sleep mask or light-blocking curtains. Use earplugs, a fan, or a white noise machine or app on your phone to block out sounds.
- Do not drink alcohol or caffeine or use nicotine for at least five hours before bedtime.
- Get regular physical activity during the daytime. Exercise or physical activity close to bedtime, or anytime in the five or six hours before sleeping, can make it harder to fall asleep.
- Do not eat heavy meals or drink a lot of liquids two to three hours before bed.
- If you still cannot sleep after about 15 minutes of getting into bed and turning out the light, get out of bed and do something relaxing until you feel sleepy.
- See your doctor or a sleep specialist if you think that you have insomnia or another sleep problem.[1]

---

[1] Office on Women's Health (OWH), "Insomnia," U.S. Department of Health and Human Services (HHS), February 22, 2021. Available online. URL: www.womenshealth.gov/a-z-topics/insomnia. Accessed May 2, 2023.

## Section 42.2 | Exploring Precision Medicine for Insomnia

Insomnia, the condition in which one has trouble falling or staying asleep, is one of the most prevalent health disorders in the United States but also one of the least understood. It is hard to pinpoint how many veterans have been diagnosed with the condition. But a large study of more than 900 former service members showed that at least 50 percent experienced major symptoms of insomnia.

Long-term insomnia is linked to a greater risk of poor health outcomes, including mental health disorders and heart disease. Symptoms of insomnia include daytime drowsiness, irritability, depression, or anxiety; attention deficits; trouble falling asleep; or an inability to sleep through the night.

Cognitive behavioral therapy I (CBT-I) is a six- to eight-session therapy that is aimed at changing sleep habits and scheduling factors, as well as misconceptions about sleep and insomnia that lead to sleep difficulties. Clinicians work one-on-one with patients to implement a series of strategies. These include finding the most suitable bedtime, restricting the amount of time spent in bed, and improving daytime habits.

Many cases of insomnia are related to poor sleep habits, depression, anxiety, lack of exercise, chronic illness, or certain drugs. The American College of Physicians recommends that behavioral programs, specifically CBT-I, because of their potential for limited side effects, be initiated prior to sleep medications.

## HOW DOES "PRECISION MEDICINE" COME INTO PLAY IN TREATING THIS CONDITION?

Precision medicine includes the choice of CBT-I versus medication. But it also involves examining whether changes to administering CBT-I may be warranted given a person's presentation, medical and mental health history, and environment. For example, people with bipolar disorder should avoid using strategies such as sleep restrictions. They would be de-emphasized in favor of something known to be highly important to bipolar disorder management, as well as sleep regulation, which is maintaining consistent daily routines. The manual for delivering CBT-I in the U.S. Department of Veterans Affairs (VA) uses a case conceptualization approach that focuses on delivering treatment according to the person's presentation and a clinical assessment of how insomnia developed, as opposed to delivering sessions in a fixed manner.

## HOW DOES A DOCTOR DECIDE WHETHER CBT-I OR MEDICATION IS THE BEST TARGETED TREATMENT METHOD FOR THE PATIENT? DOES THAT DECISION DEPEND ON THE PATIENT'S SYMPTOMS?

It is a mixture of research and clinical judgment. Based on research and recommendations by national physician groups, starting with CBT-I is the way to go. But there are things to factor into that decision, including whether the patient is a good candidate for the therapy, which, while effective, involves a lot of hard work and behavioral changes that not all people are willing or able to make. Symptoms also play a role and can help the provider know if the sleep disturbance is insomnia or is perhaps due to another sleep disorder. There are many ways in which someone can experience poor sleep, and not all of them are due to insomnia. Someone may complain of frequent awakenings in the middle of the night. But it is possible these could be due to untreated sleep apnea, a potentially serious sleep disorder in which breathing repeatedly starts and stops. In that case, a treatment program for insomnia would not be effective.

There is a growing consensus, including an official recommendation from the American Academy of Physicians (AAP), that behavioral approaches, specifically CBT-I, should be administered before sleep medications for treating insomnia. CBT-I is perhaps the most well-researched behavioral treatment for insomnia, with a high rate of efficacy. Some reports point to an 80 percent success rate. CBT-I may have short-term effects that are roughly equal to sleeping pills. However, the long-term effects tend to be superior, as sleep problems tend to return if a person stops taking a sleep aid. Add to that the risk of physical and psychological dependence on some sleep medications, and CBT-I becomes a more attractive option. CBT-I is not universally effective, however, so sleep medications may be a necessary treatment for some.

## WHAT ELSE IS IT ABOUT COGNITIVE BEHAVIORAL THERAPY THAT MAKES IT AN EFFECTIVE TREATMENT METHOD FOR INSOMNIA?

Cognitive behavioral therapy I is effective because it targets two key areas of sleep regulation thought to be disrupted in insomnia. The first target is a physical one, which is the body's homeostatic sleep drive. CBT-I works to strengthen and regularize the body's own biological drive for sleep through several behavioral strategies. The second is psychological and based on classical conditioning. When people experience night after night of poor sleep, they tend to form negative associations with their bed or their sleeping environment because they spend so much time in bed fighting for sleep. Those negative psychological associations can elicit a cascade of cognitive and physiological reactions that prevent a person from getting to sleep easily. CBT-I incorporates various strategies—collectively referred to as stimulus control—that are geared toward breaking those negative associations.

## HOW MUCH DOES STRESS PLAY A ROLE IN INSOMNIA?

Stress can play a significant role, especially if it comes along with a lot of worry. Nighttime is when most people are less distracted, and it can be a vulnerable time for succumbing to the kinds of thoughts or concerns that keep people up at night. Stress can also bring physical tension that can interfere with sleep. Managing stress effectively is not only good for your overall well-being, but it can help keep sleep disturbance from worsening.

## ARE THERE COMMON MISCONCEPTIONS OR MYTHS THAT PEOPLE HAVE ABOUT INSOMNIA? HOW TO DEAL WITH THEM?

Probably the most prevailing misconception is that if you are struggling to sleep, you just need to try harder! The reality is that the more effort you are putting into trying to force yourself to sleep, the less likely it is that you will get to sleep. You may be keeping your sleep problem going. Another myth is that we all need eight hours of sleep. Eight is a good number but not the perfect one for everyone. The National Sleep Foundation suggests a range of seven to nine hours. If you are only getting seven or so hours of sleep per night, it does not necessarily mean you have a sleep problem if you otherwise feel good about how you are functioning during the day. There are no guidelines on the time someone should go to bed. That depends on a lot of individual factors, including one's internal "biological clock." We try not to focus on specific times or numbers.

## MANY PEOPLE WITH SLEEP PROBLEMS HAVE TURNED TO ALTERNATIVE THERAPIES, SUCH AS ACUPUNCTURE, YOGA, RELAXATION, MELATONIN, AND HERBAL REMEDIES SUCH AS VALERIAN AND CHAMOMILE. WHAT DOES THE EVIDENCE SHOW ABOUT THESE THERAPIES?

The recently established VA/U.S. Department of Defense (DOD) Clinical Practice Guidelines for managing chronic insomnia and obstructive sleep apnea (OSA) have done an excellent job of examining the evidence for or against alternative methods and synthesizing that evidence to help guide clinical decision-making. For chronic insomnia, the guidelines suggest against using herbal remedies, such as valerian root or chamomile, and against taking melatonin. There is not enough evidence for or against other strategies, such as mindfulness, meditation, or yoga, to make a recommendation. However, a specific kind of acupuncture—auricular acupuncture with seed or pellet attachments—is recommended as an alternative treatment for insomnia. Auricular acupuncture can produce a range of benefits, such as calming the mind and relieving pain.[2]

---

[2] "Exploring Precision Medicine for Insomnia," U.S. Department of Veterans Affairs (VA), April 23, 2020. Available online. URL: www.research.va.gov/currents/0420-Exploring-precision-medicine-for-insomnia.cfm. Accessed May 2, 2023.

## Section 42.3 | Taking Z-Drugs for Insomnia? Know the Risks

If you are lying awake night after night, unable to sleep, you may want to talk to your health-care provider about it. She or he may prescribe insomnia medicines, such as eszopiclone (Lunesta), zaleplon (Sonata), and zolpidem (Ambien, Ambien CR, Edluar, and Zolpimist)—sometimes known as "Z-drugs"—to help you get a good night's sleep. But, as with any medication, there are risks.

Prescription-only "Z-drugs" work by slowing activity in the brain. Used properly, they can help you sleep. Quality sleep can have a positive impact on physical and mental health. But the treatments also carry the risk—though rare—of serious injuries and even death.

The U.S. Food and Drug Administration (FDA) wants you and your health-care provider to be fully aware of these risks, so the agency requires the addition of a new boxed warning—the FDA's most prominent warning—to the prescribing information, known as "labeling," and patient medication guides. In addition, the FDA is adding a contraindication, which is the agency's strongest warning, stating that patients who have experienced an episode of what is known as "complex sleep behavior" should not take these drugs.

## WHAT ARE COMPLEX SLEEP BEHAVIORS?

Complex sleep behaviors occur while you are asleep or not fully awake. Examples include sleepwalking, sleep driving, sleep cooking, or taking other medicines. The FDA has received reports of people taking these insomnia medicines and accidentally overdosing, falling, being burned, shooting themselves, and wandering outside in extremely cold weather, among other incidents. Since Ambien was approved in 1992, the FDA has identified 66 serious cases of complex sleep behaviors after a person has taken a Z-drug, 20 of which resulted in death.

Considering the large number of individuals who take the drugs, the FDA wants people to be aware of the potential dangers that can occur as a result. Patients may not remember these behaviors when they wake up the next morning. Moreover, they may experience these types of behaviors after their first dose of one of these Z-drugs or after continued use.

## YOUR HEALTH-CARE PROVIDER HAS PRESCRIBED A Z-DRUG FOR YOU: WHAT SHOULD YOU DO?

If your health-care provider prescribes a Z-drug to help you sleep, here are some things to keep in mind:

- Talk with your health-care provider about all of the benefits and risks of taking this medicine.
- Read the patient medication guide as soon as you get the prescription filled and before you start taking the medicine. If you have any questions or if there is anything you do not understand, ask your prescriber.
- If, after taking the medication, you experience a complex sleep behavior in which you engage in activities while not fully awake or take actions that you do not remember, stop taking the drug and contact your prescriber immediately.
- These events can occur on the first night you use these medicines or after a much longer period of treatment.
- Complex sleep behaviors can occur at lower dosages, as well as high dosages. It is important to carefully follow the dosing instructions in the patient medication guide.
- Do not take these medicines with any other sleep medicines, including those you can buy over-the-counter (OTC) without a prescription.
- Do not drink alcohol before or while taking these medicines. Together, they may be more likely to cause side effects.
- You may still feel drowsy the day after taking one of these drugs. Keep in mind that all medicines taken for insomnia can impair your ability to drive and activities that require alertness the morning after use.[3]

---

[3] "Taking Z-Drugs for Insomnia? Know the Risks," U.S. Food and Drug Administration (FDA), April 30, 2019. Available online. URL: www.fda.gov/consumers/consumer-updates/taking-z-drugs-insomnia-know-risks. Accessed May 1, 2023.

## Section 42.4 | Risk of Next-Morning Impairment after Use of Zolpidem and Other Insomnia Drugs

The U.S. Food and Drug Administration (FDA) is notifying the public of new information about zolpidem, a widely prescribed insomnia drug. The FDA recommends that the bedtime dose be lowered because new data show that blood levels in some patients may be high enough the morning after use to impair activities that require alertness, including driving. This announcement focused on zolpidem products approved for bedtime use, which are marketed as generics and under the brand names "Ambien," "Ambien CR," "Edluar," and "Zolpimist."

The FDA is also reminding the public that all drugs taken for insomnia can impair driving and activities that require alertness the morning after use. Drowsiness is already listed as a common side effect on the drug labels of all insomnia drugs, along with warnings that patients may still feel drowsy the day after taking these products. Patients who take insomnia drugs can experience an impairment of mental alertness the morning after use, even if they feel fully awake.

The FDA urges health-care professionals to caution all patients who use these zolpidem products about the risks of next-morning impairment for activities that require complete mental alertness. For zolpidem products, data show the risk for next-morning impairment is highest for patients taking the extended-release forms of these drugs (Ambien CR and generics). Women appear to be more susceptible to this risk because they eliminate zolpidem from their bodies more slowly than men.

Because the use of lower doses of zolpidem will result in lower blood levels in the morning, the FDA is requiring the manufacturers of Ambien, Ambien CR, Edluar, and Zolpimist to lower the recommended dose. The FDA has informed the manufacturers that the recommended dose of zolpidem for women should be lowered from 10 to 5 mg for immediate-release products (Ambien, Edluar, and Zolpimist) and from 12.5 to 6.25 mg for extended-release products (Ambien CR). The FDA also informed the manufacturers that for men, the labeling should recommend that health-care professionals consider prescribing the lower doses: 5 mg for immediate-release products and 6.25 mg for extended-release products.

## WHAT IS ZOLPIDEM?

Zolpidem is a sedative-hypnotic (sleep) medicine that is used in adults for the treatment of insomnia. Zolpidem is available as an oral tablet (Ambien and generics), an extended-release tablet (Ambien CR and generics), a sublingual (under-the-tongue) tablet (Edluar), and an oral spray (Zolpimist).

Zolpidem is also available under the brand name "Intermezzo," a lower dose sublingual tablet that is approved for use as needed for the treatment of insomnia when a middle-of-the-night awakening is followed by difficulty returning to sleep.

## WHY DOES THE FDA REQUIRE THE MANUFACTURERS OF CERTAIN ZOLPIDEM-CONTAINING PRODUCTS TO REVISE THE LABELING TO LOWER THE RECOMMENDED DOSE OF ZOLPIDEM FOR WOMEN AND TO RECOMMEND CONSIDERATION OF THE LOWER DOSE IN MEN?

The FDA is requiring the manufacturers of certain zolpidem-containing products to revise the labeling to lower the recommended dose of zolpidem-containing medicines for women and to recommend that health-care professionals consider prescribing the lower dose for men because next-morning blood levels of zolpidem may be high enough to impair activities that require alertness. Patients with high levels of zolpidem can be impaired even if they feel fully awake. Zolpidem is eliminated from the body more slowly in women, so the drug can stay in their systems longer than it does in men.

## WHAT SHOULD PATIENTS TAKING THE 10 OR 12.5 MG DOSE OF ZOLPIDEM-CONTAINING INSOMNIA MEDICINES DO NOW?

If you are taking the 10 or 12.5 mg dose of zolpidem-containing insomnia medicine, continue taking your prescribed dose as directed until you have contacted your health-care professional to ask for instructions on how to safely continue to take your medicine. Each patient and situation is unique, and the appropriate dose should be discussed with your health-care professional.

## WILL A LOWER DOSE OF ZOLPIDEM BE EFFECTIVE IN TREATING INSOMNIA?

The FDA has informed the manufacturers that the recommended dose of zolpidem for women should be lowered from 10 to 5 mg for immediate-release products (Ambien, Edluar, and Zolpimist) and from 12.5 to 6.25 mg for extended-release products (Ambien CR). For men, the FDA has informed the manufacturers that the labeling should recommend that health-care professionals consider prescribing these lower doses. These lower doses of zolpidem (5 mg for immediate-release products and 6.25 mg for extended-release products) will be effective in most women and many men.

## DOES THE FDA REQUIRE THE MANUFACTURER OF INTERMEZZO (ZOLPIDEM TARTRATE) SUBLINGUAL TABLETS TO ALSO CHANGE THE DOSING RECOMMENDATIONS?

No. When Intermezzo was FDA-approved in November 2011, the label already recommended a lower dosage in women compared to men. The recommended and maximum dose of Intermezzo is 1.75 mg for women and 3.5 mg for men, taken only once per night as needed if a middle-of-the-night awakening is followed by difficulty returning to sleep.

## DO ANY OTHER FACTORS, SUCH AS A PATIENT'S AGE, WEIGHT, OR ETHNICITY, HAVE AN EFFECT ON ZOLPIDEM LEVELS?

Based on data from pharmacokinetic trials, no relationship was evident between the zolpidem blood level and patients' body weight or ethnicity. In elderly patients, zolpidem blood levels can be higher, and lower doses are already recommended. In contrast to younger patients, zolpidem blood levels in elderly patients are not affected by sex.

## WHY IS THE FDA INFORMING THE PUBLIC ABOUT THIS SAFETY RISK NOW, AFTER ZOLPIDEM HAS BEEN ON THE MARKET FOR NEARLY 20 YEARS?

Since the approval of zolpidem, the FDA has been continually monitoring the drug's safety profile. As more data became available, the FDA continued to assess the benefits and risks of zolpidem treatment. Over the years, the FDA has received reports of possible driving impairment and motor vehicle accidents associated with zolpidem; however, in most cases, it was difficult to determine if the driving impairment was related to zolpidem or to specific zolpidem blood levels because information about the time of dosing and the time of the impairment was often not reported. Data from clinical trials and driving simulation studies have become available that allowed the FDA to better characterize the risk of driving impairment caused by specific blood levels of zolpidem and to recognize the increased risk of driving-impairing blood levels of zolpidem in women. This led the FDA to require the manufacturers of certain zolpidem-containing products to revise the dosing recommendations.

## IS NEXT-MORNING IMPAIRMENT THE SAME AS COMPLEX SLEEP-RELATED BEHAVIORS?

No, they are different. Next-morning impairment occurs when patients are awake the next morning, but levels of the insomnia medicine in their blood remain high enough to impair activities that require alertness. Complex sleep-related behaviors occur when patients get out of bed while not fully awake and sleepwalk or do an activity, such as driving a car, preparing and eating food, making phone calls, or having sex. Both problems are made worse by high levels of zolpidem.

## IS THE FDA REQUIRING THE MANUFACTURERS OF OTHER INSOMNIA MEDICINES TO REVISE THEIR DOSING RECOMMENDATIONS?

No. At this time, the FDA is only requiring the manufacturers of certain zolpidem-containing products to revise their dosing recommendations. The FDA is continuing to evaluate ways to lower the risk of next-morning impairment with other insomnia medicines.

## DO OTHER INSOMNIA MEDICINES HAVE THE SAME GENDER EFFECT AS ZOLPIDEM?

The FDA is evaluating other insomnia medicines to determine if they affect women and men differently.

## DO OVER-THE-COUNTER INSOMNIA MEDICINES THAT ARE AVAILABLE WITHOUT A PRESCRIPTION HAVE A RISK OF NEXT-MORNING IMPAIRMENT?

Yes. Over-the-counter (OTC) insomnia medicines also have a risk for next-morning impairment. The FDA is not recommending that patients who are taking prescription insomnia medicines switch to OTC insomnia medicines.

Patients who drive or perform activities that require full alertness the next morning should discuss with their health-care professional if the insomnia medicine they are using is right for them.

## WHAT CAN PATIENTS DO TO DECREASE THEIR RISK OF NEXT-MORNING IMPAIRMENT WITH INSOMNIA MEDICINES?

Patients can decrease their risk of next-morning impairment by taking the lowest dose of their insomnia medicine that treats their symptoms. It is important for patients to take their insomnia medicine exactly as prescribed. Taking a higher dose than prescribed or using more than one insomnia medicine is dangerous if patients drive or perform activities that require full alertness the next morning, even if the drugs are taken at the beginning of the night. In addition, patients should not take insomnia medicine intended for bedtime use if less than a full night's sleep (seven to eight hours) remains. Likewise, patients should not take Intermezzo, a zolpidem product that is approved for use in the middle of the night, if less than four hours of sleep remain.

## HOW MANY REPORTS OF ZOLPIDEM AND IMPAIRED DRIVING HAS THE FDA RECEIVED? WERE THESE REPORTS USED AS EVIDENCE TO SUPPORT THE PROPOSED NEW DOSING RECOMMENDATIONS FOR CERTAIN ZOLPIDEM-CONTAINING PRODUCTS?

The FDA has received about 700 reports of zolpidem and "impaired driving ability and/or road traffic accident." Following a zolpidem label change in 2007, which added information to the warnings and precautions section of the label about complex sleep-related behaviors, including sleep-driving (patients getting out of bed while not fully awake and driving), there was a great deal of media attention. Since such publicity tends to "stimulate" reporting, this led to a considerable number of reports of zolpidem and impaired driving that were submitted to the FDA's Adverse Event Reporting System (AERS) database.

However, while the adverse event reporting system reports generally can be helpful in evaluating safety concerns, these AERS reports for zolpidem lacked the information necessary to understand whether high morning blood levels of zolpidem were the cause of the reported impaired driving. Specifically, these reports often did not include the dose or time zolpidem was taken, the time of the accident, whether alcohol or other drugs were also taken, and whether and when blood levels of the drug were measured. It was not until the FDA received the new data on next-day blood levels and driving simulation studies that the apparent frequency of next-morning mental impairment was better identified.[4]

---

[4] "Questions and Answers: Risk of Next-Morning Impairment after Use of Insomnia Drugs; FDA Requires Lower Recommended Doses for Certain Drugs Containing Zolpidem (Ambien, Ambien CR, Edluar, and Zolpimist)," U.S. Food and Drug Administration (FDA), February 13, 2018. Available online. URL: www.fda.gov/drugs/drug-safety-and-avail-ability/questions-and-answers-risk-next-morning-impairment-after-use-insomnia-drugs-fda-requires-lower#q1. Accessed May 1, 2023.

# Chapter 43 | **Sleep Medication**

## **Chapter Contents**

## Section 43.1 | Prescription Sleep Aid Use among Adults

Sleep medications are a common treatment option for insomnia. Insufficient sleep is associated with many negative mental and physical health outcomes, including type 2 diabetes, heart disease, obesity, depression, and an increased risk of injury. The prevalence of sleep difficulties and the use of sleep medication has differed between women and men. This section uses 2020 National Health Interview Survey (NHIS) data to describe the percentage of women and men who used medication for sleep, defined here as taking any medication to help fall or stay asleep most days or every day in the past 30 days, by selected sociodemographic characteristics.

### OVERALL, WHAT PERCENTAGE OF ADULTS TOOK MEDICATION TO HELP THEM FALL OR STAY ASLEEP IN THE PAST 30 DAYS?

- In 2020, 6.3 percent of adults took sleep medication every day in the past 30 days; 2.1 percent took medication most days; 10.0 percent took medication some days; and 81.6 percent never took medication.

Figure 43.1 shows the percent distribution of how often adults aged 18 and over used medication in the past 30 days to help them fall or stay asleep in the United States in 2020.

### DID THE PERCENTAGE OF ADULTS WHO TOOK SLEEP MEDICATION VARY BY SEX AND AGE GROUP?

- In 2020, the percentage of adults who took medication for sleep increased with age, from 5.6 percent of those aged 18–44 to 10.1 percent of those aged 45–64 and 11.9 percent of those aged 65 and over.
- Among men, the percentage who took medication for sleep also increased with increasing age, from 4.7 percent of men aged 18–44 to 7.1 percent of men aged 45–64 and 10.1 percent of men aged 65 and over. Among women, sleep medication use was less likely among those aged

18–44 (6.5%) than those aged 45–64 (13.0%) and those aged 65 and over (13.5%).

- Men were less likely to take medication for sleep than women across all age groups.

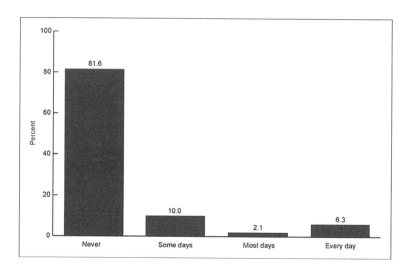

**Figure 43.1.** Percentage Distribution of How Often Adults Aged 18 and Over Used Medication in the Past 30 Days to Help Them Fall or Stay Asleep: United States, 2020

*Centers for Disease Control and Prevention (CDC)*
*Note: Use of medication for sleep frequency is based on a response to the question, "During the past 30 days, how often did you take any medication to help you fall asleep or stay asleep? Would you say never, some days, most days, or every day?" Estimates are based on household interviews with a sample of the civilian noninstitutionalized population.*

## WERE DIFFERENCES OBSERVED IN THE PERCENTAGE OF ADULTS WHO TOOK SLEEP MEDICATION BY SEX AND RACE AND HISPANIC ORIGIN?

- The percentage of adults who took medication for sleep every day or most days was highest among non-Hispanic White adults (10.4%), followed by non-Hispanic Black (6.1%) and Hispanic (4.6%) adults, and lowest among non-Hispanic Asian adults (2.8%).

- Among men, non-Hispanic White men (8.0%) were most likely to use sleep medication, and non-Hispanic Asian men (1.7%) were least likely.
- Non-Hispanic White women (12.6%) were most likely to take sleep medication, and Hispanic women (5.4%) and non-Hispanic Asian women (3.9%) were least likely.
- Across all race and Hispanic-origin groups, men were less likely than women to take sleep medication.

## WERE DIFFERENCES OBSERVED IN THE PERCENTAGE OF ADULTS WHO TOOK SLEEP MEDICATION BY SEX AND FAMILY INCOME?

- Sleep medication use decreased with increasing family income, from 10.0 percent among adults with family income less than 100 percent of the federal poverty level (FPL) to 8.7 percent of those with family income at 100 percent to less than 200 percent of FPL and 8.2 percent of those with family income at 200 percent of FPL or more.
- Among men, those with a family income of 200 percent of FPL or more (6.0%) were less likely to take sleep medication than those with a family income of less than 100 percent of FPL (8.3%) and 100 percent to less than 200 percent of FPL (8.2%).
- Among women, the observed differences in the use of sleep medication among those with family incomes less than 100 percent of FPL (11.1%), those at 100 percent to less than 200 percent of FPL (9.2%), and those at 200 percent FPL or more (10.3%) were not significant.
- Among adults with a family income of less than 100 percent of FPL and those with a family income of 200 percent of FPL or more, men were less likely to take medication for sleep than women.

Figure 43.2 shows the percentage of adults aged 18 and over who took sleep medication every day or most days in the past 30 days to help them fall or stay asleep by sex and family income in the United States in 2020.

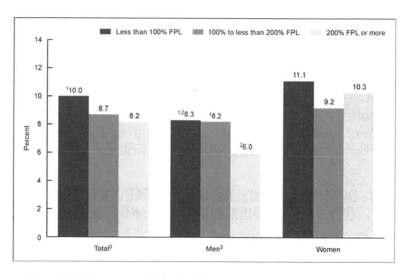

**Figure 43.2.** Percentage of Adults Aged 18 and Over Who Took Sleep Medication Every Day or Most Days in the Past 30 Days to Help Them Fall or Stay Asleep, by Sex and Family Income: United States, 2020

*Centers for Disease Control and Prevention (CDC)*
*Note: Use of medication for sleep frequency is based on a response to the question, "During the past 30 days, how often did you take any medication to help you fall asleep or stay asleep? Would you say never, some days, most days, or every day?" Estimates are based on household interviews of a sample of the civilian noninstitutionalized population.*

## SUMMARY

In 2020, 8.4 percent of adults used sleep medication every day or most days in the past 30 days to help them fall or stay asleep. In general, a greater percentage of women used sleep medication compared with men across the lifespan, races and Hispanic-origin groups, and family-income groups. Among all adults, sleep medication use increased with increasing age, decreased with increasing income, and was higher among non-Hispanic White adults compared with adults of other races and Hispanic-origin groups. Some variation was observed in the patterns between men and women. Among men, the likelihood of using sleep medication increased with increasing age, while among women, the likelihood of taking sleep medication was the same for those aged 45–64 and those aged 65 and over. Hispanic men were more likely than non-Hispanic

Asian men to take sleep medication, while among women, these groups were not different. Among men, those with family income at or above 200 percent of FPL were less likely to take sleep medication, while among women, no differences were observed across family income levels.

## DATA SOURCE AND METHODS

The NHIS is a nationally representative household survey of the civilian noninstitutionalized population. It is conducted continuously throughout the year by the National Center for Health Statistics (NCHS). Interviews are typically conducted in respondents' homes, but follow-ups to complete interviews may be conducted over the telephone. Due to the COVID-19 pandemic, data collection procedures in 2020 were disrupted. From April through June 2020, all interviews were conducted by telephone only, and from July through December 2020, interviews were attempted by telephone first, with follow-ups to complete interviews by personal visit. Questions on sleep, including the use of medication for sleep, are on the NHIS rotating core and were most recently asked in 2020.

Point estimates and corresponding variances for this analysis were calculated using SAS-callable SUDAAN software version 11.0 to account for the complex sample design of the NHIS. All estimates are based on self-report and meet NCHS data presentation standards for proportions. Differences between percentages were evaluated using two-sided significance tests at the 0.05 level. Linear and quadratic trends by age group and family income were evaluated using orthogonal polynomials in logistic regression.[1]

---

[1] "Sleep Medication Use in Adults Aged 18 and Over: United States, 2020," Centers for Disease Control and Prevention (CDC), January 25, 2023. Available online. URL: www.cdc.gov/nchs/products/databriefs/db462.htm. Accessed May 1, 2023.

## Section 43.2 | **Medicines to Help You Sleep**

Most adults need seven to eight hours of sleep each night. Not everyone gets the sleep they need. Once in a while, you may have trouble sleeping due to:

- stress
- health problems and medicines
- long work hours/shift work
- light or noise
- drinking alcohol or eating too close to bedtime

If you have trouble falling asleep or staying asleep most nights, you may have a sleep problem called "insomnia."

Some people have more serious sleep problems. Talk to your doctor if you:

- fall asleep during the day
- snore or make choking sounds in your sleep
- have odd feelings in your legs or feel like you need to move your legs

## MEDICINES TO HELP YOU SLEEP

There are medicines that may help you fall asleep or stay asleep. You need a doctor's prescription for some sleep drugs. You can get other over-the-counter (OTC) medicines without a prescription.

## Prescription

Prescription sleep medicines work well for many people, but they can cause serious side effects.

- Talk to your doctor about all the risks and benefits of using prescription sleep medicines.
- Sleep drugs taken for insomnia can affect your driving the morning after use.
- Sleep drugs can cause rare side effects such as:
  - severe allergic reactions
  - severe face swelling
  - behaviors such as making phone calls, eating, having sex, or driving while you are not fully awake

## Over-the-Counter
OTC sleep drugs have side effects, too.

## TIPS FOR BETTER SLEEP
Making some changes to your nighttime habits may help you get the sleep you need.
- Go to bed and get up at the same time each day.
- Sleep in a dark, quiet room.
- Avoid caffeine and nicotine.
- Do not drink alcohol before bedtime.
- Do something to help you relax before bedtime.
- Do not exercise before bedtime.
- Do not take a nap after 3 p.m.
- Do not eat a large meal before you go to sleep.

Talk to your health-care provider if you have trouble sleeping almost every night for more than two weeks.[2]

## PRESCRIPTION INSOMNIA DRUGS
- Ambien (zolpidem)
- Belsomra (suvorexant)
- Butisol (butabarbital)
- Doral (quazepam)
- Edluar (zolpidem)
- Estazolam
- Flurazepam
- Halcion (triazolam)
- Hetlioz (tasimelteon)
- Intermezzo (zolpidem)
- Lunesta (eszopiclone)
- Restoril (temazepam)
- Rozerem (ramelteon)

---

[2] "Sleep Problems," U.S. Food and Drug Administration (FDA), April 12, 2019. Available online. URL: www.fda.gov/consumers/free-publications-women/sleep-problems. Accessed May 3, 2023.

- Seconal (secobarbital)
- Silenor (doxepin)
- Sonata (zaleplon)
- Zolpimist (zolpidem)

## OVER-THE-COUNTER INSOMNIA DRUGS
- Benadryl (diphenhydramine)*
- Unisom (doxylamine)*

*Also, in many cold and headache combination products*[3]

## Section 43.3 | Harmful Effects of Central Nervous System Depressants

## WHAT ARE CENTRAL NERVOUS SYSTEM DEPRESSANTS?

Central nervous system (CNS) depressants, a category that includes tranquilizers, sedatives, and hypnotics, are substances that can slow brain activity. This property makes them useful for treating anxiety and sleep disorders. The following are among the medications commonly prescribed for these purposes:
- Benzodiazepines, such as diazepam, clonazepam, and alprazolam, are sometimes prescribed to treat anxiety, acute stress reactions, and panic attacks. Clonazepam may also be prescribed to treat seizure disorders and insomnia. The more sedating benzodiazepines, such as triazolam and estazolam, are prescribed for short-term treatment of sleep disorders. Usually, benzodiazepines are not prescribed for long-term use because of the high risk of developing tolerance, dependence, or addiction.

[3] "Sleep Disorder (Sedative-Hypnotic) Drug Information," U.S. Food and Drug Administration (FDA), April 30, 2019. Available online. URL: www.fda.gov/drugs/postmarket-drug-safety-information-patients-and-providers/sleep-disorder-sedative-hypnotic-drug-information. Accessed May 3, 2023.

- Nonbenzodiazepine sleep medications, such as zolpidem, eszopiclone, and zaleplon, known as "Z-drugs," have a different chemical structure but act on the same GABA type A receptors in the brain as benzodiazepines. They are thought to have fewer side effects and less risk of dependence than benzodiazepines.
- Barbiturates, such as mephobarbital, phenobarbital, and pentobarbital sodium, are used less frequently to reduce anxiety or to help with sleep problems because of their higher risk of overdose compared to benzodiazepines. However, they are still used in surgical procedures and to treat seizure disorders.

## HOW DO CENTRAL NERVOUS SYSTEM DEPRESSANTS AFFECT THE BRAIN AND BODY?

Most CNS depressants act on the brain by increasing activity at receptors for the inhibitory neurotransmitter gamma-aminobutyric acid (GABA). Although the different classes of CNS depressants work in unique ways, it is through their ability to increase GABA signaling—thereby increasing inhibition of brain activity—that they produce a drowsy or calming effect that is medically beneficial to those suffering from anxiety or sleep disorders.

## WHAT ARE THE POSSIBLE CONSEQUENCES OF CENTRAL NERVOUS SYSTEM DEPRESSANT MISUSE?

Despite their beneficial therapeutic effects, benzodiazepines and barbiturates have the potential for misuse and should be used only as prescribed. The use of nonbenzodiazepine sleep aids, or z-drugs, is less well-studied, but certain indicators have raised concerns about their misuse potential as well.

During the first few days of taking a depressant, a person usually feels sleepy and uncoordinated, but as the body becomes accustomed to the effects of the drug and tolerance develops, these side effects begin to disappear. If one uses these drugs long-term, he or she may need larger doses to achieve the therapeutic effects. Continued use can also lead to dependence and withdrawal when use is abruptly reduced or stopped. Because CNS depressants work by slowing the brain's activity, when an individual stops taking them, there can be a rebound effect, resulting in seizures or other harmful consequences.

Although withdrawal from benzodiazepines can be problematic, it is rarely life-threatening, whereas withdrawal from prolonged use of barbiturates can have life-threatening complications. Therefore, someone who is thinking about discontinuing a CNS depressant or who is suffering withdrawal after discontinuing use should speak with a physician or seek immediate medical treatment.

## WHAT ARE STIMULANTS?

Stimulants increase alertness, attention, and energy, as well as elevate blood pressure, heart rate, and respiration. Historically, stimulants were used to treat asthma and other respiratory problems, obesity, neurological disorders, and a variety of other ailments. But, as their potential for misuse and addiction became apparent, the number of conditions treated with stimulants has decreased. Now stimulants are prescribed for the treatment of only a few health conditions, including attention deficit hyperactivity disorder (ADHD), narcolepsy, and occasionally treatment-resistant depression.

## HOW DO STIMULANTS AFFECT THE BRAIN AND BODY?

Stimulants, such as dextroamphetamine and methylphenidate, act in the brain on the family of monoamine neurotransmitter systems, which include norepinephrine and dopamine. Stimulants enhance the effects of these chemicals. An increase in dopamine signaling from nonmedical use of stimulants can induce a feeling of euphoria, and these medications' effects on norepinephrine increase blood pressure and heart rate, constrict blood vessels, increase blood glucose, and open up breathing passages.

## WHAT ARE THE POSSIBLE CONSEQUENCES OF STIMULANT MISUSE?

As with other drugs in the stimulant category, such as cocaine, it is possible for people to become dependent on or addicted to prescription stimulants. Withdrawal symptoms associated with discontinuing stimulant use include fatigue, depression, and disturbed sleep patterns. Repeated misuse of some stimulants (sometimes within a short period) can lead to feelings of hostility or paranoia, or even psychosis. Furthermore, taking high doses of a stimulant may result in dangerously high body temperature and an irregular heartbeat. There is also the potential for cardiovascular failure or seizures.

## COGNITIVE ENHANCERS

The dramatic increases in stimulant prescriptions over the past two decades have led to their greater availability and to increased risk for diversion and nonmedical use. When taken to improve properly diagnosed conditions, these medications can greatly enhance a patient's quality of life. However, because many perceive them to be generally safe and effective, prescription stimulants are being misused more frequently.

Stimulants increase wakefulness, motivation, and aspects of cognition, learning, and memory. Some people take these drugs in the absence of medical need in an effort to enhance mental performance. Militaries have long used stimulants to increase performance in the face of fatigue, and the U.S. Armed Forces allow for their use in limited operational settings. The practice is now reported by some professionals to increase their productivity, by older people to offset declining cognition, and by both high school and college students to improve their academic performance.

Nonmedical use of stimulants for cognitive enhancement poses potential health risks, including addiction, cardiovascular events, and psychosis. The use of pharmaceuticals for cognitive enhancement has also sparked debate over the ethical implications of the practice. Issues of fairness arise if those with access and willingness to take these drugs have a performance edge over others, and implicit coercion takes place if a culture of cognitive enhancement gives the impression that a person must take drugs in order to be competitive.[4]

---

[4] "What Classes of Prescription Drugs Are Commonly Misused?" National Institutes of Health (NIH), June 2020. Available online. URL: https://nida.nih.gov/publications/research-reports/misuse-prescription-drugs/what-classes-prescription-drugs-are-commonly-misused. Accessed May 3, 2023.

# Chapter 44 | Other Factors That Can Improve Sleep

**Chapter Contents**

.

## Section 44.1 | Bedding and Sleep Environment

Although sleep is vital to emotional and physical health, millions of people do not get the recommended eight hours of sleep per night. Some have chronic, long-term sleep disorders, while others experience occasional trouble sleeping. Sleep deprivation can lead to daytime drowsiness, poor concentration, stress, irritability, and a weakened immune system. Among the many factors that can impact the amount and quality of sleep, bedding and the sleep environment are perhaps the easiest to control or change. Choosing a high-quality mattress, selecting the right pillow, creating a comfortable, and inviting sleep sanctuary can help people improve their sleep, as well as their overall quality of life.

Environmental factors—such as light, noise, temperature, color, accessories, and bedding—play an important role in the sleep experience. Choosing comfortable bedding, making sure the bedroom temperature is neither too hot nor too cold, and eliminating sources of distracting noise or light can make a big difference in helping people get a good night's sleep. The goal is to turn the bedroom into a soothing, relaxing, indulgent escape from the everyday pressures and hassles of life. Inviting colors and attractive accessories are available from many sources to fit any space or budget.

## CHOOSING A MATTRESS

The centerpiece of any bedroom, and the most important aspect of ensuring a comfortable, high-quality night's sleep, is the mattress. Mattresses generally have a lifespan of five to seven years, depending on usage, before the comfort and support they offer begin to decline. At this point, experts recommend evaluating the mattress and comparing it to newer models. A mattress is likely to need replacing if it shows signs of wear, such as sagging, lumps, or exposed springs. A new mattress may also be warranted if users tend to sleep better elsewhere or frequently wake up with numbness, stiffness, or pain. Research has shown that 70 percent of people report significant improvements in sleep comfort, 62 percent report improvements in sleep quality, and more than 50 percent report reductions in back pain and spine stiffness when sleeping on a new mattress rather than one that is five years old.

The search for a new mattress begins at a reputable mattress store with educated salespeople who can explain the various options and guide customers through the purchasing process. Since quality mattresses are major expenditures, it is important for customers to test different types and models to find the one that best meets their personal needs. Testing a mattress involves lying down for several minutes in various sleep positions while concentrating on the feel of each surface.

The main qualities to look for in a new mattress include comfort, support, durability, and size. Many types of cushioning materials are available to create a soft, plush feel. Beneath the surface, the mattress and foundation should provide gentle support that keeps the spine in alignment. The quality of materials and construction determine the durability of the mattress. The main mattress sizes, from smallest to largest, are as follows:

- twin (38" X 75")
- full or double (53" X 75")
- queen (60" X 80")
- California king (72" X 84")
- king (76" X 80")

Since twin- and full-sized mattresses are only 75" long, they may be too short to accommodate taller adults. If two people are sharing a bed, experts recommend buying a queen-sized or larger mattress. King-sized mattresses provide maximum sleeping space. Since an average person shifts position between 40 and 60 times per night, many people feel that a larger mattress provides them with greater freedom to move around comfortably.

The following are a few different types of mattresses to choose from:

- innerspring, which features tempered steel coils for support beneath layers of insulation and cushioning for comfort
- foam, which can be made of solid foam or layers of different kinds of foam, including viscoelastic "memory" foam that molds to individual sleepers

- airbeds, which feature an air-filled core rather than springs for support and are usually adjustable to fit sleepers' preferences
- waterbeds, which feature a water-filled core for support beneath layers of upholstery for comfort and insulation
- adjustable beds, which feature an electric motor to allow sleepers to change the position of the head and foot of the bed to increase comfort
- futons, which offer a space-saving alternative by converting into a sofa during the day

## CARING FOR A MATTRESS

After purchasing a new mattress, proper care is key to getting the most out of the investment. The first step is to ensure that the mattress and foundation are properly installed. If they have a slight "new product" odor, proper ventilation should solve the problem within a few hours. Although it is not illegal to remove the tag, it is best to leave it attached to the mattress in case it is required for a warranty claim.

Sleep sets retain their comfort and support longer if they are placed on a sturdy, high-quality bed frame. Boards should never be placed beneath the mattress to increase support. Instead, the mattress should be replaced when it reaches that stage. To keep the mattress fresh and prevent stains, it is important to use a washable mattress pad. If the mattress should require cleaning, the recommended methods are vacuuming or spot cleaning with mild soap and cold water. Mattresses should never be dry-cleaned, which can damage the material, or soaked with water.

Basic mattress care involves not allowing children to jump on the bed, which can damage its interior construction. In addition, periodically rotating the mattress from top to bottom and end to end will help extend its useful life. For other issues, it is best to follow the manufacturer's guidelines.

## CHOOSING A PILLOW

Pillows, like mattresses, need to be replaced periodically to ensure that they provide adequate support and comfort. The useful life of a pillow depends on its quality and the amount of use it receives. Most pillows should be replaced on an annual basis. A pillow generally must be replaced when it becomes lumpy or shows signs of dirt, stains, or wear and tear. An easy test to see whether a pillow has lost its capacity to support the head involves folding it in half and squeezing the air out. If it springs back to its original shape quickly, it still retains its support. If not, it may be time to buy a new pillow.

Ideally, a pillow should support the head in the same position as if the person were standing with an upright posture. Different amounts of cushioning are available for different sleeping positions. People who sleep on their side may want a firm pillow, while people who sleep on their back may want a somewhat softer pillow. A wide variety of pillows are available to fit any budget. Some of the different types of pillows include feather, down, memory foam, microbead, neck, lumbar, body, and wedge. Special pillows are also available for people who are pregnant or have sleep apnea.

### References

"The Better Sleep Guide," Better Sleep Council, May 15, 2007. Available online. URL: www.bettersleep.org/pdfs/ BetterSleepGuide_English.pdf. Accessed May 4, 2023.

"Pillows," Better Sleep Council, March 27, 2017. Available online. URL: www.bettersleep.org/mattresses-and-more/ pillows. Accessed May 4, 2023.

## Section 44.2 | Exercise and Sleep

Exercise is very important for maintaining good health. It not only promotes physical fitness, cardiovascular health, and weight management but also helps people sleep better. Regular exercise has been shown to reduce stress and anxiety, which often contribute to sleep problems. It can also improve physical health conditions that contribute to sleep disorders. For instance, exercise can help people lose weight, which can reduce the symptoms of sleep apnea. Improvements in sleep duration and quality, in turn, lead to greater energy, vitality, and mood—all of which can increase people's motivation to exercise, as well as improve their athletic performance.

The link between exercise and sleep is particularly important for people who are middle-aged or older. Around half of adults in this age group experience symptoms of chronic insomnia. Regular aerobic exercise can help this population combat insomnia without medication and improve their sleep and overall health. A 2010 study followed a group of sedentary women aged 60 or older who had been diagnosed with chronic insomnia. Half of the group remained inactive, while the other half engaged in a moderate exercise program over a four-month period. By the end of the study, the women who exercised 30 minutes per day were sleeping 45–60 minutes longer each night than the women who did not exercise. They also reported sleeping more soundly, waking up fewer times during the night, and feeling more refreshed in the morning.

## ENHANCING THE EFFECTS OF EXERCISE ON SLEEP

Although exercise has the potential to positively impact sleep, getting the full effect depends on the timing and intensity of the workout, as well as the length of time that an exercise program is sustained. The following tips can help people with sleep difficulties maximize the benefits of exercise:

- Exercising before bedtime can keep some people awake due to the release of endorphins and increased core body temperature. However, if exercise is done at least one to two hours before bed, it can promote sleepiness by decreasing endorphin levels and decreasing body temperature. Some people report no negative effects on sleep from exercising at any time of day, while others may benefit from late evening exercise. Intense workouts that elevate core temperature excessively can negatively affect sleep quality and total sleep time. The impact of exercise on sleep quality varies by individual, and avoiding intense workouts close to bedtime is recommended while allowing time for the body to relax after exercise.

- Exercise at a moderate intensity. It is not necessary to exercise at peak intensity or to the point of exhaustion to see improvements in sleep. In fact, moderate aerobic activities such as brisk walking or bicycling seem to provide the maximum benefits. Although any increase in physical activity can lead to improvements in insomnia, studies have shown that the more people exercise, the better they tend to sleep.
- Stick with the program for at least three months. For people with insomnia or other sleep issues, research has shown that it takes time for an exercise regimen to show results. At first, they may not sleep any better than they did before starting to exercise. Researchers theorize that people with existing sleep problems have highly aroused stress systems and that it may take several months for the effects of regular exercise to overcome this stress response. Eventually, however, people with insomnia can see improvements in sleep duration and quality that are better than those offered by other treatments or medications.

Finally, it is important to note that the connection between exercise and sleep works both ways. Just as exercise can help people sleep better, getting a good night's sleep can help people feel motivated to exercise and remain active. Studies have shown that people with insomnia often shorten or skip their workouts the following night when they have trouble sleeping. Sleep deprivation makes exercise feel harder and more tiring, and it can also detract from athletic performance. On the flip side, getting a good night's sleep can help athletes reach their potential. One study showed that college basketball players ran faster and made a higher percentage of shots when they got extra sleep the night before.

## References
"Exercising for Better Sleep," Johns Hopkins Medicine, June 16, 2017. Available online. URL: www.

hopkinsmedicine.org/health/wellness-and-prevention/
exercising-for-better-sleep. Accessed April 10, 2023.

Hendrick, Bill. "Exercise Helps You Sleep," WebMD,
September 16, 2010. Available online. URL: www.webmd.
com/sleep-disorders/news/20100917/exercise-helps-you-
sleep. Accessed April 10, 2023.

Pacheco, Danielle. "Exercise and Sleep," Sleep Foundation,
March 24, 2023. Available online. URL: www.
sleepfoundation.org/physical-activity/exercise-and-sleep.
Accessed April 10, 2023.

Reynolds, Gretchen. "How Exercise Can Help Us Sleep
Better," New York Times, August 21, 2013. Available
online. URL: https://archive.nytimes.com/well.blogs.
nytimes.com/2013/08/21/how-exercise-can-help-us-sleep-
better. Accessed April 10, 2023.

## Section 44.3 | Mind and Body Practices for Sleep Disorders

## SIX THINGS TO KNOW ABOUT MIND AND BODY PRACTICES FOR SLEEP DISORDERS

Do you have trouble falling or staying asleep? Many people do. An estimated 50–70 million Americans have some type of sleep disorder. Fortunately, there are treatments that can help, including psychological and behavioral therapies (mind and body practices).

Here are six things to know about mind and body practices for sleep problems:

- Experts strongly recommend multicomponent cognitive behavioral therapy for insomnia (CBT-I) for adults who have chronic insomnia. Both the American Academy of Sleep Medicine (AASM; the professional organization of sleep medicine specialists) and the American College of Physicians (ACP; the professional organization of physicians who specialize in internal medicine) strongly recommend CBT-I.

- There is evidence that relaxation techniques may be helpful for insomnia, but it is not as strong as the evidence favoring CBT-I. Relaxation techniques, such as guided imagery and progressive muscle relaxation, are safe and easy to use.
- Some studies suggest that yoga can be helpful for sleep. Studies in people with cancer, women with sleep problems, and older adults showed the beneficial effects of yoga on sleep. And, in a national survey, more than half of adults who practice yoga reported improved sleep.
- Tai chi may be helpful for people with sleep problems. Studies from several countries show that practicing tai chi may improve sleep quality.
- There is limited evidence that mindfulness meditation may help reduce insomnia and improve sleep quality. Mindfulness practices may be better than education-based treatments for sleep problems, but they do not seem to be more effective than cognitive behavioral therapy or exercise.
- If you think you may have a sleep problem, let your health-care provider know. The National Heart, Lung, and Blood Institute (NHLBI) has information that can help you prepare for your office visit.[1]

---

[1] "6 Things to Know about Mind and Body Practices for Sleep Disorders," National Center for Complementary and Integrative Health (NCCIH), December 21, 2022. Available online. URL: www.nccih.nih.gov/health/tips/things-to-know-about-mind-and-body- practices-for-sleep-disorders. Accessed April 26, 2023.

# Chapter 45 | Treating Sleep Problems of People in Recovery from Substance Use Disorders

Sleep problems are a common complaint among people with substance use disorders (SUDs). They can occur during withdrawal, but they can also last months and years into recovery and can be associated with relapse to substance use. This chapter, in brief, alerts health-care providers to the relationship between sleep disturbances and SUDs and provides guidance on how to assess and treat sleep problems in patients in recovery.

## SLEEP DISTURBANCES AND SUBSTANCE USE

Many Americans suffer from unhealthy sleep-related behaviors. The prevalence of insomnia symptoms (difficulty initiating or maintaining sleep) in the general population is estimated at 33 percent, with an estimated 6 percent having a diagnosis of insomnia. According to a 12-state survey conducted by the Centers for Disease Control and Prevention (CDC):

- 35.3 percent of survey respondents obtain less than seven hours of sleep on average during a 24-hour period.
- 48.0 percent snore.
- 37.9 percent unintentionally fall asleep during the day.

Substance use can exacerbate sleep difficulties, which in turn present a risk factor for substance use or relapse to use. The types of sleep problems vary by substance used and can include insomnia, sleep latency (the time it takes to fall asleep), disturbances in sleep cycles and sleep continuity, or hypersomnia (excessive daytime sleepiness). Specific findings on the relationship between sleep disturbances and substance use are presented below.

## Alcohol Abuse

Insomnia and other sleep disturbances are common symptoms of alcohol dependence. Many people with alcohol use disorder (AUD) have insomnia before entering treatment. Reported rates of sleep problems among people with AUD in treatment range from 25 to 72 percent. Some people recovering from AUD may continue to have sleep problems, including insomnia or sleep-disordered breathing (such as sleep apnea), for weeks, months, or sometimes years after initiating abstinence.

## Illicit Drug Use

Sleep disturbances are common among people abstaining from chronic substance use. People stopping marijuana use can experience sleep problems in the first days of withdrawal, and these problems can last for weeks. People in detoxification from opioids often report symptoms of insomnia. A study that objectively measured sleep in people who chronically use cocaine found that sleep quality deteriorated during a period of abstinence, even though the subjects perceived their sleep to be improving. Another study of people in withdrawal from cocaine found that three-quarters of the studied population experienced poor sleep quality. In a study of college students, those who reported a history of nonmedical psychostimulant use or current use reported worse subjective and overall sleep quality and more sleep disturbance compared with those who had not used such substances.

## THE EFFECTS OF SLEEP LOSS DURING RECOVERY

Sleep loss can have significant negative effects on the physical, mental, and emotional well-being of people in recovery. It can also interfere with substance abuse treatment. Persistent sleep complaints after withdrawal are associated with relapse to alcohol use. Poor sleep quality before a quit attempt from cannabis use is a risk factor for lapsing back into use within two days.

## ASSESSING SLEEP DISORDERS

If a patient initiating withdrawal from a substance or recovering from an SUD complains of a sleep disturbance, the health-care provider should assess for causes by doing the following:

- Determine the duration of recovery and medications used for SUD treatment.
- Ask questions about difficulty falling asleep, waking during the night, amount of sleep per night, snoring, sleep apnea, excessive movements during sleep, uncontrollable movements that are relieved by getting up and walking, and excessive daytime sleepiness. If possible, ask significant others the same questions about the patient.
- Rule out other causes of the sleep problem, such as stress, a life crisis, or side effects of medications the patient is taking.
- Ask the patient to write in a sleep diary or log immediately upon awakening. The patient should record the total time in bed, time of sleep onset, number of times awakened, and total time spent awake.
- Determine the frequency and duration of symptoms of insomnia. If difficulties occur two or three nights per week and last for one month or more, the patient warrants a diagnosis of insomnia.

Note that some patients tend to overestimate the quality and duration of their sleep on self-report questionnaires and in sleep logs. If warranted, a referral for an objective sleep study in a sleep laboratory can be made.

## TREATMENT FOR SLEEP DISORDERS

The association between insomnia and relapse calls for treatment that addresses insomnia during recovery. The first step in treating insomnia should focus on the status of the patient's recovery. Patients should be receiving treatment from an appropriate substance abuse treatment program. It is important to address other psychological, social, and medical problems that may contribute to insomnia, such as co-occurring mental and medical disorders, the use of medications that disturb sleep, and nicotine use.

## Nonpharmacological Treatments

Nonpharmacological treatments are preferred because many pharmacological treatments for insomnia have the potential for abuse and can interfere with SUD recovery. Research on cognitive behavioral therapy (CBT) to treat insomnia has shown positive results, generally and also in patients who are alcohol-dependent. Combining approaches may be more effective than using one approach.

Health-care providers can educate patients about simple nonpharmacological techniques that can improve sleep. Sleep education includes teaching about sleep, the effects of recovery from substance use on sleep, and health practices and environmental factors that affect sleep. Sleep can be improved by limiting bedroom activities to sleeping (e.g., refraining from activities such as reading the newspaper, paying bills, or working on electronic devices) and going to bed only when sleepy and at about the same time each day. These activities help reassociate the bed and bedroom from going to sleep. Establishing a relaxing presleep routine, which can include progressive muscle relaxation, imagery, or a warm bath, also promotes sleep. Some patients may benefit from a referral to a sleep medicine specialist.

## Pharmacological Treatments
### OVER-THE-COUNTER MEDICATIONS AND DIETARY SUPPLEMENTS

Some people who have trouble sleeping have tried over-the-counter (OTC) sleep medications or dietary supplements to help them sleep. Patients may ask about these, and care should be taken to explain their safety and efficacy. Many over-the-counter sleep medications contain antihistamines that cause sedation. They are not recommended as a long-term treatment for insomnia because they negatively affect the natural sleep cycle and have side effects, such as morning grogginess, daytime sleepiness, and impaired alertness and judgment. Furthermore, evidence supporting their long-term effectiveness is insufficient.

Popular dietary supplements taken with the intent to promote sleep include valerian and melatonin. Valerian, an herb, is thought to have sedative effects. However, studies of valerian offer mixed results, and evidence supporting the supplement's efficacy is insufficient to warrant its use. In addition, valerian could damage the liver. Melatonin is a brain hormone that helps regulate sleep patterns. Limited evidence shows that it can treat chronic insomnia in some people, and to date, there is no evidence that it is harmful.

## PRESCRIPTION MEDICATIONS WITHOUT KNOWN ABUSE POTENTIAL

Medications without known abuse potential should be the first treatment option when pharmacotherapy is necessary to treat insomnia during recovery. Ramelteon and doxepin are the only unscheduled prescription medications approved by the U.S. Food and Drug Administration (FDA) for the treatment of insomnia. Ramelteon decreases the amount of time it takes to fall asleep. Doxepin, originally FDA-approved as an antidepressant, has been approved for treating insomnia typified by problems staying asleep. These medications may be suitable for treating insomnia in patients in recovery because they do not appear to have the potential for abuse.

## OFF-LABEL MEDICATIONS

Other medications are often prescribed off-label (for purposes other than the medication's FDA-approved use) to treat insomnia. According to a survey of addiction medicine physicians, the sedating antidepressant trazodone is the medication most often prescribed for the management of sleep disorders in patients in early recovery from AUD. One study found that its use among people in recovery from AUD improved sleep efficiency. Studies of its effects on abstinence and relapse in persons with AUD are conflicting.

A 2008 study comparing trazodone with placebo for people after detoxification from alcohol showed that the trazodone group had improved sleep quality but had less improvement in the proportion of days abstinent while taking the medication. Furthermore, when the medication was discontinued, the trazodone group experienced less improvement in abstinence days and an increase in the number of drinks per drinking day. In contrast, a study published in 2011 of patients discharged from residential treatment did not find an association between trazodone use and relapse or a return to heavy drinking. A study of patients on methadone maintenance treatment found that trazodone use provided no improvement in sleep.

Other sedating antidepressants that have been used to treat insomnia include amitriptyline, mirtazapine, nefazodone, and nortriptyline. In a study of the use of mirtazapine on subjects with cocaine dependence and co-occurring depression, the medication decreased sleep latency; however, it had no measurable effect on treatment for cocaine dependence and depressive symptoms.

Gabapentin, an anticonvulsant with sedative properties, also has evidence of efficacy in treating insomnia. It has been found to be more effective in promoting sleep than lorazepam (an anxiolytic commonly prescribed to treat insomnia) among people withdrawing from alcohol. It has also been found to be more effective than trazodone in promoting sleep among those in early recovery. Acamprosate, a medication used to maintain alcohol abstinence, may also improve sleep during withdrawal from alcohol.

## PRESCRIPTION MEDICATIONS WITH KNOWN ABUSE POTENTIAL

Sedative-hypnotic medications, such as benzodiazepines and non-benzodiazepines, are commonly prescribed to treat sleep problems. However, these medications should be avoided by people with histories of SUDs, as these individuals are at an increased risk of abusing them. Benzodiazepines, such as alprazolam, diazepam, and triazolam, are especially risky for use with people with SUDs because they are potentially addicting. They can also cause residual daytime sedation, cognitive impairment, motor incoordination, and rebound insomnia. Long-term treatment of insomnia with benzodiazepines may lead to withdrawal symptoms (e.g., anxiety, irritability, seizures) when patients stop taking their medications. A careful clinical evaluation is needed to ensure appropriate prescribing. Measures to prevent abuse include the following:

- observe closely and perform ongoing evaluations
- prescribe a few tablets at a time
- schedule frequent office visits
- conduct occasional urine screenings
- use one source to dispense the medication
- occasionally taper the medication
- be attentive to risk factors, such as antisocial personality disorder and dependence on multiple substances

Alternatives to benzodiazepines include sedative-hypnotic medications, such as zaleplon, eszopiclone, and zolpidem. These medications all have the same mechanism of action as benzodiazepines but lack some of the negative side effects. However, some research indicates that at high doses, they may have the same side effects as benzodiazepines. The three medications are Schedule IV controlled substances, indicating abuse potential. For these reasons, these medications should be used only for short-term treatment of insomnia in people with a history of SUDs.[1]

---

[1] "Treating Sleep Problems of People in Recovery from Substance Use Disorders," Substance Abuse and Mental Health Services Administration (SAMHSA), 2014. Available online. URL: https://store.samhsa.gov/sites/default/files/d7/priv/sma14-4859.pdf. Accessed May 4, 2023.

# Chapter 46 | **Continuous Positive Airway Pressure**

### WHAT IS CONTINUOUS POSITIVE AIRWAY PRESSURE?

Continuous positive airway pressure (CPAP) is a machine that uses mild air pressure to keep breathing airways open while you sleep. Your health-care provider may prescribe CPAP to treat sleep-related breathing disorders, including sleep apnea. CPAP may also treat preterm infants who have underdeveloped lungs.

### WHAT DOES A CONTINUOUS POSITIVE AIRWAY PRESSURE MACHINE INCLUDE?

A CPAP machine includes the following:
- a mask or other device that fits over your nose or your nose and mouth
- straps to position the mask
- a tube that connects the mask to the machine's motor
- a motor that blows air into the tube

### HOW DOES CONTINUOUS POSITIVE AIRWAY PRESSURE WORK?

You should use your CPAP machine every time you sleep at home, while traveling, and during naps. Getting used to using your CPAP machine can take time and requires patience. Your health-care provider will work with you to find the most comfortable mask that works best for you.

You may also need help from your health-care provider to use the humidifier chamber in your machine or to adjust your pressure settings. You may also need to try a different machine that has multiple or auto-adjusting pressure settings.

For the treatment to continue to work, it is important that you clean your mask and tube every day and refill your medical device prescription at the right time to replace the mask and tube.

## WHAT ARE THE BENEFITS OF CONTINUOUS POSITIVE AIRWAY PRESSURE?

You may notice immediate improvements after starting CPAP treatment, such as better sleep quality, reduction or elimination of snoring, and less daytime sleepiness.

Equally important are the long-term benefits of CPAP, which include the following:

- helping to prevent or control high blood pressure
- lowering your risk for stroke
- improving memory and other cognitive functions

## WHAT ARE THE POSSIBLE SIDE EFFECTS OF CONTINUOUS POSITIVE AIRWAY PRESSURE?

Side effects of CPAP treatment may include congestion, runny nose, dry mouth, or nosebleeds. Some masks can cause irritation. Your health-care provider can help you find ways to relieve these symptoms and adjust to using your CPAP machine. If you experience stomach discomfort or bloating, you should stop using your CPAP machine and call your health-care provider right away.

## MEDICAL DEVICE AND INSURANCE

If your health-care provider prescribes CPAP for sleep apnea, your insurance will work with a medical device company to provide you with a CPAP machine and the mask and tube. Your provider will set up your machine with certain pressure settings. After using your machine for a while, your provider and possibly your insurance company will want to check the data card from your machine to confirm that you are using your CPAP device and to see if the machine and its pressure settings are working to reduce or eliminate apnea events while you sleep.[1]

---

[1] "CPAP," National Heart, Lung, and Blood Institute (NHLBI), March 24, 2022. Available online. URL: www.nhlbi.nih.gov/health/cpap. Accessed May 5, 2023.

# Chapter 47 | **Implantable Device for Central Sleep Apnea**

The U.S. Food and Drug Administration (FDA) approved a new treatment option for patients who have been diagnosed with moderate-to-severe central sleep apnea (CSA). The remedē® System is an implantable device that stimulates a nerve located in the chest that is responsible for sending signals to the diaphragm to stimulate breathing.

"This implantable device offers patients another treatment option for central sleep apnea," said Tina Kiang, Ph.D., acting director of the Division of Anesthesiology, General Hospital, Respiratory, Infection Control, and Dental Devices in the FDA's Center for Devices and Radiological Health. "Patients should speak with their health-care providers about the benefits and risks of this new treatment compared to other available treatments."

Sleep apnea is a disorder that causes individuals to have one or more pauses in breathing or shallow breaths during sleep. Breathing pauses can last from a few seconds to minutes. CSA occurs when the brain fails to send signals to the diaphragm to breathe, causing an individual to stop breathing during sleep for a period of 10 seconds or more before restarting again. According to the National Center on Sleep Disorders Research (NCSDR) of the National Institute of Health (NIH), CSA can lead to poor sleep quality and may result in serious health issues, including an increased risk of high blood pressure, heart attack, heart failure, stroke, obesity, and diabetes. Common treatment options for moderate-to-severe sleep apnea include medication, positive airway pressure devices (e.g., continuous positive airway pressure machine), or surgery.

The remedē® System comprises a battery pack surgically placed under the skin in the upper chest area and small, thin wires that are inserted into the blood vessels in the chest near the nerve (phrenic) that stimulates breathing. The system monitors the patient's respiratory signals during sleep and stimulates the nerve to move the diaphragm and restore normal breathing.

The FDA evaluated data from 141 patients to assess the effectiveness of the remedē® System in reducing the apnea-hypopnea index (AHI), a measure of the frequency and severity of apnea episodes. After six months, AHI was reduced by 50 percent or more in 51 percent of patients with an active remedē® System implanted. AHI was reduced by 11 percent in patients without an active remedē® System implanted.

The most common adverse events reported included concomitant device interaction, implant site infection, swelling, and local tissue damage or pocket erosion. The remedē® System should not be used by patients with an active infection or by patients who are known to require magnetic resonance imaging (MRI). This device is not intended for use in patients with obstructive sleep apnea (OSA), a condition in which the patient attempts to breathe, but the upper airway is partially or completely blocked.

The FDA granted approval of the remedē® System to Respicardia, Inc.

The FDA, an agency within the U.S. Department of Health and Human Services (HHS), protects public health by assuring the safety, effectiveness, and security of human and veterinary drugs, vaccines, and other biological products for human use and medical devices. The agency is also responsible for the safety and security of the nation's food supply, cosmetics, dietary supplements, and products that give off electronic radiation and for regulating tobacco products.[1]

---

[1] "FDA Approves Implantable Device to Treat Moderate to Severe Central Sleep Apnea," U.S. Food and Drug Administration (FDA), October 6, 2017. Available online. URL: www.fda.gov/news-events/press-announcements/fda-approves-implantable-device-treat-moderate-severe-central-sleep-apnea. Accessed May 1, 2023.

# Chapter 48 | Complementary and Alternative Medicine and Dietary Supplements for Sleep Disorders

## Chapter Contents

## Section 48.1 | Complementary and Alternative Medicine and Sleep Disorders: An Overview

### WHAT ARE SLEEP DISORDERS, AND HOW IMPORTANT ARE THEY?

There are more than 80 different sleep disorders. This section focuses on insomnia—difficulty falling asleep or difficulty staying asleep. Insomnia is one of the most common sleep disorders. Chronic, long-term sleep disorders affect millions of Americans each year. These disorders and the sleep deprivation they cause can interfere with work, driving, social activities, and overall quality of life, and they can have serious health implications. Sleep disorders account for an estimated $16 billion in medical costs each year, plus indirect costs due to missed days of work, decreased productivity, and other factors.

### IS IT A SLEEP DISORDER OR NOT ENOUGH SLEEP?

Some people who feel tired during the day have a true sleep disorder, but for others, the real problem is not allowing enough time for sleep. Adults need at least seven to eight hours of sleep each night to be well-rested, but the average adult sleeps for less than seven hours a night.

Sleep is a basic human need, such as eating, drinking, and breathing, and is vital to good health and well-being. Shortchanging yourself on sleep slows your thinking and reaction time, makes you irritable, and increases your risk of injury. It may even decrease your resistance to infections, increase your risk of obesity, and increase your risk of heart disease.

### WHAT THE SCIENCE SAYS ABOUT COMPLEMENTARY HEALTH APPROACHES AND INSOMNIA

Complementary approaches can be classified by their primary therapeutic input (how the therapy is taken in or delivered), which may be:

- nutritional (e.g., special diets, dietary supplements, herbs, probiotics, microbial-based therapies)

529

- psychological (e.g., meditation, hypnosis, music therapies, relaxation therapies)
- physical (e.g., acupuncture, massage, spinal manipulation)
- combinations such as psychological and physical (e.g., yoga, tai chi, dance therapies, some forms of art therapy) or psychological and nutritional (e.g., mindful eating)

Nutritional approaches include what the National Center for Complementary and Integrative Health (NCCIH) previously categorized as natural products, whereas psychological and/or physical approaches include what was referred to as mind and body practices.

Research has produced promising results for some complementary health approaches for insomnia, such as relaxation techniques. However, evidence of effectiveness is still limited for most products and practices, and safety concerns have been raised about a few.

## Psychological and Physical Approaches

- There is evidence that relaxation techniques can be effective in treating chronic insomnia.
  - Progressive relaxation may help people with insomnia and nighttime anxiety.
  - Music-assisted relaxation may be moderately beneficial in improving sleep quality in people with sleep problems, but the number of studies has been small.
  - Various forms of relaxation are sometimes combined with components of cognitive behavioral therapy (CBT; such as sleep restriction and stimulus control), with good results.
  - Using relaxation techniques before bedtime can be part of a strategy to improve sleep habits that also includes other steps, such as maintaining a consistent sleep schedule; avoiding caffeine, alcohol, heavy meals, and strenuous exercise too close to bedtime; and sleeping in a quiet, cool, dark room.

- Relaxation techniques are generally safe. However, rare side effects have been reported in people with serious physical or mental health conditions. If you have a serious underlying health problem, it would be a good idea to consult your health-care provider before using relaxation techniques.
- In a preliminary study, mindfulness-based stress reduction, a type of meditation, was as effective as a prescription drug in a small group of people with insomnia.
  - Several other studies have also reported that mindfulness-based stress reduction improved sleep, but the people who participated in these studies had other health problems, such as cancer.
- Preliminary studies in postmenopausal women and women with osteoarthritis (OA) suggest that yoga may be helpful for insomnia.
- Some practitioners who treat insomnia have reported that hypnotherapy enhanced the effectiveness of CBT and relaxation techniques in their patients, but very little rigorous research has been conducted on the use of hypnotherapy for insomnia.
- A small 2012 study on massage therapy showed promising results for insomnia in postmenopausal women. However, conclusions cannot be reached on the basis of a single study.
- Most of the studies that have evaluated acupuncture for insomnia have been of poor scientific quality. The current evidence is not rigorous enough to show whether acupuncture is helpful for insomnia.

## Nutritional Approaches
### MELATONIN AND RELATED DIETARY SUPPLEMENTS
- Melatonin may help with jet lag and sleep problems related to shift work.
- A 2013 evaluation of the results of 19 studies concluded that melatonin may help people with insomnia fall asleep

faster, sleep longer, and sleep better, but the effect of melatonin is small compared to that of other treatments for insomnia.

- Studies of melatonin in children with sleep problems suggest that it may be helpful, both in generally healthy children and in those with conditions such as autism or attention deficit hyperactivity disorder. However, both the number of studies and the number of children who participated in the studies are small, and all of the studies tested melatonin only for short periods of time.
- Melatonin supplements appear to be relatively safe for short-term use although the use of melatonin was linked to bad moods in elderly people (most of whom had dementia) in one study.
- The long-term safety of melatonin supplements has not been established.

- Dietary supplements containing substances that can be changed into melatonin in the body—L-tryptophan and 5-hydroxytryptophan (5-HTP)—have been researched as sleep aids.

- Studies of L-tryptophan supplements as an insomnia treatment have had inconsistent results, and the effects of 5-HTP supplements on insomnia have not been established.
- The use of L-tryptophan supplements may be linked to eosinophilia-myalgia syndrome (EMS), a complex, potentially fatal disorder with multiple symptoms, including severe muscle pain. It is uncertain whether the risk of EMS associated with L-tryptophan supplements is due to impurities in L-tryptophan preparations or to L-tryptophan itself.

## HERBS

- Although chamomile has traditionally been used for insomnia, often in the form of tea, there is no conclusive evidence from clinical trials showing whether it is helpful. Some people, especially those who are allergic to ragweed or related plants, may have allergic reactions to chamomile.

- Although kava is said to have sedative properties, very little research has been conducted on whether this herb is helpful for insomnia. More importantly, kava supplements have been linked to a risk of severe liver damage.
- Clinical trials of valerian (another herb said to have sedative properties) have had inconsistent results, and its value for insomnia has not been demonstrated. Although few people have reported negative side effects from valerian, it is uncertain whether this herb is safe for long-term use.
- Some "sleep formula" dietary supplements combine valerian with other herbs such as hops, lemon balm, passionflower, and kava or other ingredients such as melatonin and 5-HTP. There is little evidence of these preparations from studies in people.

## Other Complementary Health Approaches

- Aromatherapy is the therapeutic use of essential oils from plants. It is uncertain whether aromatherapy is helpful for treating insomnia because little rigorous research has been done on this topic.
- A 2010 systematic review concluded that current evidence does not demonstrate significant effects of homeopathic medicines for insomnia.

## IF YOU ARE CONSIDERING COMPLEMENTARY HEALTH APPROACHES FOR SLEEP PROBLEMS

- Talk to your health-care providers. Tell them about the complementary health approach you are considering and ask any questions you may have. Because trouble sleeping can be an indication of a more serious condition and because some prescription and over-the-counter (OTC) drugs can contribute to sleep problems, it is important to discuss your sleep-related symptoms with your health-care providers before trying any complementary health product or practice.

- Be cautious about using any sleep product—prescription medications, OTC medications, dietary supplements, or homeopathic remedies. Find out about potential side effects and any risks from long-term use or combining products.

- Keep in mind that "natural" does not always mean safe. For example, kava products can cause serious harm to the liver. Also, a manufacturer's use of the term "standardized" (or "verified" or "certified") does not necessarily guarantee product quality or consistency. Dietary supplements can cause health problems if not used correctly. The health-care providers you see about your sleep problems can advise you.

- If you are pregnant, nursing a child, or considering giving a child a dietary supplement, it is especially important to consult your (or your child's) health-care provider.

- If you are considering a practitioner-provided complementary health practice, check with your insurer to see if the services will be covered and ask a trusted source (such as your health-care provider or a nearby hospital or medical school) to recommend a practitioner.

- Tell all your health-care providers about any complementary health approaches you use. Give them a full picture of what you do to manage your health. This will help ensure coordinated and safe care.[1]

---

[1] "Sleep Disorders: In Depth," National Center for Complementary and Integrative Health (NCCIH), October 2015. Available online. URL: www.nccih.nih.gov/health/sleep-disorders-in-depth#hed3. Accessed May 5, 2023.

## Section 48.2 | Tai Chi

## WHAT IS TAI CHI?

Tai chi is a practice that involves a series of slow, gentle movements and physical postures, a meditative state of mind, and controlled breathing. Tai chi originated as an ancient martial art in China. Over the years, it has become more focused on health promotion and rehabilitation.

## DOES TAI CHI HELP PREVENT FALLS?

Tai chi may be beneficial in improving balance and preventing falls in older adults and people with Parkinson disease (PD). It is unknown whether tai chi can help reduce falls in people who have had a stroke or people with osteoarthritis or heart failure.

### Older Adults

A 2019 review looked at different types of exercise for preventing falls in community-dwelling older people. The duration and frequency of tai chi sessions varied among the studies. Compared to control interventions that were not thought to reduce falls, there was low-certainty evidence that tai chi may reduce the rate of falls by 19 percent (based on seven studies with 2,655 participants) and high-certainty evidence that tai chi may reduce the number of people who experience falls by 20 percent (based on eight studies with 2,677 participants). Other forms of exercise were also helpful. The authors found high-certainty evidence that balance and functional exercises—exercises that are similar to everyday actions like rising from a chair, stepping up, or rotating while standing—could reduce the rate of falls by 24 percent (based on 39 studies with 7,920 participants) and lower the number of people experiencing one or more falls by 13 percent (based on 37 studies with 8,288 participants).

### Parkinson Disease

A 2021 review analyzed three studies of tai chi's effect on falls in people with PD. The three studies included a total of 273 participants who did 60-minute tai chi sessions two to three times per week for 12 weeks to 6 months. The analysis indicated that tai chi had a significant positive effect on reducing falls when compared with both no intervention and different interventions, such as resistance training and stretching.

A 2020 summary of three reviews that included some relevant studies found that tai chi may help improve balance and reduce falls in people with PD, but the certainty of the evidence was considered to be low.

## Stroke

A 2018 review evaluated five randomized controlled trials with 346 participants who had experienced a prior stroke. (Randomized controlled trials are studies in which participants are randomly assigned to an intervention group and a control group.) Tai chi sessions were typically 60 minutes long and done two to three times weekly for 6 or 12 weeks. The review found that tai chi helped improve the participants' walking gait in the short term but not their balance when they stood and moved their upper body outside their center of gravity, such as reaching forward as much as possible while in a fixed standing position. The authors of the review said that all of the studies had high bias and were small and that large, long-term randomized controlled trials are needed to confirm the review's findings.

## Osteoarthritis

A 2015 review included nine osteoarthritis studies with a total of 543 participants. The review concluded that tai chi improved pain and stiffness in osteoarthritis, and the authors noted that the improvement may increase balance. Updated 2019 guidelines from the American College of Rheumatology and the Arthritis Foundation strongly recommend tai chi for the management of both knee and hip osteoarthritis.

## Heart Failure

A 2020 summary of one review said no definite conclusion could be drawn about using tai chi to reduce falls in people with heart failure. The authors indicated that more high-quality studies are needed. The one review, which was done in 2016, included five heart failure studies with a total of 271 participants. The review did not provide any details on tai chi's effect on balance in people with heart failure.

## DOES TAI CHI REDUCE PAIN?

A small amount of research suggests that tai may be helpful in reducing pain in people with low-back pain, fibromyalgia, and knee osteoarthritis. It is unclear whether tai chi is beneficial for alleviating pain from rheumatoid arthritis (RA).

### Low-Back Pain

A 2019 review evaluated 10 studies with 959 participants who had low-back pain. The duration of the tai chi interventions ranged from 2 to 28 weeks, with sessions done two to six times weekly and the majority lasting from 40 to 60 minutes. Because the studies used different tai chi interventions and assessment methods, the authors drew a cautious conclusion that tai chi alone or in addition to physical therapy may decrease pain intensity and improve every-day function (such as the ability to carry groceries, climb stairs, walk, and bathe and dress oneself). The authors noted a need for studies that use the same tai chi intervention and frequency.

### Rheumatoid Arthritis

A 2019 review of seven studies (345 participants) indicated uncertainty on whether tai chi reduces pain and disease activity or improves function (such as standing up from an armless chair, opening a drink or food carton, and climbing stairs) in people with RA. The tai chi sessions usually lasted one hour and were done two to three times per week for 8–12 weeks. It is also not clear how much, how intense, and for how long tai should be done to see benefits. The review authors rated the quality of the evidence very low because of concerns with study designs, a low number of participants in some studies, and a high number of people stopping their participation in some studies.

## Fibromyalgia

A 2019 review of six studies (657 participants) found that tai chi was beneficial for reducing pain scores in people with fibromyalgia. Tai chi also helped improve sleep quality, relieve fatigue, reduce depression, and increase the quality of life (QOL). The tai chi interventions typically involved 60-minute sessions done one to three times weekly for 12 weeks. The review authors said, however, that larger, higher-quality studies are needed to provide stronger evidence for these findings and to determine whether tai chi is better than conventional therapeutic exercise for people with fibromyalgia.

## Knee Osteoarthritis

The updated 2019 guidelines from the American College of Rheumatology and the Arthritis Foundation strongly recommend tai chi for the management of knee osteoarthritis.

A 2021 review of 16 studies involving 986 participants found evidence of low-to-moderate strength that tai chi was beneficial for treating and managing knee osteoarthritis. The tai chi interventions usually involved 30- to 60-minute sessions done two to four times weekly for 10–52 weeks. Participants practicing tai chi experienced improvements in pain as well as stiffness, physical function (such as walking, standing, rising from a bed, and getting in and out of a car), balance, and physiological and psychological health. The review authors noted, however, that high-quality studies are needed to confirm these findings and to determine the best type, intensity, frequency, and duration of tai chi for knee osteoarthritis.

Another 2021 review, which included 11 studies and 603 participants, found that tai chi had a positive effect on improving walking function and posture control in older adults with knee osteoarthritis. The review authors said more high-quality studies are needed to confirm the findings. In most of the studies, tai chi sessions were 60 minutes long and done two to three times per week for 8–24 weeks.

## IS TAI CHI HELPFUL FOR PEOPLE WITH CHRONIC DISEASES?
### Chronic Obstructive Pulmonary Disease

A 2021 review of 23 studies (1,663 participants) concluded that tai chi may help improve exercise capacity, lung function, and QOL in people with chronic obstructive pulmonary disease (COPD). Tai chi was better than no treatment in all areas evaluated, and it was better than breathing and walking exercises in some of the areas. The duration and frequency of the tai chi sessions varied among the included studies, and the tai chi interventions lasted from 1 to 12 months. The review authors said more high-quality studies are needed to clearly understand tai chi's effect on COPD.

### Parkinson Disease

A 2021 review looked at 26 studies of tai chi and qigong involving 1,672 participants with PD. Tai chi sessions lasted from 30 to 90 minutes and were done over 5–24 weeks, with the total number of tai chi sessions ranging from 10 to 48, depending on the study. Most of the studies showed that tai chi was more helpful than no intervention and had a positive effect that was similar to that of other therapies such as dancing, aerobic exercise, resistance training, and stretching. The authors said the overall results were limited by the different types and durations of tai chi and qigong interventions, the variety of other therapies, the small number of participants, and the different stages of PD among participants.

### Type 2 Diabetes

Some research shows that tai chi improves levels of fasting blood glucose and hemoglobin A1c (HbA1c) in people with type 2 diabetes and may improve QOL factors. Tai chi, however, does not appear to be any better than other aerobic exercises.

- A 2018 review of 14 studies (798 participants) found that tai chi was better than no exercise for managing levels of fasting blood glucose and HbA1c in adults with type 2 diabetes. Tai chi may have advantages over other aerobic exercises, such as walking and dancing, for reducing HbA1c, but the evidence was not strong. There were no differences between tai chi and other aerobic exercises for blood glucose control. Practicing tai chi for longer periods of time resulted in better results. Tai chi interventions involved 15–60-minute sessions done two to seven times per week for 4–24 weeks.

- A 2019 review of 23 studies (1,235 participants) found that tai chi was beneficial in lowering fasting blood glucose, HbA1c, insulin resistance, body mass index, and total cholesterol in people with type 2 diabetes. Tai chi was also found to improve QOL factors such as physical function, bodily pain, and social function, and it had no effect on balance. Tai chi sessions were 15–120 minutes long and were done 2–14 times weekly for 4–24 weeks. The authors said that differences between study methods and the small size of the studies might weaken the strength of the results.

## High Blood Pressure

A 2020 review looked at 28 studies (2,937 participants) and found that tai chi was better at lowering systolic and diastolic blood pressure than health education/no treatment, other exercises, or antihypertensive drugs. The time duration, weekly frequency, and total weeks of tai chi sessions varied among the included studies. However, the authors said the studies were of poor quality and had many differences among them, warranting more research to confirm the conclusions.

## Cardiovascular Disease

A 2020 review evaluated the psychological well-being of adults who were 60 years of age and older and who had cardiovascular disease (diseases of the heart and blood vessels). The review, which included 15 studies of 1,853 adults, found that tai chi was better than usual care or other types of exercise (e.g., walking, strength training) for improving QOL and psychological well-being. The length of tai chi interventions ranged from 6 to 52 weeks, with an average of 36 tai chi sessions over the duration of the studies. The specific improvements varied depending on the type of cardiovascular disease, however. For example, when compared to usual care or other exercises, tai chi participants with coronary heart disease had better mental health QOL, those with chronic heart failure experienced less depression and psychological distress, and those with high blood pressure had better physical health QOL. The authors said that the quality of the studies was, on average, acceptable and that more rigorous studies are needed.

A 2018 review of 13 studies (972 participants) found that tai chi led to large and significant improvements in aerobic capacity among people with coronary heart disease when compared to active interventions (e.g., walking, stretching) and nonactive interventions (e.g., usual medical care). The tai chi interventions involved 30–90-minute sessions done one to seven times weekly for 12 weeks to 12 months. The authors rated the quality of the studies from moderate to strong, but the studies were very small, and the authors said that more high-quality studies are needed to confirm these findings.

## DOES TAI CHI HELP WITH DEMENTIA?

A 2019 review of nine studies (656 participants) looked at the use of tai chi in the early stages of dementia in older adults (average age of 78). The short-term effect of tai chi on the overall cognition of people with mild cognitive impairment was found to be beneficial and similar to that seen with other types of exercise. The results of the studies suggested that tai chi done three times a week for 30–60 minutes per session for at least three months had a positive impact on some cognitive functions. The review authors said the quality of seven of the nine studies was rated as either good or excellent, but the studies were small.

## DOES TAI CHI IMPROVE THE QUALITY OF LIFE OF OLDER ADULTS?

A 2020 review of 13 studies (869 participants) found that tai chi had a small positive effect on the QOL and depressive symptoms of older adults with chronic conditions who lived in community settings. No significant effect was seen for mobility and physical endurance. The tai chi interventions involved 40–90-minute sessions done one to four times per week for 10–24 weeks. The authors said the studies had many differences among them, that the evidence was of low quality, and that larger high-quality studies are needed.

## CAN TAI CHI HELP REDUCE CANCER-RELATED SYMPTOMS?

Tai chi appears to be promising in improving some cancer-related symptoms and in possibly improving QOL, but researchers indicated that no definite conclusions or recommendations can be made at this point.

- A 2018 review included 22 studies of 1,283 people with different types of cancer. Three to twelve weeks of tai chi or qigong were associated with significant improvement in fatigue, sleep difficulty, depression, and overall QOL. However, the authors said that larger, higher-quality studies are needed before definitive conclusions can be drawn and before cancer- and symptom-specific recommendations can be made.

- A 2020 review included 16 studies of 1,268 participants with breast cancer. Most of the studies conducted in the United States involved 60-minute tai chi sessions done two to three times weekly for 12 weeks. Most of the studies conducted in China involved 20-minute tai chi sessions done twice daily for unknown total durations. Results showed that tai chi was no different from conventional supportive care interventions in improving fatigue, sleeping quality, depression, or body mass index at three or six months, but it was significantly better than conventional interventions at improving QOL at three months. When used with conventional supportive care interventions, tai chi was found to significantly relieve fatigue symptoms. The authors said that the studies had differences among them and that future well-designed studies with standardized protocols for a particular subgroup of breast cancer patients would be helpful.

## IS THERE ANY RESEARCH ON TAI CHI AND COVID-19?

There have been only a few studies on tai chi and COVID-19.

- A 2021 study evaluated a 10-week tai chi intervention in older adults during the COVID-19 pandemic as a possible way to help improve their mental and physical health. (Participants maintained a physical distance of 4 m from each other during the study.) The 30 participants were between the ages of 60 and 78, had not previously practiced tai chi, and had been doing fewer than two days a week of structured physical activity before the study. Half of the participants were randomly assigned to partake in two 60-minute group tai chi classes each week. The results of the study suggested that tai chi is an effective intervention that can be used under pandemic conditions to improve the psychoemotional state, cognition, and motor learning in older adults.

- A 2021 narrative review suggested that tai chi could possibly help people cope with COVID-19 and counteract the negative effect of physical inactivity, sedentary behavior, and mental disorders in the general population during the COVID-19 pandemic. The authors explained that tai chi can be practiced easily and safely at home, in isolation, or in groups, making it useful during pandemic conditions. This suggestion was not based on studies of tai chi during the COVID-19 pandemic but instead on past research about the general effects of tai chi. The authors said that future research is needed to determine the effectiveness of tai chi during the COVID-19 pandemic and to provide more valid and reliable data.

## IS TAI CHI SAFE DURING PREGNANCY?

There are no published studies on the safety of tai chi during pregnancy. However, physical activities, such as tai chi, are likely safe and desirable during pregnancy in most instances, as long as appropriate precautions are taken. If you are pregnant, talk with your health-care providers before starting tai chi.

Tai chi during pregnancy may help with blood circulation, balance, coordination, strength, relaxation, and mental health, but research in these areas is needed.

According to a 2021 review, there are no peer-reviewed studies on the effects of tai chi alone during pregnancy. The review found one study that evaluated a combined yoga and tai chi program designed for the second and third trimesters of pregnancy. In this 2013 study, 92 pregnant women with depression (46 of whom were initially in a waitlist control group) participated in a 20-minute yoga and tai chi class once a week for 12 weeks. When compared to the control group, the yoga and tai chi group had a significant reduction in levels of depression, anxiety, and sleep disturbances. Neither the 2021 review nor the 2013 study mentioned any adverse effects of tai chi during pregnancy.

## CAN TAI CHI BE HARMFUL?

Tai chi appears to be safe. A 2019 review of 24 studies (1,794 participants) found that the frequency of adverse events was similar for people doing tai chi, another active intervention, or no intervention. The review also found that in studies of people with heart failure, people in tai chi groups experienced fewer serious adverse events than people receiving no intervention. None of the serious adverse events reported in the 24 studies were thought to be caused by either tai chi or the control conditions (active interventions or no intervention). The adverse events that were reported as related to tai chi or other active interventions were minor, such as musculoskeletal aches and pain.

## WHAT KIND OF TRAINING, LICENSING, OR CERTIFICATIONS DO TAI CHI INSTRUCTORS NEED TO PRACTICE?

Tai chi instructors do not have to be licensed, and the practice is not regulated by the federal government or individual states. There is no national standard for tai chi certification. Various tai chi organizations offer training and certification programs—with differing criteria and levels of certification for instructors.[2]

## TAI CHI CHIH IMPROVES SLEEP QUALITY IN OLDER ADULTS

Poor sleep quality is a common problem among older adults. Many have moderate sleep complaints, where they experience insomnia-like symptoms but are not yet diagnosed with insomnia. Sedative medications are commonly used to treat sleep disorders but can cause harmful side effects, and behavioral interventions such as cognitive behavioral therapy (CBT) are not always practical. Few treatments focus on improving sleep quality in people with moderate complaints. Tai chi chih—the Westernized version of the Chinese slow-motion meditative exercise tai chi—may serve as an effective alternative approach.

Researchers at the University of California, Los Angeles, conducted a randomized controlled trial, funded in part by the National Center for Complementary and Alternative Medicine (NCCAM), to determine whether tai chi chih could improve sleep quality in healthy, older adults with moderate sleep complaints. In the study, 112 individuals aged 59–86 participated in either tai chi chih training or health education classes for 25 weeks. Participants rated their sleep quality based on the Pittsburgh Sleep Quality Index, a self-rate questionnaire that assesses sleep quality, duration, and disturbances.

The results of the study showed that the people who participated in tai chi chih sessions experienced slightly greater improvements in self-reported sleep quality. The researchers concluded that tai chi chih can be a useful nonpharmacologic approach to improving

[2] "Tai Chi: What You Need to Know," National Center for Complementary and Integrative Health (NCCIH), March 2022. Available online. URL: www.nccih.nih.gov/health/tai-chi-what-you-need-to-know. Accessed May 4, 2023.

sleep quality in older adults with moderate sleep complaints and may help prevent the onset of insomnia.[3]

## Section 48.3 | Melatonin

## WHAT IS MELATONIN, AND HOW DOES IT WORK?

Melatonin is a hormone that your brain produces in response to darkness. It helps with the timing of your circadian rhythms (24-hour internal clock) and with sleep. Being exposed to light at night can block melatonin production.

Research suggests that melatonin plays other important roles in the body beyond sleep. However, these effects are not fully understood.

Melatonin dietary supplements can be made from animals or microorganisms, but most often they are made synthetically. The information below is about melatonin dietary supplements.

## WHAT ARE THE HEALTH BENEFITS OF TAKING MELATONIN?

Melatonin supplements may help with certain conditions, such as jet lag, delayed sleep–wake phase disorder, some sleep disorders in children, and anxiety before and after surgery.

### Jet Lag

Jet lag affects people when they travel by air across multiple time zones. With jet lag, you may not feel well overall, and you may have disturbed sleep, daytime tiredness, impaired functioning, and digestive problems.

Research suggests that melatonin supplements may help with jet lag. This is based on medium-sized reviews from 2010 and 2014.

---

[3] "Tai Chi Chih Improves Sleep Quality in Older Adults," National Center for Complementary and Integrative Health (NCCIH), July 5, 2017. Available online. URL: https://nccih.nih.gov/research/results/spotlight/031109. htm. Accessed May 16, 2023.

- Four studies that included a total of 142 travelers showed that melatonin may be better than a placebo (an inactive substance) in reducing overall symptoms of jet lag after eastward flights. Another study of 234 travelers on eastward flights looked at only sleep quality and found low-quality evidence that melatonin may be better than a placebo for improving sleep quality.
- Two studies that included a total of 90 travelers showed that melatonin may be better than a placebo in reducing symptoms of jet lag after westward flights.

## Delayed Sleep–Wake Phase Disorder

People with delayed sleep–wake phase disorder (DSWPD) have trouble falling asleep at the usual times and waking up in the morning. They typically have difficulty getting to sleep before 2–6 a.m. and would prefer to wake up between 10 a.m. and 1 p.m.

Melatonin supplements appear to help with sleep in people with DSWPD, but it is uncertain whether the benefits outweigh the possible harms. This is based on a clinical practice guideline, a small review, and a more recent study.

- In 2015, the American Academy of Sleep Medicine (AASM) recommended melatonin supplements given at specific times for DSWPD. The recommendation was a weak one, and it came with uncertainty about whether the benefits of melatonin outweigh its potential harms.
- A 2016 review that looked at a small number of people (52) from two studies showed that melatonin supplements reduced the time it took for people with DSWPD to fall asleep when compared to placebo. On average, it took about 22 minutes less for them to fall asleep.
- A 2018 randomized controlled trial that lasted four weeks and included 307 people with DSWPD found that taking melatonin one hour before the desired bedtime combined with going to bed at a set time led to several improvements. Those improvements included

falling asleep an average of 34 minutes earlier, better sleep during the first third of the night, and better daytime functioning.

## Some Sleep Disorders in Children

Sleep problems in children can have undesirable effects on their behavior, daytime functioning, and quality of life. Children with certain conditions, such as atopic dermatitis, asthma, attention deficit hyperactivity disorder (ADHD), or autism spectrum disorder (ASD), are more prone to sleep problems than other children.

There are no overall guidelines on the best approach to improving sleep in children. However, guidelines for specific conditions recommend behavioral treatments, such as good bedtime habits and parent education, as an initial treatment that may be supplemented with medicines.

- A 2019 review looked at 18 studies on melatonin supplements that included a total of 1,021 children. Most of the studies were small, and all were relatively brief (1–13 weeks). Overall, the studies showed that melatonin was better than a placebo for improving both the time to fall asleep and total sleep. The effects of melatonin on behavior and daytime functioning, however, were not clear because the studies used different ways to measure these outcomes.
- The list below shows the review's results on melatonin's short-term effects for children with specific conditions:
  - Children with ASD fell asleep 37 minutes earlier and slept 48 minutes longer.
  - Children with ADHD fell asleep 20 minutes earlier and slept 33 minutes longer.
  - Children with atopic dermatitis fell asleep 6.8 minutes earlier and slept 35 minutes longer.
  - Children with chronic sleep-onset insomnia fell asleep 24 minutes earlier and slept 25 minutes longer.

Because there are not many studies on children and melatonin supplements, there is a lot we do not know about the use of melatonin in children. For example, there are uncertainties about what dose to use and when to give it, the effects of melatonin use over long periods of time, and whether melatonin's benefits outweigh its possible risks. Because melatonin is a hormone, it is possible that melatonin supplements could affect hormonal development, including puberty, menstrual cycles, and overproduction of the hormone prolactin, but we do not know for sure.

Because of these uncertainties, it is best to work with a health-care provider if you are considering giving a child melatonin for sleep problems.

## Anxiety before and after Surgery

Anxiety before and after surgery happens in up to 80 percent of patients.

Melatonin supplements appear to be helpful in reducing anxiety before surgery, but it is unclear if it helps to lower anxiety after surgery. This is based on a 2015 review.

- The 2015 review looked at 12 studies that involved 774 people and assessed melatonin supplements for treating anxiety before surgery, anxiety after surgery, or both. The review found strong evidence that melatonin is better than a placebo at reducing anxiety before surgery. Melatonin supplements may be as effective as standard treatment (the antianxiety medicine midazolam). However, the results on melatonin's benefits for reducing anxiety after surgery were mixed.

## IS MELATONIN HELPFUL FOR PREVENTING OR TREATING COVID-19?

Current research looking at the effects of melatonin on COVID-19 is only in the early stages. There are a few randomized controlled trials (studies evaluating melatonin in people) in progress. At this point, it is too soon to reach conclusions on whether melatonin is helpful for COVID-19.

## DOES MELATONIN HELP WITH CANCER SYMPTOMS?

Studies of the effect of melatonin supplements on cancer symptoms or treatment-related side effects have been small and have had mixed results.

Keep in mind that unproven products should not be used to replace or delay conventional medical treatment for cancer. Also, some products can interfere with standard cancer treatments or have special risks for people who have been diagnosed with cancer. Before using any complementary health approach, including melatonin, people who have been diagnosed with cancer should talk with their health-care providers to make sure that all aspects of their care work together.

## CAN MELATONIN HELP WITH INSOMNIA?

People with insomnia have trouble falling asleep, staying asleep, or both. When symptoms last a month or longer, it is called "chronic insomnia."

According to practice guidelines from the AASM (2017) and the American College of Physicians (2016), there is not enough strong evidence on the effectiveness or safety of melatonin supplementation for chronic insomnia to recommend its use. The American College of Physicians guidelines strongly recommend the use of cognitive behavioral therapy for insomnia (CBT-I) as an initial treatment for insomnia.

## DOES MELATONIN WORK FOR SHIFT WORKERS?

Shift work that involves night shifts may cause people to feel sleepy at work and make it difficult to sleep during the daytime after a shift ends.

According to two 2014 research reviews, studies on whether melatonin supplements help shift workers were generally small or inconclusive.

- The first review looked at seven studies that included a total of 263 participants. The results suggested that people taking melatonin may sleep about 24 minutes longer during the daytime, but other aspects of sleep, such as the time needed to fall asleep, may not change. The evidence, however, was considered to be of low quality.

- The other review looked at eight studies (five of which were also in the first review), with a total of 300 participants, to see whether melatonin helped promote sleep in shift workers. Six of the studies were high quality, and they had inconclusive results. The review did not make any recommendations for melatonin use in shift workers.

## IS IT SAFE TO TAKE MELATONIN?

For melatonin supplements, particularly at doses higher than what the body normally produces, there is not enough information yet about possible side effects to have a clear picture of overall safety. Short-term use of melatonin supplements appears to be safe for most people, but information on the long-term safety of supplementing with melatonin is lacking.

- interactions with medicines
  - As with all dietary supplements, people who are taking medicine should consult their health-care providers before using melatonin. In particular, people with epilepsy and those taking blood thinner medications need to be under medical supervision when taking melatonin supplements.
- possible allergic reaction risk
  - There may be a risk of allergic reactions to melatonin supplements.
- safety concerns for pregnant and breastfeeding women
  - There has been a lack of research on the safety of melatonin use in pregnant or breastfeeding women.
- safety concerns for older people
  - The 2015 guidelines by the AASM recommend against melatonin use by people with dementia.
  - Melatonin may stay active in older people longer than in younger people and cause daytime drowsiness.

- melatonin regulated as a dietary supplement
  - In the United States, melatonin is considered a dietary supplement. This means that it is regulated less strictly by the U.S. Food and Drug Administration (FDA) than a prescription or over-the-counter (OTC) drug would be. In several other countries, melatonin is available only with a prescription and is considered a drug.
- products not containing what is listed on the label
  - Some melatonin supplements may not contain what is listed on the product label. A 2017 study tested 31 different melatonin supplements bought from grocery stores and pharmacies. For most of the supplements, the amount of melatonin in the product did not match what was listed on the product label. Also, 26 percent of the supplements contained serotonin, a hormone that can have harmful effects even at relatively low levels.

## IS MELATONIN SAFE FOR CHILDREN?

In addition to the issues mentioned above, there are some things to consider regarding melatonin's safety in children.

- Parents considering giving their children melatonin should first speak with a health-care provider about melatonin use in children.
- Parents need to ensure safe storage and appropriate use of melatonin supplements.
- Use of OTC melatonin might place children and teenagers at risk for accidental or intentional overdose.
  - A 2022 study indicated that U.S. sales of melatonin—which is widely available in tablet, capsule, liquid, and gummy formulations—increased by about 150 percent between 2016 and 2020. The study authors said that the increase in sales, availability, and widespread use of melatonin in the United States has likely resulted in increased access to melatonin among children in the home.

- The 2022 study also showed that the number of reports to U.S. poison control centers about people 19 years and younger who took melatonin increased from 8,337 in 2012 to 52,563 in 2021. Over the 10-year period, the number of reports increased each year. Hospitalizations and serious outcomes from melatonin ingestion by people 19 years and younger also increased over the 10 years. Most hospitalizations involved teenagers who had intentionally taken melatonin overdoses, and the largest increase in hospitalizations occurred in children five years and younger.
- Most of the calls to poison control centers (94.3%) were for children five years and younger who accidentally consumed melatonin products in their homes.
- Data from the calls show that most of the people who had taken melatonin (82.8%) did not have any symptoms. Among those who did have symptoms, gastrointestinal, cardiovascular, or symptoms related to the central nervous system (CNS) were the most common.
- Of the 4,097 people who were hospitalized over the 10-year period, 287 needed intensive care.
- Five individuals required mechanical ventilation, and two children younger than the age of two died, but the data from the poison control centers did not show whether the two deaths were caused by a melatonin overdose or another cause.

Melatonin supplements at normal doses appear to be safe for most children for short-term use, but there are not many studies on children and melatonin. Also, there is little information on the long-term effects of melatonin use in children. Because melatonin is a hormone, it is possible that melatonin supplements could affect hormonal development, including puberty, menstrual cycles, and overproduction of the hormone prolactin, but we do not know for sure.

Possible melatonin supplement side effects reported in children have usually been mild and have included the following:

- drowsiness
- increased bedwetting or urination in the evening
- headache
- dizziness
- agitation

## WHAT ARE THE SIDE EFFECTS OF MELATONIN?

A 2015 review on the safety of melatonin supplements indicated that only mild side effects were reported in various short-term studies that involved adults, surgical patients, and critically ill patients. Some of the mild side effects that were reported in the studies included the following:

- headache
- dizziness
- nausea
- sleepiness

The possible long-term side effects of melatonin use are unclear.

## TIPS TO CONSIDER

- Remember that even though the FDA regulates dietary supplements, such as melatonin, the regulations for dietary supplements are different and less strict than those for prescription or OTC drugs.
- Some dietary supplements may interact with medicines or pose risks if you have medical problems or are going to have surgery.
- If you are pregnant or nursing a child, it is especially important to see your health-care provider before taking any medicine or supplement, including melatonin.
- If you use dietary supplements, such as melatonin, read and follow label instructions. "Natural" does not always mean "safe."

- Take charge of your health—talk with your health-care providers about any complementary health approaches you use. Together, you can make shared, well-informed decisions.[4]

## Section 48.4 | Valerian

Valerian is a plant native to Europe and Asia; it also grows in North America. It has been used medicinally since the times of early Greece and Rome. Historically, valerian was used to treat insomnia, migraine, fatigue, and stomach cramps. Today, valerian is promoted for insomnia, anxiety, depression, premenstrual syndrome (PMS), menopause symptoms, and headaches. The roots and rhizomes (underground stems) of valerian are used for medicinal purposes.

## HOW MUCH DO YOU KNOW?

Knowledge about valerian is limited because a relatively small amount of research has looked at valerian's effects on various conditions.

## WHAT HAVE YOU LEARNED?

- The evidence on whether valerian is helpful for sleep problems is inconsistent. In its 2017 clinical practice guidelines, the American Academy of Sleep Medicine (AASM) recommended against using valerian for chronic insomnia in adults.
- Two small studies suggest that valerian might be helpful for menopausal symptoms, but there is not enough evidence to know for certain.

---

[4] "Melatonin: What You Need To Know," National Center for Complementary and Integrative Health (NCCIH), July 2022. Available online. URL: www.nccih.nih.gov/health/melatonin-what-you-need-to-know#hed2. Accessed May 4, 2023.

- There is not enough evidence to allow any conclusions about whether valerian is helpful for anxiety, depression, premenstrual syndrome, menstrual cramps, stress, or other conditions.

## WHAT DO YOU KNOW ABOUT SAFETY?

- Research suggests that valerian is generally safe for short-term use by most adults. It has been used with apparent safety in studies lasting up to 28 days. The safety of long-term use of valerian is unknown.
- Little is known about whether it is safe to use valerian during pregnancy or while breastfeeding.
- Side effects of valerian include headache, stomach upset, mental dullness, excitability, uneasiness, heart disturbances, and even insomnia in some people. A few people feel drowsy in the morning after taking valerian, especially at higher doses. Some people experience dry mouth or vivid dreams.
- Because it is possible (though not proven) that valerian might have a sleep-inducing effect, it should not be taken along with alcohol or sedatives.

## KEEP IN MIND

Take charge of your health—talk with your health-care providers about any complementary health approaches you use. Together, you can make shared, well-informed decisions.[5]

---

[5] "Valerian," National Center for Complementary and Integrative Health (NCCIH), October 1, 2020. Available online. URL: www.nccih.nih.gov/health/valerian. Accessed May 4, 2023.

# Part 6 | A Special Look at Pediatric and Teen Sleep Issues

# Chapter 49 | **Safe Sleep Cribs and Infant Products**

## HOW TO PUT YOUR BABY TO SLEEP SAFELY

If you just had a baby, are expecting, or are taking care of a young infant, it is important to create a safe sleep environment for your baby. Because babies spend much of their time sleeping, the nursery should be the safest room in the house. Take a few moments to learn about safe sleep.

### Bare Is Best

With any crib, bassinet, or play yard, follow a few simple rules to keep babies sleeping safely:
- To prevent suffocation, never place pillows or thick quilts in a baby's sleep environment.
- Make sure there are no gaps larger than two fingers between the sides of the crib and the mattress.
- Proper assembly of cribs is paramount. Follow the instructions provided and make sure that every part is installed correctly. If you are not sure, call the manufacturer for assistance.
- Do not use cribs older than 10 years or broken or modified cribs. Infants can strangle to death if their bodies pass through gaps between loose components or broken slats while their heads remain entrapped.
- Set up play yards properly according to manufacturers' directions. Only use the mattress pad provided with the play yard; do not add extra padding.

- Never place a crib near a window with blind, curtain cords, or baby monitor cords; babies can strangle on cords.

## WHAT IS A FULL-SIZE BABY CRIB?

A full-size crib is a bed that:
- is designed to provide sleeping accommodations for an infant
- is intended for use in the home, in a childcare facility, in a family childcare home, or in places of public accommodation affecting commerce
- has interior dimensions of 28 ± 5/8 inches (71 ± 1.6 cm) in width x 52 3/8 ± 5/8 inches (133 ± 1.6 cm) in length

## WHAT ARE THE REQUIREMENTS FOR FULL-SIZE CRIBS?

The standard prohibits traditional drop sides and has stringent requirements for various parts of the crib, such as mattress supports, slats, and hardware. More specifically, the principal requirements for full-size cribs include the following:
- **Dynamic impact testing of the mattress support system**. This testing is intended to address incidents involving the collapse or failure of mattress support systems.
- **Impact testing of side rails and slat strength/ integrity testing**. This testing is intended to prevent slats and spindles from breaking and/or detaching during use.
- **Mattress support system testing**. This testing is intended to ensure that the mattress support does not become detached from the frame, potentially resulting in a fall.
- **Latching mechanism tests**. These tests are intended to ensure that latching and locking mechanisms work as intended, preventing unintended folding while in use.
- **Crib side configurations**. This is intended, in part, to limit movable (drop) sides and addresses the numerous incidents related to drop-side failures.

- **Label requirements**. These requirements cover numerous hazards, such as falls from the crib, suffocation on soft bedding, and strangulation on strings and cords.
- **Openings requirement for mattress support systems**. This addresses gaps in the mattress support system to reduce the possibility of entrapment.
- **Requirements for wood screws and other fasteners**. This eliminates the use of wood screws that serve as the primary method of attachment on key structural elements and also includes other fastener requirements to address incidents related to loose hardware and poor structural integrity.
- **Cyclic testing**. This testing addresses incidents involving hardware loosening and poor structural integrity.
- **Improper assembly issues**. This addresses the need to make it impossible to improperly assemble key elements or that those elements have markings that make it obvious when they have been assembled improperly.
- **Test requirement for accessories**. This is intended to address any cribs that, now or maybe in the future, include accessories, such as bassinets or changing tables.
- **Component spacing**. This is intended to prevent child entrapment between uniformly and nonuniformly spaced components, such as slats.

## WHAT IS A NON-FULL-SIZE BABY CRIB?

A non-full-size crib is a bed designed to provide sleeping accommodations for an infant, in or around the home, for travel, in a childcare facility, in a family childcare home, in a place of public accommodation affecting commerce, and for other purposes. A non-full-size crib has an interior length dimension that is either greater than 139.7 cm (55 inches) or smaller than 126.3 cm (49 3/4 inches) or an interior width dimension either greater than 77.7 cm (30 5/8 inches) or smaller than 64.3 cm (25 3/8 inches), or both. A non-full-size crib is either smaller or larger than a regular full-size crib and includes the following:

- a crib designed to be folded or collapsed without being taken apart so that it has a smaller volume than when it is in use
- a crib pen (with hard sides) that has legs that can be removed to make a playpen for a child
- a circular, hexagonal, or other unconventionally shaped cribs that have special mattresses or other unconventional parts
- a crib that does not include mesh/net/screen cribs, nonrigidly constructed cribs, cradles, car beds, baby baskets, and bassinets (Other U.S. Consumer Product Safety Commission (CPSC) standards may apply to these products.)

## WHAT ARE THE REQUIREMENTS FOR NON-FULL-SIZE CRIBS?

The principal requirements for non-full-size cribs are as follows:

- **Dynamic impact testing of the mattress support system**. This testing is intended to address incidents involving the collapse or failure of mattress support systems.
- **Impact testing of side rails and slat strength/ integrity testing**. This testing is intended to prevent slats and spindles from breaking and/or detaching during use.
- **Mattress support system testing**. This testing is intended to ensure that the mattress support does not become detached from the frame, potentially resulting in a fall.
- **Latching mechanism tests**. These tests are intended to ensure that latching and locking mechanisms work as intended, preventing unintended folding while in use, and also require that latching mechanisms be used with drop gates and movable sides.
- **Crib side configurations**. This is intended, in part, to limit movable (drop) sides and addresses the numerous incidents related to drop-side failures.

- **Label requirements**. These requirements cover numerous hazards, such as falls from the crib, suffocation on soft bedding, and strangulation on strings and cords.
- **Openings requirement for mattress support systems**. This addresses gaps in the mattress support system to minimize the possibility of entrapment.
- **Requirements for wood screws and other fasteners**. These requirements address hazards that exist when wood screws are the primary method of attachment and also include other fastener requirements to address incidents related to loose hardware and poor structural integrity.
- **Cyclic testing**. This testing addresses incidents involving hardware loosening and poor structural integrity.
- **Misassembly issues**. This addresses the need to make it impossible to misassemble key elements, or those elements must have markings that make it obvious when they have been misassembled.
- **Test requirement for accessories**. This is intended to address any cribs that, now or maybe in the future, include accessories, such as bassinets or changing tables.
- **Component spacing**. This testing is intended to prevent child entrapment between both uniformly and nonuniformly spaced components, such as slats.[1]

## CRIB SAFETY TIPS

For infants under 12 months of age, follow these practices to reduce the risk of sudden infant death syndrome (SIDS) and prevent suffocation.

---

[1] "Safe Sleep—Cribs and Infant Products," U.S. Consumer Product Safety Commission (CPSC), October 3, 2022. Available online. URL: www.cpsc.gov/SafeSleep. Accessed May 8, 2023.

## How to Use a Crib

- Place the baby on her/his back in a crib with a firm, tight-fitting mattress.
- Do not put pillows, quilts, comforters, sheepskins, pillow-like bumper pads, or pillow-like stuffed toys in the crib.
- Consider using a sleeper instead of a blanket.
- If you do use a blanket, place the baby with feet to the foot of the crib. Tuck a thin blanket around the crib mattress, covering the baby only as high as her/his chest.
- Use only a fitted bottom sheet specifically made for crib use.

## Check Your Crib for Safety

There should be:

- a firm, tight-fitting mattress so a baby cannot get trapped between the mattress and the crib
- no missing, loose, broken or improperly installed screws, brackets or other hardware on the crib, or mattress support
- no more than 2.38 inches (about the width of a soda can) between crib slats so a baby's body cannot fit through the slats and no missing or cracked slats
- no corner posts over 1/16th inch high so a baby's clothing cannot catch
- no cutouts in the headboard or footboard so a baby's head cannot get trapped

Cribs that are incorrectly assembled or have missing, loose, or broken hardware or broken slats can result in entrapment or suffocation deaths. Infants can become strangled when their head and neck become entrapped in gaps created by missing, loose, or broken hardware or broken slats.

For mesh-sided cribs or playpens, look for:

- mesh less than 1/4 inch in size, smaller than the tiny buttons on a baby's clothing
- mesh with no tears, holes, or loose threads that could entangle a baby

- mesh securely attached to the top rail and floor plate
- top rail cover with no tears or holes
- if staples are used, they are not missing, loose, or exposed[2]

## RECOMMENDATIONS FOR PARENTS/CAREGIVERS ABOUT THE USE OF BABY PRODUCTS

The U.S. Food and Drug Administration (FDA) cautions parents and caregivers against purchasing baby products with claims to prevent or reduce the chance of SIDS (sometimes called "sudden unexpected infant death" or "SUID"). These baby products can pose a risk of serious injury to a baby, including the risk of suffocation.

Common baby products with these claims include:
- infant sleep positioners—these products should not be used due to the risk of serious harm
- baby monitors
- mattresses
- crib tents
- pillows
- crib bedding, including bumpers and blankets

## What Should Parents/Caregivers Know about These Baby Products?

- Do not use infant positioners—they could harm your baby. These freestanding devices are placed in the crib or bassinet and are intended to hold an infant on their side or back while sleeping. The most common types of sleep positioners feature bolsters attached to each side of a thin mat and wedges to elevate the baby's head.
  - The FDA is aware of infant deaths from these products over the years. Infants may suffocate after rolling from a side to stomach position or after being placed on

---

[2] "Crib Safety Tips," U.S. Consumer Product Safety Commission (CPSC), October 3, 2022. Available online. URL: www.cpsc.gov/safety-education/safety-guides/cribs/crib-safety-tips. Accessed May 8, 2023.

their sides in the positioning product. Even if placed properly on their backs, infants may scoot up or downward on the positioning device and may become entrapped in the product or between the positioning device and the crib, play yard, sleep mat, or bassinet.

- Infant positioning products pose a risk of suffocation whether or not they make medical claims.

- The FDA is not aware of any clinical or scientific evidence that shows that currently available baby products prevent or reduce the chance of SIDS.

- Be aware that any product that claims to prevent or reduce the chance of SIDS has never been cleared or approved for that use by the FDA.

- The FDA discourages consumers from purchasing any product claiming to reduce a baby's SIDS risk. These products are not proven to prevent SIDS.

- Always check with your health-care professional before using any new medical product for your baby.[3]

[3] "Recommendations for Parents/Caregivers about the Use of Baby Products," U.S. Food and Drug Administration (FDA), May 3, 2023. Available online. URL: https://fda.gov/medical-devices/baby-products-sids-prevention-claims/recommendations-parentscaregivers-about-use-baby-products. Accessed May 8, 2023.

# Chapter 50 | Infants and Sleep-Related Concerns

There are about 3,500 sleep-related deaths among U.S. babies each year, including sudden infant death syndrome (SIDS), accidental suffocation, and deaths from unknown causes.

In the 1990s, there were sharp declines in sleep-related deaths following the national "Back to Sleep" safe sleep campaign. However, the declines have slowed since the late 1990s, and data from a Vital Signs (www.cdc.gov/vitalsigns/index.html) report from the Centers for Disease Control and Prevention (CDC) shows that the risk for babies persists.

"Unfortunately, too many babies in this country are lost to sleep-related deaths that might be prevented," said the CDC's Director, Brenda Fitzgerald, M.D. "We must do more to ensure every family knows the American Academy of Pediatrics (AAP) recommendations—babies should sleep on their backs, without any toys or soft bedding, and in their own crib. Parents are encouraged to share a room with the baby but not the same bed. These strategies will help reduce the risk and protect our babies from harm."

## UNSAFE SLEEP

For the Vital Signs report, the CDC analyzed Pregnancy Risk Assessment Monitoring System (PRAMS) data to describe sleep practices for babies. PRAMS, a state-based surveillance system, has monitored self-reported behaviors and experiences before, during, and after pregnancy among women with a recent U.S. live birth since the late 1980s.

The CDC examined 2015 data reported by mothers about unsafe sleep positioning, any bed sharing, and the use of soft bedding from states with available data. Unsafe sleep positioning means placing the baby on her or his side or stomach to sleep. Soft bedding includes pillows, blankets, bumper pads, stuffed toys, and sleep positioners.

In 2015, within states included in the analysis, the following are the results:

- About one in five mothers (21.6%) reported placing their baby to sleep on their side or stomach; more than half of the mothers (61.4%) reported any bed sharing with their baby, and two in five mothers (38.5%) reported using any soft bedding in the baby's sleep area.
- The percentage of mothers who reported placing their baby on her or his side or stomach to sleep varied by state, ranging from 12.2 percent in Wisconsin to 33.8 percent in Louisiana.
- Placing babies on their side or stomach to sleep was more common among mothers who were non-Hispanic Black, younger than 25 years of age, or had 12 or fewer years of education.

## SAFE SLEEP

Safe sleep practices recommended by the AAP include the following:

- placing the baby on her or his back at all sleep times—including naps and at night
- using a firm sleep surface, such as a safety-approved mattress and crib
- keeping soft objects and loose bedding out of the baby's sleep area
- sharing a room with the baby but not the same bed

"This report shows that we need to do better at promoting and following safe sleep recommendations," said Jennifer Bombard, M.S.P.H., scientist in the CDC's Division of Reproductive Health (DRH) and lead author of the analysis. "This is particularly important for populations where data show infants may be at a higher risk of sleep-related deaths."

The state public health agencies have worked with partners to promote safe sleep. These efforts include communication campaigns, messages shared during visits through Women, Infants, and Children (WIC) and through home-visiting programs; safe sleep policies; and quality improvement initiatives in hospitals and childcare centers.

Health-care providers can increase the likelihood that parents follow AAP recommendations by giving them accurate advice about safe sleep for babies. A previous study shows that only 55 percent of mothers have reported receiving correct advice about safe sleep during pregnancy and baby care visits, while 20 percent say they get no advice and 25 percent report getting incorrect advice.[1]

## INFANT SLEEP POSITIONERS AND THE RISK OF SUFFOCATION

The U.S. Food and Drug Administration (FDA) is reminding parents and caregivers not to put babies in sleep positioners. These products—sometimes also called "nests" or "antiroll" products—can cause suffocation (a struggle to breathe) that can lead to death.

The FDA regulates baby products as medical devices if, among other things, the manufacturer claims that the product is intended to cure, mitigate, treat, prevent, or reduce a disease or condition in its labeling, packaging, or advertising. A number of sleep positioners are considered medical devices because of their intended use. (This intended use can be outlined by statements made on the labels, labeling, instructions for use, or promotional materials for the products.)

Sleep positioners that do not meet the definition of a medical device may be regulated by the U.S. Consumer Product Safety Commission (CPSC). Some types of sleep positioners can feature raised supports or pillows (called "bolsters") that are attached to each side of a mat or a wedge to raise a baby's head. Products called

---

[1] "About 3,500 Babies in the US Are Lost to Sleep-Related Deaths Each Year," Centers for Disease Control and Prevention (CDC), January 9, 2018. Available online. URL: www.cdc.gov/media/releases/2018/p0109-sleep-related-deaths.html. Accessed May 8, 2023.

"nests" can feature soft, wall-like structures that surround the base. The positioners claim to keep a baby in a specific position while sleeping and are often used for babies under six months of age.

To reduce the risk of sleep-related infant deaths, including accidental suffocation and SIDS, the AAP recommends that infants sleep on their backs, positioned on a firm, empty surface. This surface should not contain soft objects, toys, pillows, or loose bedding.

## About Infant Suffocation and Other Dangers

Each year, about 4,000 infants die unexpectedly during sleep time from accidental suffocation, SIDS, or unknown causes, according to the *Eunice Kennedy Shriver* National Institute of Child Health and Human Development (NICHD).

The federal government has received reports about babies who have died from suffocation associated with their sleep positioners. In most of these cases, the babies suffocated after rolling from their sides to their stomachs.

In addition to reports about deaths, the federal government has also received reports about babies who were placed on their backs or sides in positioners but were later found in other dangerous positions within or next to these products.

To avoid these dangers, remember the following:
- The safest crib is a bare crib.
- Always put babies on their backs to sleep.

## SAFETY ADVICE

The following advice is for putting babies to sleep safely:
- Never use infant sleep positioners. Using this type of product to hold an infant on her or his side or back is dangerous.
- Never put pillows, blankets, loose sheets, comforters, or quilts under a baby or in a crib. These products can also be dangerous. Babies do not need pillows, and adequate clothing—instead of blankets—can keep them warm.
- Always keep cribs and sleeping areas bare. It means you should also never put soft objects or toys in sleeping areas.

- Always place a baby on her or his back at night and during nap time. An easy way to remember this is to follow the ABCs of safe sleep: "Alone on the Back in a bare Crib."

## Beware of Medical Claims about Sleep Positioners

Some manufacturers have advertised that their sleep positioners prevent SIDS; gastroesophageal reflux disease (GERD), in which stomach acids back up into the esophagus; or fat head syndrome (plagiocephaly), a deformation caused by pressure on one part of the skull.

Here are a few facts:

- The FDA has never cleared an infant sleep positioner that claims to prevent or reduce the risk of SIDS.
- The FDA had previously cleared some infant positioners for GERD or flat head syndrome.
- In 2010, the FDA became aware of infant positioners being marketed with SIDS claims and notified manufacturers to stop marketing these devices and submit information to support FDA clearance.

The FDA intends to take action against device manufacturers who make unproven medical claims about their products. You can do your part to keep your baby safe by not using sleep positioners.

You can report an incident or injury from an infant sleep positioner to the FDA's MedWatch program. Finally, if you have questions about how to safely put a baby to sleep or how to avoid or treat certain health issues, talk to your health-care provider.[2]

## HELPING BABIES SLEEP SAFELY

Expecting or caring for a baby? Take these steps to help your baby sleep safely and reduce the risk of sleep-related infant deaths, including SIDS.

---

[2] "Do Not Use Infant Sleep Positioners due to the Risk of Suffocation," U.S. Food and Drug Administration (FDA), April 18, 2019. Available online. URL: www.fda.gov/consumers/consumer-updates/do-not-use-infant-sleep-posi-tioners-due-risk-suffocation. Accessed May 9, 2023.

There are about 3,400 sleep-related deaths among U.S. babies each year. The CDC supports the recommendations issued by the AAP to reduce the risk of all sleep-related infant deaths, including SIDS.

Parents and caregivers can help create a safe sleep area for babies by taking the following steps:

- Place your baby on her or his back for all sleep times—naps and at night. Even if a baby spits up during sleep, babies' anatomy and gag reflexes help prevent them from choking while sleeping on their backs. Babies who sleep on their backs are much less likely to die of SIDS than babies who sleep on their sides or stomachs.

- Use a firm, flat (not at an angle or inclined) sleep surface, such as a mattress in a safety-approved crib covered only by a fitted sheet. Some parents and caretakers might feel they should place their baby on a soft surface to help them be more comfortable while sleeping. However, soft surfaces can increase the risk of sleep-related death. A firm sleep surface helps reduce the risk of SIDS and suffocation.

- Keep your baby's sleep area (e.g., a crib or bassinet) in the same room where you sleep, ideally until your baby is at least six months old. Accidental suffocation or strangulation can happen when a baby is sleeping in an adult bed or other unsafe sleep surfaces. Sharing a room with your baby is much safer than bed sharing and may decrease the risk of SIDS by as much as 50 percent. Also, placing the crib close to your bed so that the baby is within view and reach can also help make it easier to feed, comfort, and monitor your baby.

- Keep soft bedding such as blankets, pillows, bumper pads, and soft toys out of your baby's sleep area. Additionally, do not cover your baby's head or allow your baby to get too hot. Some parents may feel they should add sheets or blankets to their baby's crib to help keep their baby warm and comfortable while sleeping. However, sheets, comforters, and blankets can increase the risk of suffocation or overheat your baby. If you are worried about your baby getting cold during sleep, you can dress them in sleep clothing, such as a wearable blanket.[3]

[3] "Helping Babies Sleep Safely," Centers for Disease Control and Prevention (CDC), June 28, 2022. Available online. URL: www.cdc.gov/reproductivehealth/features/baby-safe-sleep/index.html. Accessed May 8, 2023.

# Chapter 51 | **Sudden Infant Death Syndrome**

## WHAT IS SUDDEN INFANT DEATH SYNDROME?

Sudden infant death syndrome (SIDS) is the sudden, unexplained death of a baby younger than one year of age that does not have a known cause even after a complete investigation. This investigation includes performing a complete autopsy, examining the death scene, and reviewing the clinical history.

When a baby dies, health-care providers, law enforcement personnel, and communities try to find out why. They ask questions, examine the baby, gather information, and run tests. If they cannot find a cause for the death and if the baby is younger than one year old, the medical examiner or coroner will call the death SIDS.

If there is still some uncertainty as to the cause after it is determined to be fully unexplained, then the medical examiner or coroner might leave the cause of death as "unknown."

## WHAT CAUSES SUDDEN INFANT DEATH SYNDROME?

Scientists and health-care providers are working very hard to find the cause or causes of SIDS. If we know the cause or causes, someday, we might be able to prevent SIDS from happening at all.

More and more research evidence suggests that infants who die from SIDS are born with brain abnormalities or defects. These defects are typically found within a network of nerve cells that send signals to other nerve cells. The cells are located in the part of the brain that probably controls breathing, heart rate, blood pressure, temperature, and waking from sleep. At the present time, there is no way to identify babies who have these abnormalities, but researchers are working to develop specific screening tests.

But scientists believe that brain defects alone may not be enough to cause an SIDS death. Evidence suggests that other events must also occur for an infant to die from SIDS. Researchers use the triple-risk model to explain this concept. In this model, all three factors have to occur at the same time for an infant to die from SIDS. Having only one of these factors may not be enough to cause death from SIDS, but when all three combine, the chances of SIDS are high. Even though the exact cause of SIDS is unknown, there are ways to reduce the risk of SIDS and other sleep-related causes of infant death.[1]

## MYTHS AND FACTS ABOUT SUDDEN INFANT DEATH SYNDROME AND SAFE INFANT SLEEP

- **Myth**: Babies can "catch" SIDS.
  **Fact**: A baby cannot catch SIDS. SIDS is not caused by an infection, so it cannot be caught or spread.
- **Myth**: Cribs cause "crib death" or SIDS.
  **Fact**: Cribs themselves do not cause SIDS. But features of the sleep environment—such as a soft sleep surface—can increase the risk of SIDS and other sleep-related causes of infant death. Find out more about what is a safe sleep environment for your baby.
- **Myth**: Babies who sleep on their backs will choke if they spit up or vomit during sleep.
  **Fact**: Babies automatically cough up or swallow fluid that they spit up or vomit—it is a reflex to keep the airway clear. Studies show no increase in the number of deaths from choking among babies who sleep on their backs. In fact, babies who sleep on their backs might clear these fluids better because of the way the body is built.

---

[1] "What Is SIDS?" *Eunice Kennedy Shriver* National Institute of Child Health and Human Development (NICHD), December 29, 2017. Available online. URL: https://safetosleep.nichd.nih.gov/safesleepbasics/SIDS. Accessed May 15, 2023.

## Sudden Infant Death Syndrome

- **Myth**: SIDS can be prevented.
  **Fact**: There is no known way to prevent SIDS, but there are effective ways to reduce the risk of SIDS.
- **Myth**: Shots, vaccines, immunizations, and medicines cause SIDS.
  **Fact**: Recent evidence suggests that shots for vaccines may have a protective effect against SIDS. All babies should see their health-care providers regularly for well-baby checkups and should get their shots on time as recommended by their health-care provider.
- **Myth**: SIDS can occur in babies at any age.
  **Fact**: Babies are at risk of SIDS only until they are one year old. Most SIDS deaths occur when babies are between one month and four months of age. SIDS is not a health concern for babies older than one year of age.
- **Myth**: If parents sleep with their babies in the same bed, they will hear any problems and be able to prevent them from happening.
  **Fact**: Because SIDS occurs with no warning or symptoms, it is unlikely that any adult will hear a problem and prevent SIDS from occurring. Sleeping with a baby in an adult bed increases the risk of suffocation and other sleep-related causes of infant death.

Sleeping with a baby in an adult bed is even more dangerous when:
- the adult smokes cigarettes or has consumed alcohol or medication that causes drowsiness
- the baby shares a bed with other children
- the sleep surface is a couch, sofa, waterbed, or armchair
- there are pillows or blankets on the bed
- the baby is younger than 11–14 weeks of age
- the baby shares a bed with more than one person, especially if sleeping between two adults

Instead of bed-sharing, health-care providers recommend room-sharing—keeping the baby's sleep area separate from your sleep area in the same room where you sleep. Room-sharing is known to reduce the risk of SIDS and other sleep-related causes of infant death.[2]

## SUDDEN INFANT DEATH SYNDROME AND VACCINES

Vaccines have not been shown to cause SIDS. Babies receive multiple vaccines when they are between two and four months old. This age range is also the peak age for SIDS. The timing of the two- and four-month shots and SIDS has led some people to question whether they might be related. However, studies have found that vaccines do not cause and are not linked to SIDS.

Multiple research studies and safety reviews have looked at possible links between vaccines and SIDS. The evidence accumulated over many years do not show any links between childhood immunization and SIDS.[3]

[2] "Myths and Facts about SIDS and Safe Infant Sleep," *Eunice Kennedy Shriver* National Institute of Child Health and Human Development (NICHD), December 29, 2017. Available online. URL: https://safetosleep.nichd.nih.gov/safesleepbasics/mythsfacts. Accessed May 9, 2023.
[3] "Sudden Infant Death Syndrome (SIDS) and Vaccines," Centers for Disease Control and Prevention (CDC), August 14, 2020. Available online. URL: www.cdc.gov/vaccinesafety/concerns/sids.html. Accessed May 15, 2023.

# Chapter 52 | **Schools Start Too Early**

Not getting enough sleep is common among high school students and is associated with several health risks, including being overweight, drinking alcohol, smoking tobacco, and using drugs, as well as poor academic performance. One of the reasons adolescents do not get enough sleep is early school start times. The American Academy of Pediatrics (AAP) has recommended that middle and high schools start at 8:30 a.m. or later to give students the opportunity to get the amount of sleep they need, but most American adolescents start school too early.

According to the 2014 School Health Policies and Practices Study (SHPPS), 93 percent of high schools and 83 percent of middle schools in the United States started before 8:30 a.m.

An earlier Centers for Disease Control and Prevention (CDC) study that analyzed U.S. Department of Education (ED) data from the 2011 to 2012 school year reported the following results:

- Forty-two states reported that most (75–100%) public middle and high schools started before 8:30 a.m.
- The percentage of schools starting at 8:30 a.m. or later varied greatly by state. For example:
  - No schools in Hawaii, Mississippi, and Wyoming started after 8:30 a.m.
  - Most schools in North Dakota (78%) and Alaska (76%) started after 8:30 a.m.

## ADOLESCENTS AND SLEEP

The American Academy of Sleep Medicine (AASM) recommends that teenagers aged 13–18 years should regularly sleep 8–10 hours per day for good health. Adolescents who do not get enough sleep are more likely to:

- be overweight
- not engage in daily physical activity
- suffer from symptoms of depression
- engage in unhealthy risk behaviors such as drinking, smoking tobacco, and using illicit drugs
- perform poorly in school

During puberty, adolescents become sleepy later at night and need to sleep later in the morning as a result of shifts in biological rhythms. These biological changes are often combined with poor sleep habits (including irregular bedtimes and the presence of electronics in the bedroom). During the school week, school start times are the main reason students wake up when they do. The combination of late bedtimes and early school start times results in most adolescents not getting enough sleep.

## EVERYONE CAN PLAY AN IMPORTANT ROLE
### Parents

- Model and encourage habits that help promote good sleep:
  - Set a regular bedtime and rise time, including on weekends. This is recommended for everyone—children, adolescents, and adults alike. Adolescents with parent-set bedtimes usually get more sleep than those whose parents do not set bedtimes.
  - Dim the lighting. Adolescents who are exposed to more light (such as room lighting or light from electronics) in the evening are less likely to get enough sleep.
  - Start a "media curfew." Technology use (computers, video gaming, or mobile phones) may also contribute to late bedtimes. Parents should consider banning technology use after a certain time or removing these technologies from the bedroom.

- Contact local school officials about later school start times. Some commonly mentioned barriers to keep in mind are potential increases in transportation costs and scheduling difficulties.

## Health-Care Professionals

- Educate adolescent patients and their parents about the importance of adequate sleep and the factors that contribute to insufficient sleep among adolescents.

## School Officials

- Learn more about the research connecting sleep and school start times. Good sleep hygiene, in combination with later school times, will enable adolescents to be healthier and better academic achievers.[1]

---

[1] "Schools Start Too Early," Centers for Disease Control and Prevention (CDC), October 5, 2022. Available online. URL: www.cdc.gov/sleep/features/schools-start-too-early.html. Accessed May 8, 2023.

# Chapter 53 | **Pediatric Movement Disorders in Sleep**

Babies between the ages of six and nine months sometimes begin to exhibit repetitive, rhythmic movements as part of the process of going to sleep. Some of the most common movements include body rocking, head rolling, and head banging. Children who exhibit these behaviors may roll their heads forcefully from side to side, rise up on their hands and knees, and rock back and forth vigorously, or bang their heads repeatedly on a mattress, pillow, headboard, or side rail.

Although these violent movements can be alarming for parents and caregivers to witness, they are quite common and usually harmless and tend to disappear gradually by the age of two or three. Parents often express concerns that head banging or body rocking will result in injury or brain damage, but this is rarely the case. In addition, many parents worry that these repetitive behaviors may indicate a developmental disability, yet they occur frequently among normal children. Parents should consult a pediatrician if the behaviors persist for more than a few months or if the child nods or shakes their head frequently at other times, does not interact with other people, or shows evidence of developmental delays.

Researchers are not certain why children engage in body rocking, head rolling, and head banging. They have determined that the behaviors occur three times more often in boys than in girls, and most children outgrow the habit before they reach three years of age. Some experts believe that rocking offers babies comfort or pleasure because it simulates being carried in the womb or in a parent's arms. Others theorize that the behaviors are part of the natural process of mastering movement and gaining control of the body. Some claim that rhythmic motion helps babies release stress, tension, or unspent energy and relax before going to sleep. For other children, head banging may provide a distraction from teething pain or an outlet for frustration or anger.

## COPING WITH REPETITIVE MOVEMENTS

Body rocking, head banging, and head rolling can be distressing for parents and caregivers. In addition to feeling concerned for the child's well-being, they may also feel frustrated or irritated by the noise or damage to furniture or walls. It is important to remember that babies who rock or bang their heads will usually fall asleep within a short time. Since most children simply outgrow the behavior over time, the easiest approach may be to do nothing and wait for it to go away. Reacting to the repetitive movements—even in a negative way—sometimes tends to reinforce the behavior. Other tips for dealing with body rocking, head rolling, and head banging at bedtime include the following:

- Engage in a relaxing bedtime routine that includes quiet time, cuddling, songs, nursery rhymes, or a story.
- Place a mobile above the bed or an activity center on the side of the crib to provide interest and distraction.
- Play soft, soothing music or white noise in the bedroom to promote relaxation.
- Ensure that the child does not spend too much time in bed before it is time to sleep.
- Check to make sure the child is not experiencing pain from teething, an ear infection, allergies, or other sources.
- Use a padded bumper on crib rails or headboards.
- Pull the bed away from the wall and put a thick carpet or rubber pad under the legs—or put the mattress on the floor—to reduce movement and noise.
- Try changing the bedroom in which the child sleeps.

## References

"Body-Rocking, Head-Rolling, and Head-Banging at Bedtime," Raising Children Network, August 25, 2014. Available online. URL: https://raisingchildren.net.au/preschoolers/sleep/night-time-problems/body-rocking-head-rolling-head-banging. Accessed April 25, 2023.

"Body-Rocking, Head-Rolling, and Head-Banging in Babies," World of Moms, October 10, 2014. Available online. URL: www.worldofmoms.com/articles/body-rocking-head-rolling-and-head-banging-in-babies/313/2. Accessed April 25, 2023.

"Guide to Your Child's Symptoms: Rocking/Head Banging," American Academy of Pediatrics (AAP), 2001. Available online. URL: www.springspediatrics.com/headbanging.htm. Accessed April 25, 2023.

# Chapter 54 | **Tonsil Surgery Improves Some Behaviors in Children with Sleep Apnea Syndrome**

A study funded by the National Institutes of Health (NIH) found that children with sleep apnea syndrome who have their tonsils and adenoids removed sleep better, are less restless and impulsive, and report a generally better quality of life (QOL). However, the study found that cognitive abilities did not improve when compared with children who did not have surgery, and researchers say that the findings do not mean surgery is an automatic first choice.

"This is the first rigorous, controlled evaluation of a commonly performed treatment for childhood sleep apnea, in terms of looking at functional outcomes," said Susan Shurin, M.D., a pediatrician and deputy director of the NIH's National Heart, Lung, and Blood Institute (NHLBI). "This study provides additional data that can help parents and providers make more informed decisions about treating children with this disorder, and it identifies additional areas of research."

Obstructive sleep apnea (OSA) syndrome is a common disorder in which the airway becomes blocked during sleep, causing shallow breathing or breathing pauses. The sleep disturbances that result can lead to many issues in children, including learning difficulties and behavioral problems.

Enlarged or swollen tonsils are a major risk factor for pediatric sleep apnea syndrome, and surgery to remove them and the nearby adenoid can help open up blocked airways. Over 500,000 adenotonsillectomies are performed annually on children, primarily for sleep apnea. However, the extent that surgery can improve cognition and behavior previously had not been rigorously studied.

The Childhood Adenotonsillectomy Trial (CHAT) enrolled 464 children between the ages of five and nine with OSA syndrome from seven sleep centers across the United States and randomly assigned them into two groups. One received adenoid and tonsil surgery within a month after enrollment, while the other received supportive medical care and careful monitoring or watchful waiting. At enrollment, both groups of children were evaluated by psychometricians—people trained to administer and interpret psychological tests—on their cognition (primarily attention and organizational skills); they were also evaluated by caregivers and teachers on their behavior and QOL, and they had sleep studies to assess their breathing and sleep parameters. After seven months, the children were reevaluated.

The researchers found no differences in cognitive skills between the two groups, but the children who underwent surgery showed improved sleep quality, behavioral regulation, and QOL measures, such as being more active and experiencing less daytime sleepiness. Beneficial effects were observed even among overweight children, in whom there has been particular uncertainty about the role of surgery in sleep apnea treatment.

Overall, 79 percent of children in the surgery group had a resolution of their sleep apnea after seven months, compared to 46 percent in the watchful waiting group.

"While more of the children who underwent early surgery had improvements in their sleep apnea measures, nearly half of the children without surgery also had improvements during the seven months of observation," said senior author Susan Redline, M.D., M.P.H., of Brigham and Women's Hospital and Beth Israel Deaconess Medical Center, both in Boston. "This and the lack of significant cognitive decline in the watchful waiting group suggest that reassessing a child after a period of observation may be a valid therapeutic option for some children, especially those with mild symptoms."

Dr. Redline added that these results should not be applied to children with the most severe sleep apnea syndrome or very young children, who were not included in this study.[1]

[1] "Tonsil Surgery Improves Some Behaviors in Children with Sleep Apnea Syndrome," National Heart, Lung, and Blood Institute (NHLBI), May 21, 2013. Available online. URL: www.nhlbi.nih.gov/news/2013/tonsil-surgery-im-proves-some-behaviors-children-sleep-apnea-syndrome. Accessed May 9, 2023.

# Chapter 55 | **Bed-Wetting**

Children may have a bladder control problem—also called "urinary incontinence" (UI)—if they leak urine by accident and are past the age of toilet training. A child may not stay dry during the day, called "daytime wetting," or through the night, called "bed-wetting."

Children normally gain control over their bladders somewhere between the ages of two and four—each in their own time. Occasional wetting is common even in children between the ages of four and six. By four years of age, when most children stay dry during the day, daytime wetting can be very upsetting and embarrassing. By five or six years of age, children might have a bed-wetting problem if the bed is wet once or twice a week over a few months.

Most bladder control problems disappear naturally as children grow older. When needed, a health-care professional can check for conditions that may lead to wetting.

Loss of urine is almost never due to laziness, a strong will, emotional problems, or poor toilet training. Parents and caregivers should always approach this problem with understanding and patience.

## WHAT ARE THE TYPES OF BLADDER CONTROL PROBLEMS IN CHILDREN?

Children usually have one of two main bladder control problems:
- daytime wetting, also called "diurnal enuresis"
- bed-wetting, also called "nocturnal enuresis"

Some children may have trouble controlling their bladders both day and night.

591

## Daytime Wetting

For infants and toddlers, wetting is a normal part of development. Children gradually learn to control their bladders as they grow older. Problems that can occur during this process and lead to daytime wetting include the following:

- **Holding urine too long**. Your child's bladder can overfill and leak urine.
- **Overactive bladder**. Your child's bladder squeezes without warning, causing frequent runs for the toilet and wet clothes.
- **Underactive bladder**. Your child uses the toilet only a few times a day, with little urge to do so. Children may have a weak or interrupted stream of urine.
- **Disordered urination**. Your child's bladder muscles and nerves do not work together smoothly. Certain muscles cut off urine flow too soon. Urine left in the bladder may leak.

## Bed-Wetting

Children who wet the bed fall into two groups: those who have never been dry at night and those who started wetting the bed again after staying dry for six months.[1]

## HOW COMMON IS URINARY INCONTINENCE IN CHILDREN?

By five years of age, more than 90 percent of children can control urination during the day. Nighttime wetting is more common than daytime wetting in children, affecting 30 percent of 4-year-olds. The condition resolves itself in about 15 percent of children each year; about 10 percent of 7-year-olds, 3 percent of 12-year-olds, and 1 percent of 18-year-olds continue to experience nighttime wetting.

---

[1] "Definition & Facts for Bladder Control Problems and Bedwetting in Children," National Institute of Diabetes and Digestive and Kidney Diseases (NIDDK), September 2017. Available online. URL: www.niddk.nih.gov/health-information/urologic-diseases/bladder-control-problems-bedwetting-children/definition-facts. Accessed May 9, 2023.

# WHAT CAUSES NIGHTTIME URINARY INCONTINENCE?

The exact cause of most cases of nighttime UI is not known. Though a few cases are caused by structural problems in the urinary tract, most cases probably result from a mix of factors, including slower physical development, an overproduction of urine at night, and the inability to recognize bladder filling when asleep. Nighttime UI has also been associated with attention deficit hyperactivity disorder (ADHD), obstructive sleep apnea (OSA), and anxiety. Children may also inherit genes from one or both parents that make them likely to have nighttime UI.

## Slower Physical Development

Between the ages of 5 and 10, bed-wetting may be the result of a small bladder capacity, long sleeping periods, and an underdevelopment of the body's alarms that signal a full or emptying bladder. This form of UI fades away as the bladder grows, and the natural alarms become operational.

## Overproduction of Urine at Night

The body produces antidiuretic hormone (ADH), a natural chemical that slows down the production of urine. More ADH is produced at night, so the need to urinate lessens. If the body does not produce enough ADH at night, the production of urine may not slow down, leading to bladder overfilling. If a child does not sense the bladder filling and awaken to urinate, wetting will occur.

## Structural Problems

A small number of UI cases are caused by physical problems in the urinary tract. Rarely, a blocked bladder or urethra may cause the bladder to overfill and leak. Nerve damage associated with the birth defect spina bifida can cause UI. In these cases, UI can appear as a constant dribbling of urine.

## Attention Deficit Hyperactivity Disorder

Children with ADHD are three times more likely to have nighttime UI than children without ADHD. The connection between ADHD and bed-wetting has not been explained, but some experts theorize that both conditions are related to delays in central nervous system (CNS) development.

## Obstructive Sleep Apnea

Nighttime UI may be one sign of OSA. Other symptoms of OSA include snoring, mouth breathing, frequent ear and sinus infections, sore throat, choking, and daytime drowsiness. Experts believe that when the airway in people with OSA closes, a chemical may be released in the body that increases water production and inhibits the systems that regulate fluid volume. Successful treatment of OSA often resolves the associated nighttime UI.

## Anxiety

Anxiety-causing events that occur between two and four years of age—before total bladder control is achieved—might lead to primary enuresis. Anxiety experienced after the age of four might lead to secondary enuresis in children who have been dry for at least six months. Events that cause anxiety in children include physical or sexual abuse; unfamiliar social situations, such as moving or starting at a new school; and major family events, such as the birth of a sibling, a death, or divorce. UI itself is an anxiety-causing event. Strong bladder contractions resulting in daytime leakage can cause embarrassment and anxiety that lead to nighttime wetting.

## Genetics

Certain genes have been found to contribute to UI. Children have a 30 percent chance of having nighttime UI if one parent was affected as a child. If both parents were affected, there is a 70 percent chance of bed-wetting. Figures 55.1 and 55.2 show the side view of females' and males' urinary tract, respectively.

# Bed-Wetting

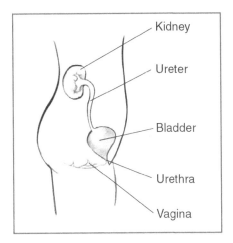

**Figure 55.1.** Female Urinary Tract

*National Institute of Diabetes and Digestive and Kidney Diseases (NIDDK)*

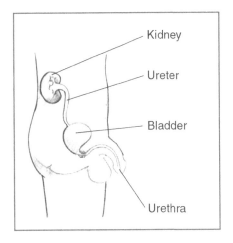

**Figure 55.2.** Male Urinary Tract

*National Institute of Diabetes and Digestive and Kidney Diseases (NIDDK)*

## HOW IS BED-WETTING CURED?

Most UI fades away naturally as a child grows and develops and does not require treatment. When treatment is needed, options include bladder training and related strategies, moisture alarms, and medications.

### Growth and Development

As children mature, the following will happen:
- Bladder capacity increases.
- Natural body alarms become activated.
- An overactive bladder settles down.
- Production of ADH becomes normal.
- Response to the body's signal that it is time to void improves.

### Bladder Training and Related Strategies

Bladder training consists of exercises to strengthen the bladder muscles to better control urination. Gradually, lengthening the time between trips to the bathroom can also help by stretching the bladder, so it can hold more urine. Additional techniques that may help control daytime UI include:
- urinating on a schedule—timed voiding—such as every two hours
- avoiding food or drinks with caffeine
- following suggestions for healthy urination, such as relaxing muscles and taking enough time to allow the bladder to empty completely

Waking children up to urinate can help decrease nighttime UI. Ensuring children drink enough fluids throughout the day so they do not drink a lot of fluids close to bedtime may also help. A healthcare provider can give guidance about how much a child needs to drink each day, as the amount depends on a child's age, physical activity, and other factors.

## MOISTURE ALARMS

At night, moisture alarms can wake children when they begin to urinate. These devices use a water-sensitive pad connected to an alarm that sounds when moisture is first detected. A small pad can clip to the pajamas, or a larger pad can be placed on the bed. For the alarm to be effective, children must awaken as soon as the alarm goes off, stop the urine stream, and go to the bathroom. Children using moisture alarms may need to have someone sleep in the same room to help wake them up.

## MEDICATIONS

Nighttime UI may be treated by increasing ADH levels. The hormone can be boosted by a synthetic version known as "desmopressin" (DDAVP), which is available in pill form, nasal spray, and nose drops. DDAVP is approved for use in children. Another medication called "imipramine" (Tofranil) is also used to treat nighttime UI though the way this medication prevents bedwetting is not known. Although both of these medications may help children achieve short-term success, relapse is common once the medication is withdrawn. UI resulting from an overactive bladder may be treated with oxybutynin (Ditropan), a medication that helps calm the bladder muscle and control muscle spasms.[2]

---

[2] "Urinary Incontinence in Children," National Institute of Diabetes and Digestive and Kidney Diseases (NIDDK), June 2012. Available online. URL: www.niddk.nih.gov/-/media/7831DE2FDE4C4F11823138E15DA45BD1.ashx. Accessed May 9, 2023.

# Chapter 56 | **Sleepwalking in Children**

Sleepwalking, or "somnambulism," is when a child unconsciously walks and performs actions while asleep. It is most common in kids between four and eight years old and usually happens within the first few hours of falling asleep. Sleepwalking can involve more than just walking and can last from a few seconds to 30 minutes. Although it is usually harmless, it can be dangerous if the child wanders outside or does something inappropriate. Most children outgrow sleepwalking by their teen years, and keeping them safe during episodes is essential.

## CAUSES OF SLEEPWALKING

Sleepwalking is more common in children and may run in families. Different factors can cause sleepwalking. These can include the following:

- not getting enough sleep
- having an irregular sleep schedule
- feeling stressed or anxious
- being in a new sleep environment
- having a fever or illness
- taking certain medications
- having a family history of sleepwalking

Sleepwalking can sometimes be a symptom of an underlying condition such as migraines, sleep apnea, head injuries, or restless legs syndrome (RLS).

## SYMPTOMS OF SLEEPWALKING

The most common symptom of sleepwalking is walking during sleep, but there are also other actions associated with this condition. Some of the other symptoms of sleepwalking are as follows:
- moving around the house after waking up
- repeating actions sitting up in bed
- making awkward movements
- speaking or muttering while asleep
- not reacting or responding when spoken to
- doing habitual or repetitive actions, such as opening and closing doors
- urinating in inappropriate locations

Sleepwalkers might also exhibit other symptoms, such as difficulty waking up, seeming dazed, and having no memory of sleepwalking.

## COMPLICATIONS OF SLEEPWALKING

Sleepwalking may co-occur with night terrors. The complications of sleepwalking are as follows:
- **Injury**. The sleepwalking person may hurt themselves or others during the episode.
- **Embarrassment**. Due to sleepwalking, the affected individual may feel embarrassed, or they may experience problems with relationships. This can lead to depression or anxiety if left untreated for a long time.
- **Sleep deprivation**. Excess daytime sleepiness and tiredness may be a result of sleepwalking.

## DIAGNOSIS OF SLEEPWALKING

A health-care provider can diagnose sleepwalking through various methods. Typically, the health-care provider will first gather information from family members who have observed the child's behavior during sleep. A physical and psychological assessment might be conducted to eliminate other possible reasons for sleepwalking. If another underlying medical issue is causing the child's sleepwalking, that issue must be treated first.

If a health-care provider suspects a child has a sleep disorder, they might suggest a particular test called a "sleep study," where the child would spend a night in a special sleep study room to measure parameters such as how they breathe, their heart rate, and how their muscles move. The child might also be monitored on video during the whole process of sleep. This would help the health-care provider diagnose the underlying causes of sleepwalking in children.

While tests such as a physical exam, sleep study, or electroencephalogram (EEG) can be used to diagnose sleepwalking, they are not always necessary. In many cases, health-care providers rely on the accounts of family members and other symptoms to diagnose sleepwalking.

## WHEN TO SEEK MEDICAL INTERVENTION

It is advisable to contact the physician if:

- sleepwalking happens frequently and severely or puts the child in danger
- the child gets injured repeatedly during sleepwalking events or leaves the house while sleepwalking
- sleepwalking occurs after the teenage years and causes daytime sleepiness or psychological factors such as stress or anxiety contribute to sleep disturbances
- there is suspicion of a medical cause such as sleep apnea, seizure disorder, or a limb movement disorder

Usually, sleepwalking does not need treatment, but if it happens often and causes problems or if the child is sleepy during the day, talking to a health-care provider is necessary. In such cases, a treatment called "scheduled awakening" may be recommended, where the child is woken up before the usual sleepwalking time, which can help reset their sleep cycle and control sleepwalking behavior to prevent sleepwalking. In rare cases, the health-care provider may prescribe medicine to aid sleep.

## TREATMENT FOR SLEEPWALKING

Treatment options for sleepwalking include the following:

- **Treating any underlying condition**. If sleepwalking is associated with an underlying condition, treatment is focused on that medical condition.
- **Adjusting medication**. If medications are found to be the cause of sleepwalking, those medications are adjusted accordingly.
- **Resolving stress**. Relaxation therapies, biofeedback, hypnosis, and cognitive behavioral therapy (CBT) are recommended to reduce stress or other mental health conditions and improve sleep quality.
- **Anticipatory awakenings**. This treatment option involves waking a person 15 minutes before she or he sleepwalks.
- **Medications**. Medications are not initially recommended; however, the health-care provider may recommend them after diagnosis.

## PREVENTION OF SLEEPWALKING

Sleepwalking and its complications can be prevented by the following steps:

- **Get adequate sleep**. Fatigue can lead to sleepwalking. Put your child to bed early to avoid sleepwalking.
- **Establish a relaxing activity**. Complete calming activities before sleep, such as reading a book, taking a warm bath, meditating, solving puzzles, or completing relaxing exercises.
- **Find a pattern**. Take note of the time when sleepwalking occurs. If there is a pattern within the timings, it may be used for anticipatory awakenings.
- **Make a quiet bedroom**. A calm atmosphere can improve your child's quality of sleep.
- **Avoid caffeine**. It is recommended to avoid caffeine and sugar before bedtime.

## WHAT TO DO IF YOUR CHILD SLEEPWALKS

When your child sleepwalks, do the following:

- **Do not wake your child**. Try not to wake your child during a sleepwalking episode; waking your child from sleepwalking may cause them to feel confused and disorientated.
- **Get your child back to bed**. Guide your child safely back to bed by repeating soothing statements and reassuring them that they are at home.
- **Offer comfort**. Provide them with physical comfort.
- **Take safety measures**. Make the environment safe by locking doors and windows and putting fragile objects away in order to prevent any injuries during sleepwalking episodes.

To effectively manage a child's sleepwalking problem and ensure their safety and comfort throughout the night, parents can establish a consistent sleep routine, promote relaxation before bedtime, and steer clear of caffeine and late-night beverages. These measures can be effectively helpful in managing the child's sleepwalking issues.

## References

"Kids and Sleepwalking," CHOC Children's, February 3, 2016. Available online. URL: www.choc.org/health-topics/kids-and-sleepwalking. Accessed April 11, 2023.

Martel, Janelle. "Pediatric Sleepwalking," Healthline Media, May 21, 2018. Available online. URL: www.healthline.com/health/sleep/sleepwalking-and-children. Accessed April 11, 2023.

"Sleepwalking," Cleveland Clinic, January 22, 2020. Available online. URL: https://my.clevelandclinic.org/health/diseases/14292-sleepwalking. Accessed April 11, 2023.

"Sleepwalking," Mayo Foundation for Medical Education and Research (MFMER), July 21, 2017. Available online. URL: www.mayoclinic.org/diseases-conditions/sleepwalking/symptoms-causes/syc-20353506. Accessed April 11, 2023.

"Sleepwalking," The Nemours Foundation, August 22, 2018. Available online. URL: https://kidshealth.org/en/parents/sleepwalking.html. Accessed April 11, 2023.

"Sleepwalking (Somnambulism)," WebMD LLC., November 15, 2021. Available online. URL: www.webmd.com/sleep-disorders/sleepwalking-causes. Accessed April 11, 2023.

# Chapter 57 | **Bruxism and Sleep**

Bruxism is a movement disorder in which a person grinds, clenches, or gnashes their teeth. Many people may unconsciously grind or clench their teeth, but whether it is diagnosed as bruxism depends on the pain level and frequency. The marked absence of clinical symptoms makes it difficult to estimate the prevalence of bruxism. Most cases go unreported since the majority of "bruxers" remain unaware of their problem until a diagnosis can be made by visible signs of teeth wear. Bruxism is thought to affect an estimated 30–40 million people in the United States and tends to occur episodically during certain periods of a person's life. Bruxism can be either diurnal (daytime) or nocturnal (night). When people unconsciously clench their jaws during the day, it is called "awake bruxism," and when they grind or clench their teeth while they are asleep, it is called "sleep bruxism."

## PREVALENCE OF SLEEP BRUXISM

Sleep bruxism occurs during the night and is classified as a type of sleep disorder. This means that it can be more challenging to manage because individuals are not aware of it happening while they are asleep. While many people who grind their teeth during the night are not even aware of it, severe cases of sleep bruxism can have serious health consequences. According to the Cleveland Clinic's report, as many as 15 percent of children and around 10 percent of adults are impacted by bruxism. However, the exact number of people with sleep bruxism may be higher since many people are unaware that they grind their teeth during sleep. Sleep bruxism can occur at any age but is more common in children and decreases with age.

## RISK FACTORS OF SLEEP BRUXISM

Bruxism can be caused by various factors that increase your risk. Among the peripheral factors studied, the most important one is dental occlusion, which refers to the misalignment of the teeth in the upper and lower jaws.

Among all the factors that may contribute to sleep bruxism, the ones most extensively studied have been psychosocial factors, which include stress and anxiety. Bruxing in children may often be traced to their emotional and psychological state. For instance, anxiety in children stemming from causes such as school exams, bullying, scolding from parents, or moving to a new neighborhood may be a significant risk factor for sleep bruxism.

For adults, common sources of stress include workplace tensions, family problems, relationship issues, or anxiety about health conditions. Certain personality types tend to be more vulnerable to stress-related bruxism, including those who are highly aggressive, competitive, or hyperactive.

The risk of developing bruxism can be increased by certain lifestyle factors, such as smoking, alcohol consumption, and drug use. Bruxism may also develop as a side effect of certain medications, such as certain antidepressants, or as a symptom of neurological disorders, such as Parkinson disease, epilepsy, dementia, night terrors, sleep apnea, and attention deficit hyperactivity disorder (ADHD). Studies have also shown that bruxism is often related to other sleep disorders, such as excessive snoring, pauses in breathing, or obstructive sleep apnea (OSA).

## SYMPTOMS AND DIAGNOSIS OF SLEEP BRUXISM

While mild-to-moderate muscle activity in bruxers may not cause any issues, severe cases could lead to dental problems, such as the premature wearing of the teeth and dental implants. Tightness or fatigue can be felt in the jaw muscles, and sometimes, the jaw can get locked or stuck. This can cause pain or soreness in the jaw, neck, or face, and it may even feel like there is an earache. One could also experience a dull headache starting in their temples or damage from chewing on the inside of their cheek due to bruxism. This condition can also disrupt one's sleep, causing further discomfort and potential health issues.

Bruxism is usually diagnosed through a visit to a dentist. During a regular checkup, the dentist will look for and inquire about the following symptoms:

- damaged teeth
- unusual teeth sensitivity
- swelling and pain in the jaw or facial muscles around the mouth
- tongue indentations
- headaches or earaches
- frequent awakening or poor quality of sleep

## TREATMENT FOR SLEEP BRUXISM

Treatments for bruxism should be selected to best fit the individual patient and the underlying cause of the disorder. When a dental problem is determined to be the cause of bruxism, a dental appliance, such as a splint or mouth guard, might alleviate the condition. These devices help prevent the teeth from grinding together and also protect the tooth enamel from further damage.

In addition, there are some dental procedures that can be done to fix issues with the alignment of the teeth and jaw or to repair damage caused by clenching and grinding. These procedures can help improve the way the teeth and jaw work together, which can also help alleviate pain and discomfort. Correcting the position and placement of the tongue, teeth, and lips can bring about a significant improvement in the condition. Biofeedback is another treatment method used to assess and alter the movement of the muscles around the mouth and jaw. The doctor may use monitoring equipment to help guide the patient toward overcoming the habit of clenching the jaw or grinding the teeth.

If the reason for teeth grinding is related to the mind, then there are some therapies and techniques that can help stop grinding the teeth and feel better. Stress management is the foremost issue to be addressed in people with bruxism. Cognitive behavioral therapy (CBT) can help people who have problems with the way their mouth and jaw are aligned. It can teach them ways to cope with these problems and improve their overall well-being. Counseling sessions with experts can help patients develop coping strategies. Other common means of reducing stress include meditation, relaxation, exercise, and music. Hypnosis has also proven to be an effective treatment for people who grind their teeth at night. Most patients with bruxism tend to respond well to the proper treatment prescribed by the appropriate professional.

## References

"Bruxism," The Johns Hopkins Medicine, September 16, 2015. Available online. URL: www.hopkinsmedicine.org/health/conditions-and-diseases/bruxism. Accessed April 10, 2023.

"Bruxism (Teeth Grinding)," Cleveland Clinic, May 7, 2021. Available online. URL: https://my.clevelandclinic.org/health/diseases/10955-teeth-grinding-bruxism. Accessed April 10, 2023.

"Bruxism (Teeth Grinding)," Mayo Foundation for Medical Education and Research (MFMER), August 10, 2017. Available online. URL: www.mayoclinic.org/diseases-conditions/bruxism/symptoms-causes/syc-20356095. Accessed April 10, 2023.

"Bruxism (Teeth Grinding or Clenching)," The Nemours Foundation/KidsHealth, n.d. Available online. URL: https://kidshealth.org/en/parents/bruxism.html. Accessed April 10, 2023.

"Causes of Bruxism," The Bruxism Association, n.d. Available online. URL: www.bruxism.org.uk/causes-of-bruxism.php. Accessed April 10, 2023.

"Epidemiology of Bruxism in Adults: A Systematic Review of the Literature," National Center for Biotechnology Information (NCBI), 2013. Available online. URL: https://pubmed.ncbi.nlm.nih.gov/23630682. Accessed April 10, 2023

Shilpa Shetty et al. "Bruxism: A Literature Review," *The Journal of Indian Prosthodontic Society Volume 10 (3): 141-148*, National Center for Biotechnology Information (NCBI), U.S. National Library of Medicine (NLM), January 22, 2011. Available online. URL: www.ncbi.nlm.nih.gov/pmc/articles/PMC3081266. Accessed April 10, 2023.

# Chapter 58 | **Caffeine and Teens' Sleep**

## WHAT IS CAFFEINE?

Caffeine is a bitter substance that occurs naturally in more than 60 plants, including:

- coffee beans
- tea leaves
- kola nuts, which are used to flavor soft drink colas
- cacao pods, which are used to make chocolate products

There is also synthetic (man-made) caffeine, which is added to some medicines, foods, and drinks. For example, some pain relievers, cold medicines, and over-the-counter (OTC) medicines for alertness contain synthetic caffeine. So do energy drinks and "energy-boosting" gums and snacks.

Most people consume caffeine from drinks. The amount of caffeine in different drinks can vary a lot, but it is generally:

- an 8-ounce cup of coffee: 95–200 mg
- a 12-ounce can of cola: 35–45 mg
- an 8-ounce energy drink: 70–100 mg
- an 8-ounce cup of tea: 14–60 mg

## WHAT ARE CAFFEINE'S EFFECTS ON THE BODY?

Caffeine has many effects on your body's metabolism that include the following:

- stimulating your central nervous system (CNS), which can make you feel more awake and give you a boost of energy
- being a diuretic, meaning that it helps your body get rid of extra salt and water by urinating more

- increasing the release of acid in your stomach, sometimes leading to an upset stomach or heartburn
- maybe interfering with the absorption of calcium in the body
- increasing your blood pressure

Within one hour of eating or drinking caffeine, it reaches its peak level in your blood. You may continue to feel the effects of caffeine for four to six hours.

## WHAT ARE THE SIDE EFFECTS OF TOO MUCH CAFFEINE?

For most people, it is not harmful to consume up to 400 mg of caffeine a day. If you do eat or drink too much caffeine, it can cause health problems, such as:

- restlessness and shakiness
- insomnia
- headaches
- dizziness
- fast heart rate
- dehydration
- anxiety
- dependency, so you need to take more of it to get the same results

Some people are more sensitive to the effects of caffeine than others.

## WHAT ARE ENERGY DRINKS, AND WHY CAN THEY BE A PROBLEM?

Energy drinks are beverages that have added caffeine. The amount of caffeine in energy drinks can vary widely, and sometimes, the labels on the drinks do not give you the actual amount of caffeine in them. Energy drinks may also contain sugars, vitamins, herbs, and supplements.

Companies that make energy drinks claim that the drinks can increase alertness and improve physical and mental performance.

This has helped make the drinks popular with American teens and young adults. There is limited data showing that energy drinks might temporarily improve alertness and physical endurance. There is not enough evidence to show that they enhance strength or power. But what we do know is that energy drinks can be dangerous because they have large amounts of caffeine. And, since they have lots of sugar, they can contribute to weight gain and worsen diabetes.

Sometimes, young people mix their energy drinks with alcohol. It is dangerous to combine alcohol and caffeine. Caffeine can interfere with your ability to recognize how drunk you are, which can lead you to drink more. This also makes you likely to make bad decisions.

## WHO SHOULD AVOID OR LIMIT CAFFEINE?

You should check with your health-care provider about whether you should limit or avoid caffeine if you:

- are pregnant since caffeine passes through the placenta to your baby
- are breastfeeding since a small amount of caffeine that you consume is passed along to your baby
- have sleep disorders, including insomnia
- have migraines or other chronic headaches
- have anxiety
- have gastroesophageal reflux disease (GERD) or ulcers
- have arrhythmia (a problem with the rate or rhythm of your heartbeat)
- have high blood pressure
- take certain medicines or supplements, including stimulants, certain antibiotics, asthma medicines, and heart medicines (Check with your health-care provider about whether there might be interactions between caffeine and any medicines and supplements that you take.)
- are a child or teen (Neither should have as much caffeine as adults. Children can be especially sensitive to the effects of caffeine.)

## WHAT IS CAFFEINE WITHDRAWAL?

If you have been consuming caffeine on a regular basis and then suddenly stop, you may have caffeine withdrawal. Symptoms can include:

- headaches
- drowsiness
- irritability
- nausea
- trouble concentrating

These symptoms usually go away after a couple of days.[1]

## IF A COFFEE OR TEA SAYS "DECAFFEINATED," DOES THAT MEAN IT CONTAINS NO CAFFEINE?

No. Decaf coffees and teas have less caffeine than their regular counterparts, but they still contain some caffeine. For example, decaf coffee typically has 2–15 mg in an 8-ounce cup. If you react strongly to caffeine in a negative way, you may want to avoid these beverages altogether.

## HOW MUCH CAFFEINE IS TOO MUCH?

For healthy adults, the U.S. Food and Drug Administration (FDA) has cited 400 mg a day—that is about four or five cups of coffee—as an amount not generally associated with dangerous, negative effects. However, there is wide variation in both how sensitive people are to the effects of caffeine and how fast they metabolize it (break it down).

Certain conditions tend to make people more sensitive to caffeine's effects, as can some medications. In addition, if you are pregnant, trying to become pregnant, or breastfeeding or are concerned about another condition or medication, you are recommended to talk to your health-care provider about whether you need to limit caffeine consumption.

---

[1] MedlinePlus, "Caffeine," National Institutes of Health (NIH), April 30, 2019. Available online. URL: https://medlineplus.gov/caffeine.html. Accessed May 5, 2023.

The FDA has not set a level for children, but the American Academy of Pediatrics (AAP) discourages the consumption of caffeine and other stimulants by children and adolescents.

## IS IT OKAY FOR KIDS TO CONSUME CAFFEINE?

You are recommended to consult with your health-care provider for advice regarding your child's caffeine consumption.

## IS DRINKING A LOT OF CAFFEINE A SUBSTITUTE FOR SLEEP?

No. Caffeine is a stimulant, which may cause you to be more alert and awake, but it is not a substitute for sleep. Typically, it can take four to six hours for your body to metabolize half of what you consumed. So a cup of coffee at dinner may keep you awake at bedtime.

## HOW CAN YOU CUT BACK ON CAFFEINE WITHOUT CAUSING UNPLEASANT SIDE EFFECTS?

If you are used to drinking caffeine-containing beverages every day and want to cut back, it is best to do so gradually. Stopping abruptly can cause withdrawal symptoms such as headaches, anxiety, and nervousness. Unlike opioid or alcohol withdrawal, caffeine withdrawal is not considered dangerous, but it can be unpleasant. You may want to talk to your health-care provider about how to cut back.[2]

---

[2] "Spilling the Beans: How Much Caffeine Is Too Much?" U.S. Food and Drug Administration (FDA), December 12, 2018. Available online. URL: www.fda.gov/consumers/consumer-updates/spilling-beans-how-much-caffeine-too-much. Accessed May 5, 2023.

# Part 7 | Additional Help and Information

# Chapter 59 | **Glossary of Terms Related to Sleep Disorders**

**acupuncture:** A technique in which practitioners stimulate specific points on the body—most often by inserting thin needles through the skin. It is one of the practices used in traditional Chinese medicine.

**addiction:** A chronic, relapsing disease characterized by compulsive drug seeking and use despite serious adverse consequences and by long-lasting changes in the brain.

**alcohol:** A chemical substance found in drinks such as beer, wine, and liquor. It is also found in some medicines, mouthwashes, household products, and essential oils (scented liquid taken from certain plants). It is made by a chemical process called "fermentation" that uses sugars and yeast.

**allergy:** A condition in which the body has an exaggerated response to a substance (e.g., food or drug). It is also known as "hypersensitivity."

**antibiotic:** A drug that kills or stops the growth of bacteria. Antibiotics are a type of antimicrobial. Penicillin and ciprofloxacin are examples of antibiotics.

**anticonvulsant:** A drug or other substance used to prevent or stop seizures or convulsions. It is also called "antiepileptic."

**antidepressant:** A name for a category of medications used to treat depression.

This glossary contains terms excerpted from documents produced by several sources deemed reliable.

**antigen:** Any substance that causes the body to make an immune response against that substance. Antigens include toxins, chemicals, bacteria, viruses, or other substances that come from outside the body.

**antihistamine:** Drugs that are used to prevent or relieve the symptoms of hay fever and other allergies by preventing the action of a substance called "histamine," which is produced by the body. Histamine can cause itching, sneezing, runny nose, and watery eyes and sometimes can make breathing difficult. Some of these drugs are also used to prevent motion sickness, nausea, vomiting, and dizziness. Since they may cause drowsiness as a side effect, some of them may be used to help people go to sleep.

**apnea:** Cessation of breathing.

**arthritis:** A term used to describe more than 100 rheumatic diseases and conditions that affect joints, the tissues which surround the joints, and other connective tissues.

**assessment:** The process of gathering evidence and documentation of a student's learning.

**asthma:** A chronic disease in which the bronchial airways in the lungs become narrowed and swollen, making it difficult to breathe.

**benzodiazepine:** A central nervous system (CNS) depressant.

**biological clock:** It times and controls a person's sleep–wake cycle and will attempt to function according to a normal day/night schedule even when that person tries to change it.

**biomarkers:** A biological molecule found in blood, other body fluids, or tissues that is a sign of a normal or abnormal process or of a condition or disease.

**bladder:** The organ in the human body that stores urine. It is found in the lower part of the abdomen.

**bruxism:** A movement disorder characterized by grinding and clenching of teeth.

**calcium:** A mineral that is an essential nutrient for bone health. It is also needed for the heart, muscles, and nerves to function properly and for blood to clot.

**calorie:** A unit of energy in food. Carbohydrates, fats, protein, and alcohol in the foods and drinks we eat provide food energy or "calories."

**cancer:** A term for diseases in which abnormal cells in the body divide without control. Cancer cells can invade nearby tissues and can spread to other parts of the body through the blood and lymphatic system, which is a network of tissues that clears infections and keeps body fluids in balance.

**cataplexy:** A sudden loss of motor tone and strength.

**central nervous system (CNS):** Comprises the nerves in the brain and spinal cord. These nerves are used to send electrical impulses throughout the body, resulting in voluntary and reflexive movement. Information about the environment is received by the senses and sent to the central nervous system (CNS), which causes the body to respond appropriately.

**central sleep apnea (CSA):** It is caused by irregularities in the brain's normal signals to breathe.

**chronic insomnia:** A condition in which sleep problems occur at least three nights a week for more than a month.

**circadian rhythms:** Physical, mental, and behavioral changes that follow a roughly 24-hour cycle, responding primarily to light and darkness in an organism's environment.

**clinical trial:** A research study in which one or more human subjects are prospectively assigned to one or more interventions (which may include placebo or other control) to evaluate the effects of those interventions on health-related biomedical or behavioral outcomes.

**cognitive behavioral therapy (CBT):** A blend of two therapies: cognitive therapy (CT) and behavioral therapy. It focuses on a person's thoughts and beliefs and how they influence a person's mood and actions and aims to change a person's thinking to be more adaptive and healthy.

**complementary and alternative medicine (CAM):** It is the term for medical products and practices that are not part of standard medical care.

**continuous positive airway pressure:** A treatment that uses mild air pressure to keep the airways open.

**corticosteroids:** Powerful anti-inflammatory hormones made naturally in the body or by humans for use as medicine. Corticosteroids may be injected into the affected joints to temporarily reduce inflammation and relieve pain.

**culture:** A test to see whether there are tuberculosis (TB) bacteria in your phlegm or other body fluids. This test can take two to four weeks in most laboratories.

**diabetes:** A disease in which blood glucose (blood sugar) levels are above or below normal.

**diet:** What a person eats and drinks. Any type of eating plan.

**dopamine:** A neurotransmitter present in regions of the brain that regulate movement, emotion, motivation, and feelings of pleasure.

**enuresis:** Involuntary urination during sleep.

**enzyme:** A protein that speeds up chemical reactions in the body.

**exercise:** A type of physical activity that involves planned, structured, and repetitive bodily movement done to maintain or improve one or more components of physical fitness.

**exposure:** Contact with infectious agents (bacteria or viruses) in a manner that promotes transmission and increases the likelihood of disease.

**genes:** Genes, which are made up of deoxyribonucleic acid (DNA), are the basic units that define the characteristics of every organism. Genes carry information that determines traits, such as eye color in humans and resistance to antibiotics in bacteria.

**genetics:** The study of particular genes, deoxyribonucleic acid (DNA), and heredity.

**genome:** A genome is an organism's complete set of genes that carry the genetic instructions for building and maintaining that organism.

**hormone:** Substance produced by one tissue and conveyed by the bloodstream to another to affect a function of the body, such as growth or metabolism.

**hypersomnia:** A complaint of excessive daytime sleep or sleepiness.

**hypertension:** Also called "high blood pressure," it is having blood pressure greater than 140 over 90 millimeters of mercury (mmHg). Long-term high blood pressure can damage blood vessels and organs, including the heart, kidneys, eyes, and brain.

**hypnosis:** A trance-like state in which a person becomes more aware and focused on particular thoughts, feelings, images, sensations, or behaviors.

**hypothalamus:** The area of the brain that controls body temperature, hunger, and thirst.

**immune system:** A complex system of cellular and molecular components having the primary function of distinguishing self from not self and defense against foreign organisms or substances.

**immunity:** Protection against a disease. Immunity is indicated by the presence of antibodies in the blood and can usually be determined with a laboratory test.

## Glossary of Terms Related to Sleep Disorders

**inflammation:** Redness, swelling, heat, and pain resulting from injury to tissue (parts of the body underneath the skin). It is also known as "swelling."

**insomnia:** Not being able to sleep.

**jet lag:** A sleep disorder caused by traveling across different time zones.

**Kleine-Levin syndrome:** It is characterized by recurring but reversible periods of excessive sleep.

**lesion:** An area of abnormal tissue. A lesion may be benign (not cancer) or malignant (cancer).

**light therapy:** It is used to treat seasonal affective disorder.

**melatonin:** A natural hormone that plays a role in sleep.

**metabolism:** The chemical changes that take place in a cell or an organism. These changes make energy and the materials cells and organisms need to grow, reproduce, and stay healthy. Metabolism also helps get rid of toxic substances.

**multiple sleep latency test (MSLT):** This is a daytime sleep study that measures how sleepy you are. It is typically done the day after a polysomnography (PSG).

**muscles:** Bundles of specialized cells that contract and relax to produce movement when stimulated by nerves.

**mutation:** A change in a DNA sequence that can result from DNA copying mistakes made during cell division, exposure to ionizing radiation, exposure to chemical mutagens, or infection by viruses.

**narcolepsy:** A disorder that causes periods of extreme daytime sleepiness. The disorder may also cause muscle weakness.

**neuron:** A nerve cell that is the basic working unit of the brain and nervous system, which processes and transmits information.

**nightmare:** A bad dream that brings out strong feelings of fear, terror, distress, or anxiety.

**nocturia:** Frequent urination of two or more times per night.

**non-rapid eye movement (non-REM) sleep:** Stages of sleep ranging from light sleep to deep sleep.

**nutrition:** The taking in and use of food and other nourishing material by the body. Nutrition is a three-part process. First, food or drink is consumed. Second, the body breaks down the food or drink into nutrients. Third, the nutrients enter the bloodstream and travel to different parts of the body where they are needed to keep you healthy.

**obesity:** It refers to excess body fat. Because body fat is usually not measured directly, a ratio of body weight to height is often used instead.

**obstructive sleep apnea (OSA) (syndrome):** In this condition, the airway collapses or becomes blocked during sleep.

**organ:** A part of the body that performs a specific function. For example, the heart is an organ.

**organism:** Any living thing, including humans, animals, plants, and microbes.

**osteoarthritis:** The most common form of arthritis. It is characterized by the breakdown of joint cartilage, leading to pain, stiffness, and disability.

**over-the-counter (OTC):** Refers to a medicine that can be bought over-the-counter without a prescription (doctor's order). Examples include analgesics (pain relievers), such as aspirin and acetaminophen. Also called "nonprescription" and "over-the-counter."

**overweight:** It refers to an excessive amount of body weight that includes muscle, bone, fat, and water. A person who has a body mass index (BMI) of 25–29.9 is considered overweight.

**parasomnia:** It is defined as undesirable behavioral, physiological, or experiential events that accompany sleep.

**perception (hearing):** Process of knowing or being aware of information through the ear.

**periodic limb movement disorder (PLMD):** It causes repetitive jerking movements of the limbs, especially the legs. These movements occur every 20 to 40 seconds and cause repeated awakening and severely fragmented sleep.

**physical activity:** Any bodily movement that is produced by the contraction of skeletal muscle and that substantially increases energy expenditure.

**polysomnogram:** A sleep study that records brain activity, eye movements, heart rate, and blood pressure.

**pregnancy:** The condition between conception (fertilization of an egg by a sperm) and birth, during which the fertilized egg develops in the uterus. In humans, pregnancy lasts about 288 days.

**prevalence:** The number of disease cases (new and existing) within a population over a given time period.

# Glossary of Terms Related to Sleep Disorders

**prevention:** Actions that reduce exposure or other risks, keep people from getting sick, or keep disease from getting worse.

**prognosis:** The likely outcome or course of a disease; the chance of recovery or recurrence.

**protein:** A molecule made up of amino acids. Proteins are needed for the body to function properly. They are the basis of body structures, such as skin and hair, and of other substances, such as enzymes, cytokines, and antibodies.

**quarantine:** The isolation of a person or animal who has a disease (or is suspected of having a disease) in order to prevent further spread of the disease.

**radiation:** Energy moving in the form of particles or waves. Familiar radiations are heat, light, radio, and microwaves.

**rapid eye movement (REM) sleep:** It is the active or paradoxical phase of sleep in which the brain is active.

**restless legs syndrome (RLS):** A disorder that causes a powerful urge to move your legs. Your legs become uncomfortable when you are lying down or sitting. Some people describe it as a creeping, crawling, tingling, or burning sensation. Moving makes your legs feel better, but not for long.

**rheumatoid arthritis:** A form of arthritis in which the immune system attacks the tissues of the joints, leading to pain, inflammation, and eventually joint damage and malformation. It typically begins at a younger age than osteoarthritis does, causes swelling and redness in joints, and may make people feel sick, tired, and feverish. Rheumatoid arthritis may also affect skin tissue, the lungs, the eyes, or the blood vessels.

**sleep cycle:** It is defined as a segment of non-rapid eye movement (non-REM) sleep followed by a period of rapid eye movement (REM) sleep.

**sleep debt:** It develops when daily sleep time is less than an individual needs.

**sleep deprivation:** Sleep deprivation is a condition that occurs if you do not get enough sleep.

**sleep hygiene:** The promotion of regular sleep is known as "sleep hygiene."

**sleep medicine:** The specialty concerned with conditions characterized by disturbances of usual sleep patterns or behaviors.

**sleepwalking:** It refers to doing other activities when you are asleep such as eating, talking, or driving a car.

**snoring:** Snoring is an example of sleep-disordered breathing—a condition that makes it more difficult to breathe during sleep.

**sodium:** A mineral and an essential nutrient needed by the human body in relatively small amounts (provided that substantial sweating does not occur).

**stage 2 sleep:** When we enter stage 2 sleep, our eye movements stop, and our brain waves (fluctuations of electrical activity that can be measured by electrodes) become slower, with occasional bursts of rapid waves called "sleep spindles."

**stage 3 sleep:** In stage 3, extremely slow brain waves called "delta waves" begin to appear, interspersed with smaller and faster waves.

**steroid:** Any of a group of lipids (fats) that have a certain chemical structure. Steroids occur naturally in plants and animals, or they may be made in the laboratory.

**stimulants:** Stimulants increase alertness, attention, and energy, as well as elevate blood pressure, heart rate, and respiration.

**stroke:** It is also known as a "cerebrovascular accident" (CVA), caused by a lack of blood to the brain, resulting in the sudden loss of speech, language, or the ability to move a body part and, if severe enough, death.

**tobacco:** A plant with leaves that have high levels of the addictive chemical nicotine. After harvesting, tobacco leaves are cured, aged, and processed in various ways. The resulting products may be smoked (in cigarettes, cigars, and pipes), applied to the gums (as dipping and chewing tobacco), or inhaled (as snuff).

**vaccine:** A product made from very small amounts of weak or dead germs that can cause diseases—for example, viruses, bacteria, or toxins. It prepares your body to fight the disease faster and more effectively so you will not get sick. Vaccines are administered through needle injections, by mouth, and by aerosol.

**yoga:** A mind and body practice with origins in ancient Indian philosophy. The various styles of yoga typically combine physical postures, breathing techniques, and meditation or relaxation.

# Chapter 60 | **Directory of Resources Providing Information about Sleep Disorders**

## GENERAL

**American Academy of Dental Sleep Medicine (AADSM)**
901 Warrenville Rd., Ste. 180
Lisle, IL 60532
Phone: 630-686-9875
Fax: 630-686-9876
Website: www.aadsm.org
Email: info@aadsm.org

**American Academy of Sleep Medicine (AASM)**
2510 N. Frontage Rd.
Darien, IL 60561
Phone: 630-737-9700
Fax: 630-737-9790
Website: www.aasm.org
Email: contact@aasm.org

**American Association of Sleep Technologists (AAST)**
330 N. Wabash Ave., Ste. 2000
Chicago, IL 60611
Phone: 312-321-5191
Website: www.aastweb.org
Email: info@aastweb.org

**American Sleep Medicine**
7900 Belfort Pkwy., Ste. 300
Jacksonville, FL 32256
Toll-Free: 855-875-3372
Phone: 904-517-5500
Fax: 904-517-5501
Website: www.
americansleepmedicine.com
Email: info@
americansleepmedicine.com

Resources in this chapter were compiled from several sources deemed reliable; all contact information was verified and updated in May 2023.

## American Thoracic Society (ATS)

25 Bdwy., 4th Fl.
New York, NY 10004
Phone: 212-315-8600
Fax: 212-315-6498
Website: www.thoracic.org
Email: atsinfo@thoracic.org

## Better Sleep Council (BSC)

Website: bettersleep.org
Email: info@sleepproducts.org

## The Center for Sleep & Wake Disorders

5454 Wisconsin Ave., Ste. 1725
Chevy Chase, MD 20815
Phone: 301-654-1575
Fax: 301-654-5658
Website: www.sleepdoc.com
Email: mail@sleepdoc.com

## Cleveland Clinic

9500 Euclid Ave.
Cleveland, OH 44195
Toll-Free: 800-223-2273
Phone: 216-444-2200
Website: my.clevelandclinic.org

## Eastern Iowa Sleep Center (ESIC)

275 10th St. S.E., Ste. 3330
Cedar Rapids, IA 52403
Toll-Free: 877-361-4433
Phone: 319-362-4433
Fax: 319-362-4466
Website: www.eisleep.com
Email: info@eisleep.com

## *Eunice Kennedy Shriver* National Institute of Child Health and Human Development (NICHD)

P.O. Box 3006
Rockville, MD 20847
Toll-Free: 800-370-2943
Toll-Free Fax: 866-760-5947
Website: www.nichd.nih.gov
Email:
NICHDInformationResource
Center@mail.nih.gov

## MedBridge LLC

536 Old Howell Rd.
Greenville, SC 29615
Toll-Free: 866-527-5970
Fax: 864-527-5971
Website: www.
medbridgehealthcare.com
Email: info@medbridgegroup.com

## Michigan Academy of Sleep Medicine (MASM)

P.O. Box 942
Southfield, MI 48037
Phone: 313-874-1360
Fax: 313-874-1366
Website: www.masm.wildapricot.org
Email: kcarter@wcmssm.org

## National Heart, Lung, and Blood Institute (NHLBI)

31 Center Dr. Bldg. 31
Bethesda, MD 20892
Toll-Free: 877-645-2448
Website: www.nhlbi.nih.gov/about/
divisions/division-lung-diseases/
national-center-sleep-disorders-
research
Email: nhlbiinfo@nhlbi.nih.gov

## National Institute of Neurological Disorders and Stroke (NINDS)
P.O. Box 5801
Bethesda, MD 20824
Toll-Free: 800-352-9424
Website: www.ninds.nih.gov

## The Nemours Foundation/ KidsHealth®
10140 Centurion Pkwy.,
N.Jacksonville, FL 32256
Toll-Free: 800-472-6610
Website: kidshealth.org

## Nocturna Sleep Center, LLC
9077 S. Pecos Rd., Ste. 3700
Henderson, NV 89074
Toll-Free: 866-990-8762
Phone: 702-896-7378
Website: www.nocturnasleep.com
Email: Scheduling@nocturnasleep.
net

## Ohio Sleep Medicine Institute (OSMI)
4975 Bradenton Ave.
Dublin, OH 43017
Phone: 614-766-0773
Fax: 614-766-2599
Website: www.sleepohio.com
Email: info@sleepmedicine.com

## The Sleep Doctor
1414 N.E. 42nd St., Ste. 400
Seattle, WA 98105
Website: thesleepdoctor.com
Email: contact@thesleepdoctor.
com

## Sleep Foundation
1414 N.E. 42nd St., Ste. 400
Seattle, WA 98105
Toll-Free: 877-672-8966
Website: www.sleepfoundation.org

## Sleep Medicine Center, Washington University in St. Louis
1600 S. Brentwood Blvd., Ste. 600
St. Louis, MO 63144
Phone: 314-362-4342
Fax: 314-747-3813
Website: sleep.wustl.edu

## Sleep Research Society (SRS)
2510 N. Frontage Rd.
Darien, IL 60561
Phone: 630-737-9702
Website: www.sleepresearchsociety.
org
Email: coordinator@srsnet.org

## Spectrum Health
100 Michigan St., N.E.
Grand Rapids, MI 49503
Toll-Free: 866-989-7999
Phone: 616-391-1774
Website: www.spectrumhealth.org

## UT Sleep Disorders Center
1928 Alcoa Hwy.
Bldg. B, Ste. 303
Knoxville, TN 37920
Phone: 865-305-8761
Website: www.utmedicalcenter.org/
medical-care/specialty-practices/
ut-sleep-disorders-center

## Valley Sleep Center

P.O. Box 30388
Mesa, AZ 85275-0388
Phone: 480-830-3900
Fax: 480-830-3901
Website: www.valleysleepcenter.com
Email: sleep@valleysleepcenter.com

## CIRCADIAN RHYTHM DISORDERS

### Circadian Sleep Disorders Network

4619 Woodfield Rd.
Bethesda, MD 20814
Website: www.
circadiansleepdisorders.org
Email: csd-n@csd-n.org

## HYPERSOMNIA

### Hypersomnia Foundation

4514 Chamblee Dunwoody Rd.,
Ste. 229
Atlanta, GA 30338
Phone: 404-301-1924
Website: www.
hypersomniafoundation.org
Email: info@
hypersomniafoundation.org

## KLEINE-LEVIN SYNDROME

### Kleine-Levin Syndrome Foundation, Inc.

P.O. Box 5382 San Jose, CA
95150-5382
Phone: 714-394-9817
Website: klsfoundation.org
Email: info@klsfoundation.org

## NARCOLEPSY

### Narcolepsy Network

3242 N.E. Third Ave., Ste. 1101
Camas, WA 98607
Toll-Free: 888-292-6522
Phone: 401-667-2523
Website: www.narcolepsynetwork.
org
Email: info@narcolepsynetwork.org

### Wake Up Narcolepsy, Inc.

P.O. Box 60293
Worcester, MA 01606
Phone: 978-751-3693
Website: www.wakeupnarcolepsy.
org
Email: info@wakeupnarcolepsy.org

## RESTLESS LEGS SYNDROME

### Restless Legs Syndrome (RLS) Foundation, Inc.

3006 Bee Caves Rd., Ste. D206
Austin, TX 78746
Phone: 512-366-9109
Fax: 512-366-9189
Website: www.rls.org
Email: info@rls.org

## SLEEP APNEA

### American Sleep Apnea Association (ASAA)
1250 Connecticut Ave.
N.W., Ste. 700
Washington, DC 20036
Toll-Free: 888-293-3650
Toll-Free Fax: 888-293-3650
Website: www.sleephealth.org
Email: asaa@sleephealth.org

### The Infant & Children Sleep Apnea Awareness Foundation, Inc.
New Smyrna Beach, FL 32170
Phone: 386-426-5858
Website: www.kidssleepdisorders.org
Email: terrilynn@kidssleepdisorders.org

## OTHER DISORDERS AFFECTING SLEEP

### Alzheimer's Association
225 N. Michigan Ave., 17th Fl.
Chicago, IL 60601
Toll-Free: 800-272-3900
Website: www.alz.org

### American Gastroenterological Association (AGA)
4930 Del Ray Ave.
Bethesda, MD 20814
Phone: 301-654-2055
Fax: 301-654-5920
Website: www.gastro.org
Email: member@gastro.org

### American Parkinson Disease Association (APDA)
P.O. Box 61420
Staten Island, NY 10306
Toll-Free: 800-223-2732
Fax: 718-981-4399
Website: www.apdaparkinson.org
Email: apda@apdaparkinson.org

### Anxiety and Depression Association of America (ADAA)
8701 Georgia Ave., Ste. 412
Silver Spring, MD 20910
Phone: 240-485-1001
Fax: 240-485-1035
Website: www.adaa.org
Email: information@adaa.org

### COPD Foundation
3300 Ponce de Leon Blvd.
Miami, FL 33134
Toll-Free: 866-731-2673
Website: www.copdfoundation.org
Email: info@copdfoundation.org

### National Center for Posttraumatic Stress Disorder (NCPTSD)
215 N. Main St.
White River Junction, VT 05009
Phone: 802-296-6300
Fax: 802-296-5135
Website: www.ptsd.va.gov
Email: ncptsd@va.gov

**National Institute of Mental Health (NIMH)**
6001 Executive Blvd.
Rm. 6200, MSC 9663
Bethesda, MD 20892-9663
Toll-Free: 866-615-6464
Phone: 301-443-4513
TTY: 301-443-8431
Toll-Free TTY: 866-415-8051
Fax: 301-443-4279
Website: www.nimh.nih.gov
Email: nimhinfo@nih.gov

**National Multiple Sclerosis Society**
900 S. Bdwy., Ste. 250
Denver, CO 80209
Toll-Free: 800-344-4867
Website: www.nationalmssociety.
org

# INDEX

# INDEX

Page numbers followed by "n" refer to citation information; by "t" indicate tables; and by "f" indicate figures.

# Index

# Index

# Index

computed tomography (CT),
  headache 352
confusional arousals, parasomnias 269
congenital central hypoventilation
  syndrome (CCHS)
  overview 212–215
  sleep apnea 192
constipation
  cancer 389
  congenital central hypoventilation
    syndrome (CCHS) 213
  fibromyalgia 343
  nicotine 428
  nocturia 404
continuous positive airway pressure
  (CPAP)
  obstructive sleep apnea (OSA) 203
  overview 523–524
  sleep disorders 91, 165
  sleep deprivation 128, 465
COPD Foundation, contact
  information 631
cortex
  Alzheimer disease (AD) 332
  rapid eye movement (REM) 38, 67
  sleep anatomy 9
  sleep deprivation 182
corticosteroids
  cancer 390
  multiple sclerosis (MS) 332
cortisol
  chronic fatigue syndrome
    (CFS) 378
  circadian rhythm disorder 225
  neurotransmitters 14
  shift works 457
  sleep deprivation 138
CPAP *see* continuous positive airway
  pressure
cradles, safe sleep 562
cribs, overview 559–566

*Cryptochrome* genes, circadian
  rhythms 20
CSBs *see* complex sleep behaviors
CSF *see* cerebrospinal fluid
CT *see* computed tomography
CVD *see* cardiovascular disease

# D

daylight
  importance of sleep 7
  napping 58
  posttraumatic stress disorder
    (PTSD) 316
  sleep and work 445
  sleep disorders in men 107
  sleep disorders in women 98
  sleep habits 33
  sleep sufficiency 122
daylight savings
  napping 58
  sleep deprivation 452
daytime drowsiness
  central sleep apnea (CSA) 205
  food and alcohol 428
  insomnia 478
  obstructive sleep apnea (OSA) 594
  sleep environment 507
daytime sleepiness
  central sleep apnea (CSA) 205
  circadian rhythm disorders 220
  idiopathic hypersomnia (IH) 244
  insomnia 92
  jet lag 158
  narcolepsy 261
  night terrors 79
  sleep apnea 189
  sleep apnea syndrome 588
  sleep myths 24
  sleepwalking 285, 600
  substance use disorders (SUDs) 519
  tension-type headache 359

# Index

# Index

# Index

# Index

# Index

# Index

# Index

# Index

# Index

# Index

# Index

# Index

# Index